Workbook to Accompany
Medical Assisting:
Administrative and Clinical Competencies

Fourth Edition

Lucille Keir, CMA-A

Barbara A. Wise, BSN, RN, MA(Ed)

Connie Krebs, CMA-C, BGS

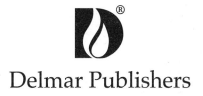

Delmar Publishers

an International Thomson Publishing Company

Albany • Bonn • Boston • Cincinnati • Detroit • London • Madrid
Melbourne • Mexico City • New York • Pacific Grove • Paris • San Francisco
Singapore • Tokyo • Toronto • Washington

COPYRIGHT © 1998
Delmar is a division of Thomson Learning. The Thomson Learning logo is a registered trademark used herein under license.

Printed in the United States of America
    14 15 16   XXX   06 05 04 03

For more information, contact Delmar, 3 Columbia Circle, PO Box 15015, Albany, NY 12212-0515; or find us on the World Wide Web at http://www.delmar.com

International Division List

Japan:
Thomson Learning
Palaceside Building 5F
1-1-1 Hitotsubashi, Chiyoda-ku
Tokyo 100 0003 Japan
Tel: 813 5218 6544
Fax: 813 5218 6551

Australia/New Zealand
Nelson/Thomson Learning
102 Dodds Street
South Melbourne, Victoria 3205
Australia
Tel: 61 39 685 4111
Fax: 61 39 685 4199

UK/Europe/Middle East:
Thomson Learning
Berkshire House
168-173 High Holborn
London
WC1V 7AA United Kingdom
Tel: 44 171 497 1422
Fax: 44 171 497 1426

Latin America:
Thomson Learning
Seneca, 53
Colonia Polanco
11560 Mexico D.F. Mexico
Tel: 525-281-2906
Fax: 525-281-2656

Canada:
Nelson/Thomson Learning
1120 Birchmount Road
Scarborough, Ontario
Canada M1K 5G4
Tel: 416-752-9100
Fax: 416-752-8102

Asia:
Thomson Learning
60 Albert Street, #15-01
Albert Complex
Singapore 189969
Tel: 65 336 6411
Fax: 65 336 7411

Library of Congress Catalog Card No: 97-16219

ISBN: 0-8273-7713-4

TABLE OF CONTENTS

To the Learner   v

SECTION 1
MEDICAL HEALTH CARE ROLES AND RESPONSIBILITIES   1

CHAPTER 1
Health Care Providers   1
Unit 1   A Brief History of Medicine   1
Unit 2   The Health Care Team   3
Unit 3   Medical Practice Specialties   5

CHAPTER 2
The Medical Assistant   9
Unit 1   Training, Job Responsibilities,
         and Employment Opportunities   9
Unit 2   Personal Characteristics   11
Unit 3   Professionalism   11

CHAPTER 3
Medical Ethics and Liability   15
Unit 1   Ethical and Legal Responsibilities   15
Unit 2   Professional Liability   18

CHAPTER 4
The Office Environment   20
Unit 1   Safety, Security, and Emergency
         Provisions in the Medical Office   20
Unit 2   Efficient Office Design   23
Unit 3   Office Management Equipment   25
Unit 4   Ergonomics in the Medical Office   28
Unit 5   Preparing for the Day   31

CHAPTER 5
Interpersonal Communications   35
Unit 1   Verbal and Nonverbal Messages   35
Unit 2   Behavioral Adjustments   39
Unit 3   Patients and Their Families   42
Unit 4   Office Interpersonal Relationships   44

SECTION 2
THE ADMINISTRATIVE ASSISTANT   46

CHAPTER 6
Oral and Written Communications   46
Unit 1   Telephone Communications   46

Unit 2   Schedule Appointments   60
Unit 3   Written Communications   65
Unit 4   Receiving and Sending
         Office Communications   74

CHAPTER 7
Records Management   78
Unit 1   The Patient's Medical Record   78
Unit 2   Filing   81

CHAPTER 8
Collecting Fees   87
Unit 1   Medical Care Expenses   87
Unit 2   Credit Arrangements   89
Unit 3   Bookkeeping Procedures   91
Unit 4   Computer Billing   104
Unit 5   Collecting Overdue Payments   105

CHAPTER 9
Health Care Coverage   111
Unit 1   Fundamentals of Managed Care   114
Unit 2   Health Care Plans   114
Unit 3   Preparing Claims   116

CHAPTER 10
Medical Office Management   124
Unit 1   The Language of Banking   124
Unit 2   Currency, Cash, and Petty Cash   127
Unit 3   Salary, Benefits, and Tax Records   133
Unit 4   General Management Duties   135

SECTION 3
STRUCTURE AND FUNCTION OF THE BODY   137

CHAPTER 11
Anatomy and Physiology of the Human Body   137
Unit 1   Anatomical Descriptors and
         Fundamental Body Structure   137
Unit 2   The Nervous System   146
Unit 3   The Senses   151
Unit 4   Integumentary System   158
Unit 5   The Skeletal System   162
Unit 6   The Muscular System   169
Unit 7   The Respiratory System   175

Unit 8	The Circulatory System	181
Unit 9	The Immune System	188
Unit 10	The Digestive System	194
Unit 11	The Urinary System	204
Unit 12	The Endocrine System	210
Unit 13	The Reproductive System	214

SECTION 4
THE CLINICAL MEDICAL ASSISTANT 224

CHAPTER 12
Preparing for Clinical Duties 224

Unit 1	Guidelines for the Personal Safety and Well-being of Staff and Patients	224
Unit 2	Infection Control	226

CHAPTER 13
Beginning the Database 232

Unit 1	Medical History	232
Unit 2	Triage	235
Unit 3	Vital Signs	236

CHAPTER 14
Preparing Patients for Examinations 246

Unit 1	Procedures of the Eye and Ear	246
Unit 2	Positioning and Draping for Examinations	250
Unit 3	Preparing Patients for Examinations	255
Unit 4	Assisting with Special Examinations	258

CHAPTER 15
Specimen Collection and Laboratory Procedures 261

Unit 1	The Microscope	261
Unit 2	Capillary Blood Tests	265
Unit 3	Venous Blood Tests	270
Unit 4	Body Fluid Specimens	273
Unit 5	Bacterial Smears and Cultures	276

CHAPTER 16
Diagnostic Tests, X-Rays, and Procedures 279

Unit 1	Diagnostic Tests	279
Unit 2	Cardiology Procedures	282
Unit 3	Diagnostic Procedures	290
Unit 4	Diagnostic Radiological Examinations	293

CHAPTER 17
Minor Surgical Procedures 296

CHAPTER 18
Assisting with Medications 303

Unit 1	Prescription and Nonprescription Medications	303
Unit 2	Methods of Administering Medications	312
Unit 3	Injections and Immunizations	314

CHAPTER 19
Emergencies, Acute Illness, and Accidents 320

Unit 1	Managing Emergencies in the Medical Office	320
Unit 2	Acute Illness	322
Unit 3	First Aid in Accidents and Injuries	327

SECTION 5
BEHAVIORS AND HEALTH 329

CHAPTER 20
Behaviors Influencing Health 329

Unit 1	Nutrition, Exercise, and Weight Control	329
Unit 2	Mobility Assistance	332
Unit 3	Habit-Forming Substances	333
Unit 4	Stress and Time Management	336

SECTION 6
EMPLOYABILITY SKILLS 339

CHAPTER 21
Achieving Satisfaction in Employment 339

Unit 1	The Job Search	339
Unit 2	Getting the Job and Keeping It	344

PERFORMANCE EVALUATION CHECKLIST SECTION P1–P235

CERTIFICATE OF COMPLETION P237

TO THE LEARNER

This workbook has been written to help you review the concepts and information presented in the textbook and provide a means for you to achieve competency in your performance of the procedures. Each unit in the text can be correlated to a unit in the workbook. The material in the workbook contains many different types of exercises to provide a variety of things to be completed.

Assignment sheets have been developed to help you review the information concerning the theory and skill contents, the general technical content, and the basic anatomy content. These sheets ask you to answer questions, fill in blanks, define terms, match answers, work puzzles, etc. When the sheets for each chapter have been completed, they can be removed and given to your teacher for evaluation. Always be sure to fill in your name and the date everywhere it is indicated on the sheets. The answers to the questions have been included in your teacher's Instructor's Manual.

Another feature of your workbook is the Performance Evaluation Checklists. You will find one in the back of this workbook for each procedure in your textbook. These sheets are prepared to provide a means for you to achieve a measurement of your ability to perform the procedure. You should practice the procedures following the steps as identified in your text, keeping the Terminal Performance Objective in mind. You will notice procedure competency involves using the correct equipment and materials, accurate performance of the procedure steps, and completion within an acceptable period of time. In those procedures where a period of time for completion has not been identified in the objective, it is because of the great amount of variability of the task and/or equipment and materials available to you. Spaces have been provided on the Performance Evaluation Checklists to document the time required to complete the procedure, as well as the time the procedure began and ended. In procedures where no standards for time and accuracy are provided, your instructor will inform you of the required standards based on the actual conditions in your classroom situation.

When you feel you have mastered the skill, ask one of your classmates (if you are in a school situation) to observe your technique following the procedure evaluation requirements. When you are confident of your ability, sign the evaluation form and give it to your teacher. This will inform the teacher that you are ready for evaluation. The teacher will then observe your performance of the procedure or may delegate the responsibility to another person.

In many units, you will find "situations" for which you are asked to respond. There are no specific right or wrong answers. Think about the things you have read in your text in order to arrive at your answer. You will encounter many similar actual situations in and out of the office. When family members, friends, and neighbors know you are a medical assistant, they will look for information and advice. These simulated situations will be very helpful, but remember, you are not qualified to diagnose an illness or prescribe treatment. Your role is to recognize potential problems, advise, facilitate care and treatment, and provide information within the limits of your knowledge and experience.

It is suggested that you obtain a large 3-ring notebook in which to keep your completed assignment and evaluation sheets. Insert the sheets into their original position and maintain your complete workbook for reference and review.

The authors hope you will find the workbook to be both challenging and interesting. It is our desire that you master the content of the text to the best of your ability and we believe this workbook will assist you in that process. We wish you success as you complete your assignments and prepare to be a medical assistant.

ASSIGNMENT SHEET

Section I: MEDICAL HEALTH CARE ROLES AND RESPONSIBILITIES
Chapter 1: HEALTH CARE PROVIDERS
Unit 1: A BRIEF HISTORY OF MEDICINE

Review the objectives and text for each unit before completing the assignment sheet for that unit in this chapter. When all sheets for the chapter have been completed, remove them from this workbook and give them to the instructor for evaluation.

A. SPELLING: Each line contains three different spellings of a word. Underline the correctly spelled word.

1.	anesthesha	anesthesia	anethesha
2.	aprenticeship	apprentiship	apprenticeship
3.	aceptic	aseptic	aseptec
4.	caughtery	cauterey	cautery
5.	disease	desease	deseace
6.	epedemic	epidemic	epidemik
7.	ethere	ether	ethir
8.	gilds	guelds	guilds
9.	infectious	infectuous	enfectuous
10.	physican	psychian	physician
11.	plaque	plage	plague
12.	practitioners	practioners	practitoners
13.	scintific	scientific	sientific
14.	surgeon	sirgin	sergeon
15.	vakcination	vaccination	vacsination

B. MATCHING: Read the definition in Column I and then find the matching answer in Column II. Place the letter of the correct answer in the space provided.

COLUMN I

_____ 1. Symbol of medical profession
_____ 2. Father of modern medicine
_____ 3. Invented stethoscope
_____ 4. A physician in Rome who wrote over 500 books
_____ 5. First successful heart transplant
_____ 6. Discovered the pap test
_____ 7. First reported studies of circulation of blood by heart
_____ 8. Built over 200 microscopes and first to see RBCs
_____ 9. Founder of scientific surgery
_____ 10. Introduced use of ether as anesthetic in 1800s
_____ 11. Writer and physician who coined word anesthesia
_____ 12. Pasteurization
_____ 13. Foundation for aseptic technique
_____ 14. Discovered X rays
_____ 15. Developed the smallpox vaccine
_____ 16. Nobel Prize in 1912 for research joining blood vessels
_____ 17. Early female physician; author of "Diseases of Women"
_____ 18. Nurse who formed American Red Cross

COLUMN II

a. Anton van Leeuwenhoek
b. George Papanicolaou
c. Willian Harvey
d. Wilhelm Roentgen
e. W.T.G. Morton
f. caduceus
g. Edward Jenner
h. Galen
i. Oliver Wendell Holmes
j. Alexis Carrel
k. Louis Pasteur
l. Hippocrates
m. Christian Bernard
n. Joseph Lister
o. John Hunter
p. Rene Laennec
q. Marie Curie
r. Grace Goldsmith

_____ 19. First woman to qualify as Physician in United States
_____ 20. Founder of modern nursing
_____ 21. Discovered polio virus and discovered a vaccine
_____ 22. First world-famous woman scientist whose work led directly to treatment of cancer with radium
_____ 23. Developed first mercury thermometer
_____ 24. In 1940s instituted first nutrition training for medical students anywhere in the world

s. Clara Barton
t. Gabriel Fahrenheit
u. Elizabeth Blackwell
v. Trotula Platearius
w. Jonas Salk
x. Florence Nightingale

C. BRIEF ANSWER

During the ancient medical history period, several things were believed responsible for illness and some unusual treatments were used.

1. What was credited as the cause of disease? _____

2. How were migraines, epilepsy, insanity, and head injuries treated? _____

3. How did the Egyptians solve "clogged" body canals? _____

4. The Greeks believed in a god of healing. What did they use for treatments? _____
_____

In Medieval history, other beliefs and methods of treatment were held.

5. What did Anglo-Saxons in Britain believe caused illness? _____
_____

6. How did the priests cure the sick in about 400 AD? _____
_____

7. In 1277 AD, how was tuberculosis treated? _____

8. In 1352, what different things were believed to be the cause of the plagues? _____
_____
_____

9. The practice of medicine in the beginning of the seventeenth century was divided among three guilds. Name and briefly describe their education and area of practice.

a. _____

b. _____
_____

c. _____

10. As late as the 1600s what were some of the old practices still being used in the colonies and was the unusual prescription ordered for Queen Anne? _____
_____

11. What sciences aided medical science in making rapid advances in the eighteenth century? _____
_____

12. What did *Ebony* Magazine report in 1993 regarding the accomplishments of Drs. Alexa Canady and Deborah Hyde-Rowan? _____
_____

After your instructor has returned your work to you, make all necessary corrections and place in a 3-ring notebook for future reference.

ASSIGNMENT SHEET

Chapter 1: HEALTH CARE PROVIDERS
Unit 2: THE HEALTH CARE TEAM
A. MULTIPLE CHOICE: Place the correct letter on the blank line for each of the following questions.

_____ 1. One whose primary duty is obtaining a medical history and other important information from patients in the hospital is termed a(n):
   a. Unit Clerk   c. Dietician
   b. Admissions Clerk   d. Office Manager

_____ 2. A _____ performs specialized chemical, microscopic, and bacteriological tests of blood, tissue, and other bodily fluids.
   a. Nurse Practitioner   c. Laboratory Technician
   b. Physician Assistant   d. Accessioning Technician

_____ 3. One who practices skills most often in the hospital setting to assist patients in many ways through purposeful activity is called:
   a. Physician Assistant   c. Physical Therapist
   b. Pharmacist   d. Occupational Therapist

_____ 4. A member of the health care team who helps patients with their diets, usually in a hospital or clinic, is called a:
   a. Nurse Practitioner   c. Dietician
   b. Pharmacist   d. Nutritionist

_____ 5. One who is trained by physicians, instructed in certain aspects of medicine, and practices under their direct supervision is called a:
   a. Registered Nurse   c. Physician Assistant
   b. Licensed Practical Nurse   d. Paramedic

_____ 6. The _____ is trained in the art of drawing blood for diagnostic purposes.
   a. Paramedic   c. Physician Assistant
   b. Physical Therapist   d. Phlebotomist

_____ 7. A qualified person who has been trained in assisting patients in rehabilitation programs following accident or injury is called a(n):
   a. Occupational Therapist   c. Registered Nurse
   b. Physical Therapist   d. Podiatrist

_____ 8. One who is a licensed specialist in formulating and dispensing medications is a:
   a. Pharmacist   c. Registered Nurse
   b. Paramedic   d. Physician

_____ 9. A professional who is highly trained and skilled in mechanical manipulation of the spinal column is a(n):
   a. Occupational Therapist   c. Licensed Practical Nurse
   b. Chiropractor   d. Physical Therapist

_____ 10. A member of the health care team who performs procedures to improve the ventilatory functions of a patient is a(n):
   a. Phlebotomist   c. Radiology Technician
   b. Electrocardiogram Technician   d. Respiratory Therapist

_____ 11. A _____ provides testing and counseling services to patients in private or group practice.
      a. Podiatrist   c. Paramedic
      b. Dietician   d. Psychologist

B. SPELLING: Each line contains four different spellings of a word. Underline the correctly spelled word.

1. dietitian	dietician	deititian	dietision
2. phlebatomist	plebotamist	phlebotomist	pflebotomist
3. therapast	theirapist	therapist	tharapist
4. technicien	technician	technision	tecnician
5. chiropractor	chiropracter	chyroprakder	chirupractor
6. nutricionist	nutrionist	nutritionist	newtritionist
7. ocupational	occupattional	occupational	occupationale
8. licensed	licenced	licensced	licensead
9. professional	preffessional	profesional	professionel
10. physiciaan	physichian	pysican	physician

C. MATCHING: Read the Subspecialties in Column I and then find the matching answer in Column II. Place the letter of the correct answer in the space provided.

COLUMN I

_____ 1. Immunology
_____ 2. Preventive Medicine
_____ 3. Acupuncture
_____ 4. Hypnosis
_____ 5. Rheumatology
_____ 6. Nutrition
_____ 7. Surgery
_____ 8. Cardiovascular Disease
_____ 9. Hypertension
_____ 10. Aerospace Medicine

COLUMN II

a. Mainly used in psychotherapy
b. Treats high blood pressure
c. How body utilizes nutrients
d. Deals with allergies
e. Originated in the Far East
f. Stresses keeping healthy
g. Research effects of space environment
h. Treats inflammatory disorders
i. Many specialized areas
j. Heart and circulatory problems

D. FILL IN THE BLANK

1. The Podiatrist or _____ deals with diseases and disorders of the _____.
2. The business office manager should have good _____ skills.
3. The Licensed Practical Nurse may perform basic nursing skills under the direct supervision of a physician or _____.
4. The _____ is one who is specialized in the microscopic identification of cells and tissues.
5. Emergency Medical Technicians must _____ every two years.
6. An R.N. is defined as a _____ nurse who has completed a school of nursing and passed the NCLEX-RN.
7. A _____ is sometimes called an administrative specialist or a ward secretary.
8. A registered nurse who has acquired expert knowledge in a special branch of practice is called a nurse _____.
9. The _____ acts as an assistant to, or in place of, the physician especially in the military.
10. The _____ of the x-ray technician must be provided by the American Registry of Radiologic Technologists.

After your instructor has returned your work to you, make all necessary corrections and place in a 3-ring notebook for future reference.

ASSIGNMENT SHEET

Chapter 1: HEALTH CARE PROVIDERS
Unit 3: MEDICAL PRACTICE SPECIALTIES

Review the objectives and text for each unit before completing the assignment sheet for that unit in this chapter. When all sheets for this chapter have been completed, remove them from this workbook and give them to the instructor for evaluation.

A. FILL IN THE BLANKS

1. _____ dedicate their lives to the practice of medicine or to acquiring skill sin the art and science of treating disease and maintaining health.

2. A physician may have an area of special interest that may be referred to as a _____.

3. The term _____ is derived from the Latin word meaning "to teach."

4. Persons who hold _____ , or _____ are entitled to be addressed as Doctor.

5. A _____ contributes specific expert skills and knowledge in serving patients.

6. The type of practice that covers the broadest spectrum is called _____.

7. Three types of medical specialties that are hospital based are _____ , _____ , and emergency or traumatic medicine.

B. MATCHING

COLUMN I		COLUMN II
_____	1. OD	a. Doctor of Osteopathy
_____	2. PhD	b. Doctor of Dental Surgery
_____	3. DPM	c. Doctor of Medicine
_____	4. DC	d. Doctor of Divinity
_____	5. DO	e. Doctor of Optometry
_____	6. DDS	f. Doctor of Veterinary Medicine
_____	7. MD	g. Doctor of Philosophy
		h. Doctor of Chiropractic
		i. Doctor of Podiatric Medicine

C. MULTIPLE CHOICE: Place the correct letter on the blank line for each of the following questions.

_____ 1. One who specializes in the treatment of diseases and disorders of the stomach and intestines is a/an
    a. Gerontologist.   c. Gastroenterologist.
    b. Endocrinologist.   d. Allergist.

_____ 2. The field of medicine that deals with diagnosing and treating diseases and disorders of the female reproductive tract is
    a. Gerontology.   c. Nephrology.
    b. Gynecology.   d. Obstetrics.

_____ 3. Measuring the accuracy of vision to determine if corrective lenses (eyeglasses) are needed describes the field of
    a. Orthopedics.   c. Optometry.
    b. Oncology.   d. Obstetrics.

_____ 4. A specialty that deals with the diagnosis and treatment of diseases and disorders of the CNS (central nervous system) is
    a. Psychology.   c. Nuclear Medicine.
    b. Neurology.   d. Nephrology.

_____ 5. Treatment and diagnosis of acute illnesses or injuries is a specialty called
    a. Surgery.   c. Pathology.
    b. Physical Medicine.   d. Traumatic Medicine.

6. One who specializes in the treatment and diagnosis of pronounced manifestation of emotional problems or mental illnesses which may have an organic causative factor is called a
   a. Psychiatrist.
   b. Psychologist.
   c. Neurologist.
   d. Podiatrist.

7. Analysis of tissue samples to confirm diagnosis is performed by a/an
   a. Urologist.
   b. Hematologist.
   c. Pathologist.
   d. Nephrologist.

8. One who specializes in the diagnosis and treatment of the foot is called a
   a. Surgeon.
   b. Podiatrist.
   c. Pathologist.
   d. Chiropractor.

9. Sports medicine is a medical specialty which deals with diagnosing and treating
   a. emotional problems.
   b. injuries sustained in athletic events.
   c. disorders and diseases of the urinary system.
   d. conditions of altered immunological

10. A radiologist specializes in diagnosing and treating diseases and disorders
    a. by manual or operative methods.
    b. with the use of radionuclides.
    c. with roentgen rays and other forms of radiant energy.

11. Dermatology is the specialty of medicine which deals with diagnosis and treatment of diseases and disorders of the
    a. glands of internal secretion.
    b. skin.
    c. teeth and gums.
    d. kidneys.

12. Nephrology is the medical specialty which deals with the diagnosis and treatment of
    a. blood and blood forming tissue.
    b. the internal organs.
    c. stomach and intestines.
    d. the kidneys.

13. One who is a specialist in the diagnosis and treatment of problems in conceiving and maintaining pregnancy is a(n)
    a. Pediatrician.
    b. Family Practitioner.
    c. Endocrinologist.
    d. Infertility Specialist.

14. A hematologist specializes in the diagnosis and treatment of disorders and diseases of
    a. the internal organs.
    b. bones.
    c. blood and blood forming tissue.
    d. the central nervous system.

15. The field of medicine which provides direct care to pregnant females during pregnancy, child birth, and immediately thereafter is called
    a. Obstetrics.
    b. Infertility.
    c. Pediatrics.
    d. Gynecology.

16. Anesthesiology is the medical specialty which deals with
    a. manual or operative methods.
    b. the use of radionuclides.
    c. administering anesthetic agents prior to and during surgery
    d. altered immunological reactivity.

17. A cardiologist specializes in the diagnosis and treatment of abnormalities, diseases, and disorders of the
    a. glands.
    b. aging.
    c. heart.
    d. central nervous system

18. One who specializes in diagnosing and treating diseases and malfunctions of the glands of internal secretion is called a/an
    a. Cardiologist.
    b. Chiropractor.
    c. Endocrinologist.
    d. Otorhinolaryngologist.

D. CROSSWORD PUZZLE: Using your text and TABLE 1-1 complete this crossword puzzle:

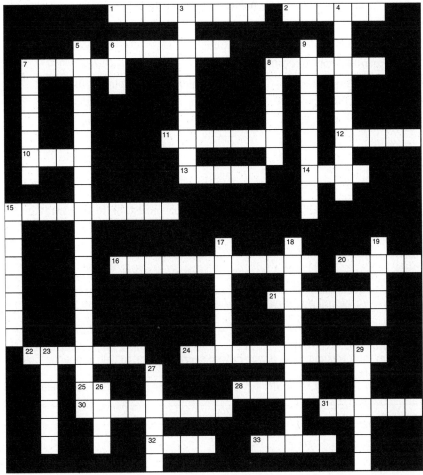

ACROSS

1. urgency
2. responsibilities
6. altered immune reaction
7. common name for physician
8. branch of medicine that uses radionuclides
10. A Dermatologist treats problems of the _____
11. renewed periodically
12. Pulmonary specialists treat diseases/disorders of the _____
13. expertise in a certain area
14. a surgeon cuts _____ skin
15. field of medicine dealing with small children
16. deals with pregnancy/childbirth
20. anesthetics make you _____
21. pathology is the study of _____
22. operation
24. commonly known as a counselor
25. abbreviation for symptoms
28. opposite of chronic
30. _____ medicine is practiced in the emergency room
31. combining form that refers to the heart
32. The Health care _____ works together
33. orthopedics

DOWN

3. field of medicine that deals with senior citizens
4. specialist who helps childless couples
5. ENT specialist
6. practicing medicine is an _____ and science
7. deals with problems of the teeth and gums
8. a Neurologist is expert in this specific anatomical area
9. career/work
15. branch of medicine that treats problems of the feet
17. field of medicine that treats genitourinary problems
18. Chiropractic
19. from general practice to a specialist
23. emergency
26. Radiologists use these in diagnosing
27. blood (combining form)
29. Endocrinologists study about what glands _____

E. SPELLING: Each line contains four different spellings of a word. Underline the correctly spelled word.

1. allargist	allergest	allergist	alergist
2. anesthesiology	annesthesiology	anesthisology	anasthesiology
3. gastrointerologist	gastroenterologist	gastronterologist	gastranologist
4. geriatricks	gariacktrics	giractrics	geriatrics
5. ophthalmology	opthalmology	optamology	ophthalamalagy
6. obstitrician	obstetrician	obstatrician	obstetrecian
7. psychiatrist	psychiotrist	psyciatrist	psychatrist
8. pediatrist	padiatrist	podiatrist	podatrist
9. pediatician	pediatrician	peditrician	pedeatrician
10. urologist	uriologist	urologest	urolgist

F. CRITICAL THINKING SCENARIOS: What would your response be in the following situations?

1. Your neighbor asks you the difference between an internal medicine specialist and an endocrinologist.

   _____

   _____

2. You are attending a family reunion and overhear a discussion where there is an obvious uncertainty about the use of the title "Dr." _____

3. A female patient, whom the physician has never before seen, phones to ask about the possibility of having a food allergy. This patient tells you that a fine red rash is all over her body. _____

   _____

   _____

After your instructor has returned your work to you, make all necessary corrections and place in a 3-ring notebook for future reference.

ASSIGNMENT SHEET

Chapter 2: THE MEDICAL ASSISTANT
Unit 1: TRAINING, JOB RESPONSIBILITIES, AND EMPLOYMENT OPPORTUNITIES

Review the objectives and text for each unit before completing the assignment sheet for that unit in this chapter. When all sheets for the chapter have been completed, remove them from this workbook and give them to the instructor for evaluation.

A. BRIEF ANSWER

1. Why did health care occupations develop? _____
_____

2. Name the seven fastest growing occupations in the health service industry. _____
_____
_____

3. Why have health occupations grown? _____
_____

4. Looking at Table 2-2 on page 25 in the text, identify the following:
   A. Which occupation showed a surplus in 1994 and is projected in 2005? _____
   B. Which occupation shows the greatest number of job openings? _____
   C. How many projected new medical assistants will be needed by 2005? (remember the listings are in thousands) _____
   D. How many medical secretaries were employed in 1994 and how many more will be needed by 2005?
   _____
   E. What is the most significant source of training for medical records technicians? _____
5. Where can training for medical assisting be obtained? _____
_____

6. In the discussion of the seven "hottest jobs", under CAREER LADDERING, determine the amount of training and licensure (if needed) required to obtain the following jobs.
   A. Licensed practical nurse _____
   B. Emergency medical technician _____
   _____
   C. Recreational therapist _____
   _____
   D. Respiratory therapist _____
   _____
   E. Dental Hygienist _____
   _____
   F. Nuclear Medicine Technologist _____
   G. Physician Assistant _____

B. FILL IN THE BLANK: In the list below, using "A" or "C", identify which tasks are considered administrative and which are clinical.

_____ 1. Complete insurance forms
_____ 2. Maintain medical records
_____ 3. Take vital signs
_____ 4. Schedule appointments
_____ 5. Take medical histories
_____ 6. Prepare and give injections
_____ 7. Assist with medical procedures

_____ 8. Prepare medications
_____ 9. Handle mail
_____ 10. Prepare correspondence
_____ 11. Perform ECGs
_____ 12. Handle telephone calls

C. MATCHING: Read the definition in Column II and then find the matching answer in Column I. Place the letter of the correct answer in the space provided.

COLUMN I

_____ 1. administrative
_____ 2. analysis
_____ 3. clinical
_____ 4. competency
_____ 5. compliance
_____ 6. confidential
_____ 7. methodical
_____ 8. professional
_____ 9. proprietary
_____ 10. technologist
_____ 11. therapist
_____ 12. therapeutic

COLUMN II

a. Conformity to formal or official requirements
b. Following a plan or method
c. One trained and skilled in the methods of a profession
d. A person trained in the technical aspect of an area of study
e. Business and management tasks of a practice
f. Non-public educational institutions
g. An examination to determine something's content
h. Tasks dealing with patient examination and treatment
i. Having medicinal or healing properties
j. A person who provides restorative treatments
k. Being capable, able to perform at an acceptable level
l. Held in strict confidence, secretive

D. WORD PUZZLE: Fill in the puzzle to spell out health occupations terms

```
1.            _ _ O _ _ _ _ _ _ _
2.          _ _ _ _ _ C _ _ _ _
3.            _ _ C _ _ _ _ _
4.              _ _ _ U _
5.           _ _ _ _ _ P _ _ _ _ _ _ _
6.              H E A L T H
7         _ _ _ _ _ T _ _ _
8.  _ _ _ _ _ _ _ I _ _
9.       _ _ _ _ _ O _ _ _ _ _ _
10.                N _ _ _ _
11. _ _ _ _ _ _ S _ _ _ _ _
```

1. Individual responsible for maintaining financial records
2. A doctor
3. Legal permit to engage in a certain activity
4. AAMA occupational analysis
5. A person who greets or welcomes
6. A state of freedom from disease
7. Individual responsible for office correspondence
8. An individual who provides a remedy
9. A person who applies scientific or mechanical methods
10. A person who provides care for the sick or injured
11. A person trained and skilled in a profession

After your instructor has returned your work to you, make all necessary corrections and place in a 3-ring notebook for future reference.

ASSIGNMENT SHEET

Chapter 2: THE MEDICAL ASSISTANT
Unit 2: PERSONAL CHARACTERISTICS
A. MATCHING: Read the definition in Column II and then find the matching answer in Column I. Place the letter of the correct answer in the space provided.

COLUMN I

_____	1. Accuracy
_____	2. Adaptable
_____	3. Conservative
_____	4. Courteous
_____	5. Dependable
_____	6. Discreet
_____	7. Empathy
_____	8. Enthusiasm
_____	9. Honesty
_____	10. Initiative
_____	11. Patience
_____	12. Perseverance
_____	13. Punctual
_____	14. Reliable
_____	15. Respectful
_____	16. Self control
_____	17. Tact

COLUMN II

a. Can be relied upon, responsible
b. Ambition, hustle; set something in motion
c. Detailed correctness, exactness
d. Trustworthy, the quality of being truthful
e. Show restraint
f. Calmness in waiting; tolerant
g. Delicate skill in saying or doing the right thing
h. In exact agreement with appointed time
i. Zeal, intense interest
j. The ability to adjust
k. Showing regard for, considerate
l. Trying to identify one's feelings with those of another
m. To be cautious, handle with care, not wasteful
n. Prudent, cautious, especially in speech
o. To be polite, well-mannered
p. Trustworthy, dependable, responsible
q. Persistent effort, prolong

B. BRIEF ANSWER

Five personality qualities were identified in the text. List each one and give a brief definition.

1. _____
2. _____
3. _____
4. _____
5. _____

C. TRUE OR FALSE: Place a "T" for True or "F" for False in the space provided.

To be perceived as a professional, you must look like a professional. The following statements apply to your image. Indicate if they are true or false.

_____ 1. A skin rash on your body should not cause concern to a patient.
_____ 2. Being grossly overweight is beneficial when dealing with dieting patients who need to identify with a role model.
_____ 3. Personal illness requires prompt attention.
_____ 4. Deodorant will cover the odor from old perspiration.
_____ 5. Refrain from using hand cream because it attracts organisms.
_____ 6. Care should be taken to keep your hands out of your hair.
_____ 7. Chewing gum while working is unprofessional.
_____ 8. It is best to wear white underwear under a white uniform.
_____ 9. Your posture affects your energy level.
_____ 10. Chapped, cracked hands may allow organisms to enter the body.

_____ 11. Wearing a fragrance with a strong aroma helps soften the medicinal environment in the physician's office.

_____ 12. For women, vivid cosmetics and nailpolish are nice accents to a white uniform.

D. WORD PUZZLE

Enter letters to complete the puzzle from the words in "Words to Know.".

```
 1.               _ _ C _ _ _ _ _
 2.          _ _ _ _ _ H _
 3.    _ _ _ _ _ _ A _ _ _
                 P  E  R  S  O  N  A  L
 4.         _ _ _ _ A _ _ _
 5.           _ _ _ C _ _ _ _
 6.            _ _ T _ _ _ _ _
 7.        _ _ _ _ _ E _ _ _
 8.         _ _ _ _ _ R _ _ _
 9.          _ _ _ _ I _ _ _ _ _
10.        _ _ _ _ _ S _ _ _ _
11.            _ _ T _ _ _ _ _
12.          _ _ _ _ I _ _ _
13.      _ _ _ _ _ C _ _ _ _
14.          _ _ _ _ S _ _
```

1. Correct
2. Identify with the feelings of another
3. Visible presence
4. Dependable
5. Prudent, cautious
6. Tolerant
7. Polite
8. Act together
9. Set in motion
10. Intense interest
11. Feelings toward
12. Willing to adjust
13. Show regard for
14. Trustworthy

After your instructor has returned your work to you, make all necessary corrections and place in a 3-ring notebook for future reference.

ASSIGNMENT SHEET

Chapter 2: THE MEDICAL ASSISTANT
Unit 3: PROFESSIONALISM
A. FILL IN THE BLANK

1. The pioneers in medicine often were paid with the family's goods or valuables which is called _____.

2. _____ of every transaction between physician and patient is a must.

3. In _____, medical assistants from _____ states met in Kansas City, and adopted the name _____.

4. The primary purpose of the AAMA was to raise the standards of the medical assistant to a _____

_____.

5. The Maxine Williams Scholarship fund was established to assist those interested in pursuing a career in medical assisting and are based on _____.

6. The American Registry of Medical Assistants (ARMA) was established in _____ and operates with continual support and guidance from the _____.

7. The purpose of the ARMA is to advance the standards and profession of medical assisting and to

_____.

8. A _____ year revalidation process has been developed through the American Medical Technologists Institute for Education (AMTIE) for ARMA members.

9. One who interprets and transcribes patient information from oral to printed form by typing or with the use of a word processor is known as a _____.

10. In _____, the American Association for Medical Transcription (AAMT) was incorporated in _____ for the advancement of medical transcription.

11. _____ is the registered service mark for the rating that has become the recognized standard of measurement of secretarial proficiency.

12. The American Medical Technologists outline the requirements of professionalism in their

_____.

13. Both the AAMA national certification exam and the ARMA registry exam are designed to evaluate _____ competency in medical assisting.

14. Continuing education is available through professional medical assistant organizations which offer _____ to those who successfully complete seminars, workshops, publications, and home-study programs.

B. MATCHING: Read the definition in Column II and then find the matching answer in Column I. Place the letter of the correct answer in the space provided.

COLUMN I

_____ 1. evaluation
_____ 2. competent
_____ 3. professionalism
_____ 4. accreditation
_____ 5. registry

_____ 6. revalidation
_____ 7. certification
_____ 8. reputation
_____ 9. initiative

COLUMN II

a. process of evaluating competency in a specific area of expertise
b. reconfirmation of one's competency in a specific area of expertise
c. to start on one's own; to begin
d. assessment; judgment concerning worth of a person
e. the assignment of credentials; approval given for meeting established standards
f. what is generally believed about one's character
g. one who is trained and skilled in the methods of the profession
h. place where the listing of competent individuals is kept
i. fit, able, capable in a specific area

C. ESSAY: Write an essay answer for each of the following questions:

1. When, where, and why did the medical assistant profession begin? _____
   _____
   _____

2. a. Write the AAMA approved definition of medical assisting: _____
   _____
   _____

   b. Write the ARMA approved definition of medical assisting: _____
   _____

3. State the purpose of the AMT Standards of Practice and what members must recognize in themselves. _____
   _____
   _____
   _____

4. List the ten competencies outlined in the AAMA Role Delineation that demonstrate professionalism.
   _____
   _____
   _____

5. Explain why it is important for professionals to certify or recertify according to the guidelines set by the
   professional medical assistant organizations. _____
   _____

6. List the professional organizations that would be beneficial to the medical assistant.
   _____
   _____
   _____
   _____

   After your instructor has returned your work to you, make all necessary corrections and place in a 3-ring
notebook for future reference.

ASSIGNMENT SHEET

Chapter 3: MEDICAL ETHICS AND LIABILITY

Unit 1: ETHICS AND LEGAL RESPONSIBILITIES

Review the objectives and text for each unit before completing the assignment sheet for that unit in this chapter. When all sheets for the chapter have been completed, remove them from this workbook and give them to the instructor for evaluation.

A. BRIEF ANSWER

1. Complete the missing licensure requirements for physicians in the following list:

   a. _____

   b. be of good moral character

   c. _____

   d. have completed an approved residency program or its equivalent

   e. _____

   f. have passed the oral and written examinations administered by the Board of Medical Examiners of the state.

2. What are the exceptions to the need for a license to practice medicine? _____

   _____

3. What are the two basic elements that constitute the practice of medicine? _____

   _____

4. Identify the areas of medical ethics that are of particular concern to the medical assistant. _____

   _____

5. Which of the five primary elements of the American Association of Medical Assistants Code of Ethics stresses continuing education? (list it below) _____

   _____

   _____

6. How can DRGs cause ethical issues for physicians? _____

   _____

7. What is the most common transplant? _____

8. Explain what the term "emancipated minor" means? _____

   _____

9. What is the recommended statement that should be made to the patient by the medical assistant responsible for obtaining the consent form for invasive, experimental, and high risk medical services? _____

   _____

10. What does privileged communication mean? _____

    _____

11. Describe the conditions for revocation or suspension of a medical license. _____

    _____

    _____

12. Describe unprofessional conduct. _____

    _____

    _____

B. MATCHING: Read the definition in Column II and then find the matching answer in Column I. Place the letter of the correct answer in the space provided.

COLUMN I

_____ 1. offer
_____ 2. contract law
_____ 3. reciprocity
_____ 4. ethics
_____ 5. tort
_____ 6. implied consent
_____ 7. civil laws
_____ 8. endorsement
_____ 9. acceptance
_____ 10. consideration

COLUMN II

a. deals with what is morally right and wrong
b. deals with findings of negligence; most common basis for lawsuits against physicians
c. takes place when appointment is given and the doctor examines the patient
d. written consent for medical services
e. pass exam administered by the National Board of Medical Examiners
f. takes place when a competent individual indicates desire to be a patient
g. payment given in exchange for services
h. license granted in new state because of equal requirements of original license
i. patient enters into agreement by coming to see physician
j. patient/doctor relationship considered contract
k. defines powers of government and its citizens
l. deals with laws governing property ownership, corporation, and inheritance

C. FILL IN THE BLANK

1. A medical license may be revoked for _____ .
2. A license may be revoked because of proven _____ in the application for the license.
3. Physicians who are found to be incompetent to practice because of _____ may have their license revoked.
4. The ethical standards established by a profession are administered by _____ .
5. The physician must release patient information when the patient authorizes the release or if the release of information is _____ .
6. With proper documentation, any person of sound mind and legal age may give any part of the body after death for _____ .
7. Human organs should never be _____ .
8. Copies of the living will document should be filed with the _____ .
9. Every member of the medical care team should be currently certified in _____ .
10. Under the _____ patients must receive written information explaining their right-to-die options according to their state laws.
11. A _____ is defined as any number of actions done by one person or group of persons that causes injury to another or others.
12. The negligent causing of an injury, when committed by a physician in the course of professional duties, is commonly referred to as _____ .
13. Libel and slander are two forms of _____ .
14. A deliberate attempt or threat to touch without consent is called _____ .
15. _____ is the unauthorized touching of another person.

16

D. WORD PUZZLE: Use the following definitions to fill in the blanks for words to know and words found in the unit.

1.   __ __ P __ __ __ __
2.   __ R __ __ __ __
3. __ __ __ __ __ __ __ O __
4.   __ __ C __ __ __ __ __
5.   __ __ __ __ R __ __ __
6.   __ __ __ A __ __ __ __ __ __
7. __ __ __ __ __ __ S __
8.   __ __ __ __ __ T __
9.   __ __ I __ __ __ __
10.   N __ __ __ __ __ __ __ __
11.   __ __ A __ __ __ __ __ __ __
12.   __ __ __ T
13.   __ I __ __ __ __ __ __ __
14.   __ __ __ O __ __ __ __ __ __
15.   __ __ __ __ N __ __ __

1. Definite, specific
2. Violation of a law, contract, or other agreement
3. A standard of criticism or judgment
4. The principles of any branch of knowledge
5. To count separately; name one by one
6. Injury done to a person's reputation by or through slanderous statements
7. To surround, enclose
8. To bind legally or morally
9. Feebleness of body or mind caused by old age
10. Malpractice
11. Characterized by cheating and deceit; obtain by dishonest means
12. An injurious, harmful action, not involving a breach of contract, for which a civil action can be brought
13. Anything to which a person is liable, responsible, legally bound
14. To cancel; withdraw; to take back
15. A legal permit to engage in an activity

After your instructor has returned your work to you, make all necessary corrections and place in a 3-ring notebook for future reference.

ASSIGNMENT SHEET

Chapter 3: MEDICAL ETHICS AND LIABILITY

Unit 2: PROFESSIONAL LIABILITY

A. ESSAY

1. Describe the correct procedure for terminating the physician-patient contract.

_____

_____

_____

_____

_____

_____

2. Explain the term "abandonment", and give an example.

_____

_____

_____

_____

3. What is professional negligence? Give an example of professional negligence.

_____

_____

_____

4. In what situations could a medical assistant be charged with malpractice?

_____

_____

5. What is the purpose of the Good Samaritan Act?

_____

_____

6. List the reasons for keeping medical records.

_____

_____

7. Who owns medical office records?

_____

8. Do patients have the right to the information in their medical records?

_____

_____

9. What special precautions should be taken when giving written instructions to a patient?

_____

_____

10. What kinds of notes are inappropriate in a patient's chart? Why?

_____

_____

_____

11. Describe the acceptable method for making changes in medical records.

_____

_____

_____

B. TRUE OR FALSE: Place a "T" for True or "F" for False in the space provided.

_____ 1. Physicians have no right to determine whom they will see as patients.

_____ 2. Patients have the right to receive care equal to the standards of care in the community as a whole.

_____ 3. A physician may choose to withdraw from the care of a patient who does not follow instructions for treatment or follow-up appointments or who leaves a hospital against advice to stay.

_____ 4. The medical assistant has the right to be free from sexual discrimination.

_____ 5. The victim of sexual harassment must be of the opposite sex.

_____ 6. The testimony of a physician as an expert medical witness is never necessary in a case of negligence.

_____ 7. The doctrine, *res ipsa loquitur,* means the thing speaks for itself.

_____ 8. The physician's liability is expressed in the doctrine of *respondeat superior.*

_____ 9. The medical assistant is considered an agent for the physician under the law of agency.

_____ 10. The Good Samaritan law covers physicians even if they receive compensation for the emergency care given.

_____ 11. An implied agreement is considered to be a legal contract in a medical office.

_____ 12. The medical assistant should never attempt to perform a procedure without having been properly trained.

C. FILL IN THE BLANK

1. Statements regarding patients may be considered _____ of character and a breach of confidentiality.

2. An attorney may agree to take the testimony of the physician by _____.

3. A medical assistant may also receive a _____ to appear in court with patient records.

4. A _____ is a law that designates a specific limit of time during which a claim may be filed in malpractice suits or in the collection of bills.

5. _____ cannot be tolerated in handling medical records.

6. Each office should have a _____ regarding the release of information from a medical record.

7. The requirement of confidentiality regarding the medical record is no longer recognized when the patient _____ against the physician.

8. When in doubt about disclosing patient information, _____ by not disclosing rather than by disclosing.

9. The _____ to disclose information should be placed in the patient's chart with a copy of the information released.

10. Corrections in the medical record should appear in _____.

After your instructor has returned your work to you, make all necessary corrections and place in a 3-ring notebook for future reference.

ASSIGNMENT SHEET

Chapter 4: THE OFFICE ENVIRONMENT
Unit 1: SAFETY, SECURITY, AND EMERGENCY PROVISIONS IN THE MEDICAL OFFICE

Review the objectives and text for each unit before completing the assignment sheet for that unit in this chapter. When all sheets for the chapter have been completed, remove them from this workbook and give them to the instructor for evaluation.

A. BRIEF ANSWER

1. List four things to check every morning to assure a safe environment in the medical office.

   1. _____   3. _____
   2. _____   4. _____

2. Identify four hazards to which you should be alert in the business area of an office.

   1. _____   3. _____
   2. _____   4. _____

3. Name five things in an examining room which might cause an unsafe situation.

   1. _____   4. _____
   2. _____   5. _____
   3. _____

4. What eight things in a medical office are under the OSHA regulations?

   1. _____   5. _____
   2. _____   6. _____
   3. _____   7. _____
   4. _____   8. _____

5. What does the term "fire triangle" mean? _____
   _____
   _____

6. Name seven things that might start a fire in an office.

   1. _____   5. _____
   2. _____   6. _____
   3. _____   7. _____
   4. _____

7. What types of natural disasters require an established office policy regarding appropriate action to take?
   _____
   _____

8. Why are severe weather drills necessary? _____

9. How does knowing what to do or how to act affect a person's response to a crisis? _____
   _____
   _____

10. How would you clean up the following?
    1. Body fluids _____
    2. Glass fragments _____

11. Name the eight telephone numbers which might be posted near each office telephone.

    1. _____   5. _____
    2. _____   6. _____
    3. _____   7. _____
    4. _____   8. _____

12. Using your local phone directory, complete the "card" below listing the service and its appropriate number.

```
┌─────────────────────────────────────────────┐
│                                             │
│             EMERGENCY NUMBERS               │
│                                             │
│  _____  _____    _____  _____          │
│                                             │
│  _____  _____    _____  _____          │
│                                             │
│  _____  _____    _____  _____          │
│                                             │
│  _____  _____    _____  _____          │
│                                             │
└─────────────────────────────────────────────┘
```

13. What can you do to protect yourself from skin and mucous membrane exposure to harmful organisms?

_____

_____

B. CROSSWORD PUZZLE

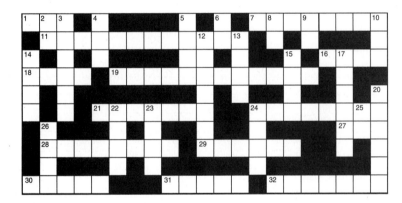

ACROSS

1. A pair
7. To leave
11. Device to put out fire
16. Entranceway
18. Floor coverings
19. Contaminated material
21. Obstruction, a guard
24. Potentially dangerous
28. Holder for soap
29. Reducing danger
30. Remains, left over
31. Covering for hand
32. A disease prevention substance

DOWN

2. Us
3. An essential element for life and combustion
4. The virus associated with AIDS
5. A federal agency
6. Myself
8. Virginia (abbr.)
9. California (abbr.)
10. Assists with hearing
12. Dangerous
13. Unusual, not common
14. A section, place
15. Combustible material
17. Place of employment
20. Safe, protected from dange
22. The eventual result of HIV
23. Dangerous chance
24. Able to see
25. Learning disabled (abbr.)
26. A federal agency

Name _____

After your instructor has returned your work to you, make all necessary corrections and place in a 3-ring notebook for future reference.

ASSIGNMENT SHEET

Chapter 4: THE OFFICE ENVIRONMENT
Unit 2: EFFICIENT OFFICE DESIGN
A. WORD PUZZLE: Complete the blanks using the definitions below.

1. _ _ _ I _ _
2. _ _ _ _ _ M _ _ _
3. _ _ _ _ _ _ P _ _ _ _ _
4. _ _ _ _ _ _ L _ _ _
5. _ _ _ E _ _ _ _ _ _ _
6. _ _ _ _ M _ _ _ _ _ _
7   _ E _ _ _ _ _ _
8. _ _ _ _ _ N _ _ _ _ _ _
9. _ _ _ T _ _ _ _ _
10. _ _ _ _ A _ _
11. _ _ _ T _ _ _ _ _ _ _ _ _ _
12. _ _ _ I _ _ _
13. _ _ _ O _ _ _ _
14. _ _ _ N _ _

1. layout, arrangement
2. to act out
3. foresight
4. limitation, physical handicap
5. translator
6. to serve
7. practicable/workable
8. infectious
9. nurture
10. order by law
11. to infect
12. printing/writing system for the blind
13. sleeplessness
14. action/gestures used to convey information

B. ESSAY

1. Explain the ADA and state when it became effective.

_____
_____
_____
_____

2. What specifically is mandated by the ADA of 1990?

_____
_____
_____
_____

3. Where in a medical facility should provisions be made for disabled persons?

_____

_____

4. Explain in your own words what is meant by "efficient office design"?

_____

_____

_____

5. Discuss what can make patients feel comfortable and satisfied when visiting a medical facility?

_____

_____

6. Discuss the reasons for separating well-visit and sick patients in the reception area.

_____

_____

7. Where should rest rooms, public phones, water fountains be located for patient use in the medical facility?

_____

_____

8. Explain the proper way to speak to a hearing impaired (deaf) person.

_____

_____

_____

9. What may happen if the daily schedule is more often than not backed up? Why?

_____

_____

10. Describe how one should speak to a person in a wheelchair.

_____

_____

11. Where can information be obtained regarding regulations concerning persons with disabilities?

_____

_____

C. TRUE OR FALSE: Place a "T" for True or "F" for False in the space provided.

_____   1. Patients who are hearing impaired or deaf should have a signer available to communicate their needs

_____   2. You should talk directly to the interpreter to communicate information for the handicapped patient.

_____   3. Proper ventilation and moderate temperature is necessary for comfort in a public facility.

_____   4. All patients waiting for appointments are placed at risk for possible contamination of communicable diseases.

_____   5. The management of the schedule is not a vital part of the medical practice.

After your instructor has returned your work to you, make all necessary corrections and place in a 3-ring notebook for future reference.

ASSIGNMENT SHEET

Chapter 4: THE OFFICE ENVIRONMENT
Unit 3: OFFICE MANAGEMENT EQUIPMENT

A. COMPLETION:

1. Demonstrate the use of a calculator, with emphasis on accuracy in determining the total on each column of figures:

a. 85.00	b. 40.00	c. 70.00
10.00	16.00	25.00
10.00	-12.00	65.00
-15.00	100.00	-125.00
4.00	18.00	37.00
10.00	-35.00	-54.00
Total _____	Total _____	Total _____

2. Use a calculator to determine the balance due on the following patient account—total each appointment and payment, list monthly balances and final balance due. (Insurance filing charge not reimbursable)

		Charges	Receipts	Balance
6/1/97	Office consult—extensive	105.00		
	Diagnostic x/ray testing	67.00		
	Laboratory	35.00		
6/10/97	Office, follow-up, extensive	85.00		_____
	ECG	65.00		
	Culture	40.00		
	Injection, antibiotic	30.00		_____
7/1/97	Office, intermediate	65.00		_____
7/21/97	Office intermediate	65.00		_____
8/1/97	Insurance filed (Medicare, Travelers)	10.00		_____
9/15/97	Medicare payment		272.16	
	Medicare write off		226.80	_____
9/25/97	Travelers payment		58.04	_____

B. COMPLETION

1. List the nine examples of items frequently copied which are identified in the text. _____

_____

_____

_____

2. What is microfilming? _____

_____

_____

3. How can microfiche material be read? _____

_____

_____

4. You are having difficulty transcribing dictation due to the following possible reasons. What could you say to the physician to improve the quality of the content?

   a. You are not sure what type of dictation is to be transcribed or when it was recorded. _____

_____

_____

b. The message is clear but you do not know to whom it goes or where to send it. _____

_____

c. You can't tell if a pause is the end of the sentence or a break in dictation. _____

_____

d. The dictation seems to be muffled and slurred at times and often barely audible because of background noise. _____

_____

e. You are never sure if the dictation is finished or it's a break in the message. _____

_____

5. List 4 features of a word processor. _____

_____

6. What is a computer? _____

_____

_____

7. Name three types of printers _____

8. Give ten examples of medical management software uses. _____

_____

_____

_____

_____

C. MATCHING: Read the definition in Column II and then find the matching answer in Column I. Place the letter of the correct answer in the space provided.

COLUMN I

COLUMN II

_____ 1. Batch   a. A readable paper copy or printout

_____ 2. Bug   b. Information that can be processed or produced by a computer

_____ 3. Cursor   c. A single stored unit of information that is named

_____ 4. Data   d. Formatting

_____ 5. Disk   e. Video display unit with a screen

_____ 6. File   f. To move the cursor up, down, right, or left

_____ 7. Font   g. An error in a program

_____ 8. Hard copy   h. Anything plugged into a computer

_____ 9. Initialize   i. A set of instructions written in computer language

_____ 10. Memory   j. An accumulation of data to be processed

_____ 11. Modem   k. Data held in storage

_____ 12. Monitor   l. Process or code that prevents overwriting data or a program on a disk

_____ 13. Peripheral   m. A marker on the screen showing where the next character will be placed

_____ 14. Program   n. An assortment of characters of a given size and style

_____ 15. Scroll   o. A magnetic storage device made of plastic

_____ 16. Write-protect   p. A peripheral device that enables a computer to communicate over phone lines

D. WORD SEARCH: FIND THE FOLLOWING WORDS IN THE PUZZLE.

1. ACRONYM
2. CALCULATOR
3. COMPUTER
4. DICTATION
5. ELECTRONIC
6. HARDWARE
7. MENU
8. MICROFICHE
9. MICROFILM
10. PAYEE
11. PROCESSOR
12. PROGRAM
13. SOFTWARE
14. TECHNOLOGY
15. TRANSCRIPTION

```
E C P G T O U R A D W Y C M I B
X T R A C Q S P R O G R A M C T
U D O D B W C M I C R O F I L M
H R C D I C T A T I O N L C G E
A V E T O M E N U R P C S R Q Y
R X S A D L C U Z F G O O O H K
D J S L M Z H T S P C M F F W F
W B O T R A N S C R I P T I O N
A K R A C R O N Y M G U W C H J
R C A L C U L A T O R T A H K L
E L E C T R O N I C M E R E N P
S V A D C O G G H F C R E T R O
D G V K P A Y E E R H P Z W C A
```

After your instructor has re turned your work to you, make all necessary corrections and place in a 3-ring notebook for future reference.

ASSIGNMENT SHEET

Chapter 4: THE OFFICE ENVIRONMENT
Unit 4: ERGONOMICS IN THE OFFICE

A. BRIEF ESSAY

1. A. What is ergonomics; and B. Who does it affect in the workplace?

   A. _____

   _____ .

   _____

   B. _____

   _____ . _____

   _____

2. Why is ergonomics so important?

   _____

   _____

   _____

3. What should be done if an office staff has problems with patient flow and other scheduling issues and cannot seem to remedy them?

   _____

   _____

   _____

4. List the main considerations for an efficient medical office layout.

   _____

   _____

   _____

   _____

5. What are the two most important points to consider in a medical office layout design?

   _____

   _____

   _____

6. Comment on room size in an office plan.

   _____

   _____

   _____

7. Why is room temperature so important in a medical facility?

   _____

   _____

   _____

8. How can foul odors be kept in check?

   _____

   _____

   _____

9. Discuss lighting and how it relates to safety.

   _____

   _____

   _____

   _____

10. What is ocular accommodation and what can be done to prevent it?

_____

_____

11. How can computer operators prevent conditions such as carpal tunnel syndrome and cumulative trauma disorder?

_____

_____

12. List items that can absorb sound to keep noise at a moderate level.

_____

_____

13. Why should soft instrumental music be played in a medical office?

_____

14. How is a TV best used in a medical office reception room (if at all)?

_____

_____

15. Why is the decor in a medical facility important?

_____

_____

16. What is the goal of ergonomics in general?

_____

_____

17. (Refer to Figure 4-32) Why is the work station in this picture ergonomically correct?

_____

_____

_____

18. What can result in a crowded facility where someone is always in your way.

_____

_____

_____

B. UNSCRAMBLE

1. _ _ _ _ _   KOVEE
2. _ _ _ _ _ _ _ _   RMETLANI
3. _ _ _ _ _   REGLA
4. _ _ _ _ _ _   MARUAT
5. _ _ _ _ _ _ _ _ _   SDIICEILNP
6. _ _ _ _ _ _   NUTLEN
7 _ _ _ _ _ _ _   YLASPDI
8. _ _ _ _ _ _ _ _   VANOREET

C. COMPLETION

1. A varied schedule of duties can help you stay _____ .

2. The avoidance of _____ is advised with all lighting as it can impair one's vision and is uncomfortable as well.

3. _____ may signal problems such as overheating of equipment, chemical leaks, or other serious potential health hazards.

4. The _____ of the VDT properly will prevent glare from incoming light from windows and artificial lights in the room.

5. For those who work with computers routinely, a _____ should be used.

6. Most everyone feels more _____ in bright and colorful rooms.

7. For those who sit most of the day at work, _____ is necessary in order to avoid back and other work-related conditions.

8. An adjustable chair is desirable for comfort and _____ of the back.

9. Using _____ may help in avoiding posture problems.

10. The _____ is the most critical for an ergonomically sound workplace.

After your instructor has returned your work to you, make all necessary corrections and place in a 3-ring notebook for future reference.

ASSIGNMENT SHEET

Chapter 4: THE OFFICE ENVIRONMENT
Unit 5: PREPARING FOR THE DAY

COMPLETION

1. Prepare a checklist for opening the office. (Refer to the procedure.) _____
   _____
   _____

2. What is the role of the receptionist? _____

3. Why is the reception room atmosphere important? _____
   _____

4. Name six things to check in the reception room. _____
   _____
   _____

5. List information that might be included in a practice information brochure. _____
   _____
   _____

6. Complete one sample new patient information form in this workbook yourself, then role play being a
   receptionist and interview.

7. Why should social climate be monitored? _____
   _____

8. List desirable characteristics for a receptionist. _____
   _____
   _____

9. Complete a copy of the form on page 32 to reflect the following situation—use yourself as the patient.
   Insurance company—Health Care One
   Insurance ID—123-45-6789-A Coverage Code S—Group-II
   You have been ill for the past week: fever, chills, coughing, pain over LL chest area, expectorating, blood tinged
    mucous
   Description Section: new patient, high complexity ($110) culture for strep ($35) therapeutic injection ($25)
   EKG ($50) respiratory function ($70) misc. drugs ($20)
   Diagnosis: acute bronchitis; pneumonia (viral), otitis media
   Doctor: use your physician's name - office visit accept assignment

10. Complete a copy of the form on page 33 to reflect the following situation—use yourself as the patient, today's
    date, and the same insurance information as in the previous situation.
    For interview—about one week ago you began having abdominal discomfort and occasional diarrhea. The pain
     and frequency of diarrhea have intensified.
    Diagnosis: abdominal pain—diarrhea—diverticulitis
    Description: extended exam—established patient ($85) antibiotic injection ($25)
    Procedure: high sigmoidoscopy ($90)
    Misc.: Review x-ray report ($15)
    Next appt.: 1 month
    Doctor: use your personal physician

11. What tasks should you do when closing the office for the day? _____
    _____
    _____
    _____

Name _____

PATIENT'S LAST NAME	FIRST	INITIAL	BIRTHDATE	SEX ☐ MALE ☐ FEMALE	TODAY'S DATE
ADDRESS	CITY	STATE	ZIP	RELATIONSHIP TO SUBSCRIBER	INJURY DATE
SUBSCRIBER OR POLICYHOLDER				INSURANCE CARRIER	
ADDRESS	CITY	STATE	ZIP	INS. I.D.　COVERAGE CODE　GROUP	

ASSIGNMENT AND RELEASE: I HEREBY AUTHORIZE MY INSURANCE BENEFITS TO BE PAID DIRECTLY TO THE UNDERSIGNED PHYSICIAN. I AM FINANCIALLY RESPONSIBLE FOR NON-COVERED SERVICES. I ALSO AUTHORIZE THE PHYSICIAN TO RELEASE ANY INFORMATION REQUIRED.

IDENTIFY

OTHER HEALTH COVERAGE ☐ YES ☐ NO

DISABILITY RELATED TO:
☐ ACCIDENT　☐ INDUSTRIAL　☐ ILLNESS　☐ OTHER

SIGNED
(PATIENT, OR PARENT, IF MINOR) _____ Date _____

DATE SYMPTOMS APPEARED, INCEPTION OF PREGNANCY, OR ACCIDENT OCCURRED:

✓	DESCRIPTION	CPT/MD	FEE	✓	DESCRIPTION	CPT/MD	FEE	✓	DESCRIPTION	CPT/MD	FEE
	OFFICE VISITS	NEW PT			LABORATORY (Cont'd.)				PROCEDURES		
	Moderate Complex	99203			Wet Mount	87210			EKG　93000	93005	
	Moderate/High Comp.	99204			Pap Smear	88150			Resp. Function Test	94010	
	High Complexity	99205			Handling	99000			Ear Lavage	69210	
	OFFICE VISITS	EST. PT			Hemocult Stool	82270			Injection Inter. Jt.*	20605	
	Minimal	99211			Glucose	82948			Injection Major Jt.*	20610	
	Self Limited Comp.	99212			INJECTIONS				Anoscopy	46600	
	Low/Moderate Comp.	99213			Vitamin B12/B Complex	J3420			Sigmoidoscopy	45355	
	Moderate Complex	99214			ACTH	J0140			I & D*	10060	
	High Complexity	99215			Depo-Estradiol	J1000			Electrocautery*	17200	
	CONSULTATIONS	OFFICE			Depo Testosterone	J1070			Thromb Hemor.*	46320	
	Moderate Complexity	99243			Imferon	J1760			Inj. Tendon*	20550	
	Mod. to High Comp.	99244			Tetanus Toxoid	J3180					
	HOME	EST. PT			Influenza Vaccine - Flu	90724			MISCELLANEOUS		
	Moderate Complexity	99352			Pneumococcal Vaccine	90732			Drugs, Supplies, Materials	99070	
	ER				TB Tine Test	86585			Special Reports	99080	
	Moderate Severity	99283			Aminophyllin	J0280			Services After Hrs.	99050	
	High Severity	99284			Terbutaline Sulf.	J3105			Services 10pm - 8am	99052	
	LABORATORY				Demerol HCL	J0990			Services Sun. & Holidays	99054	
	Urinalysis - Complete	81000			Compazine	J0780			Counseling	99403	
	Hemoglobin	85018			Injection Therapeutic	90782					
	Culture, Strep/Monilia	87081			Estrone Susp.	J1410					

DIAGNOSIS:

☐ Allergic Rhinitis 477.9	☐ Chronic Fatigue Synd. 300.5	☐ Hemorrhoids 455.6
☐ Anemia 280.9	☐ COPD 496	☐ Hiatal Hernia 553.3
☐ Angina Pectoris 413	☐ Costochondritis 733.99	☐ Hiatal Hernia & Reflux 530.1
☐ Anxiety 300.00	☐ CVA 431	☐ HVD 402.10
☐ Aortic Stenosis 424.1	☐ Cystitis 595.9	☐ Hyperlipidemia 272.4
☐ ASCVD 429.2	☐ Deg. Disc. Disease, CX 722.4	☐ Hypoestrogenism 256.3
☐ ASHD 414.9	☐ Deg. Disc. Dis., Lumbar 722.52	☐ Hypothyroidism 244.9
☐ Asthma 493.9	☐ Depression, Endogenous 296.2	☐ Impacted Cerumen 380.4
☐ Atrial Fibrillation 427.31	☐ Dermatitis 692.9	☐ Influenza, Viral 487.1
☐ Bigeminy 427.89	☐ Diabetes Mellitus, Adult 250.0	☐ Irritable Bowel Syndrome 564.1
☐ BPH 600	☐ Diarrhea 558.9	☐ Laryngitis 464.0
☐ Bronchitis, Acute 466.1	☐ Diverticulitis 562.11	☐ Menopausal Syndrome 627.2
☐ Bronchitis, Chronic 491.9	☐ Esophagitis 530.1	☐ Mitral Insufficiency 396.2
☐ Bursitis 726	☐ Fibrocystic Breast Disease 610.11	☐ Moniliasis 112
☐ Cardiomyopathy 425.4	☐ Fissure in Ano 565.0	☐ Myocardial Infarction 410.9
☐ Carotid Artery Disease 433.1	☐ Gastroenteritis 558.9	☐ Neuritis 729.2
☐ Cerebral Vascular Disease 437.9	☐ Gout 274.9	☐ Osteoarthritis 715.9
☐ CHF 428.0	☐ HCVD 429.2	☐ Osteoporosis 733.0
☐ Cholecystitis 575.1	☐ Headache, Vascular 784.0	☐ Otitis Media 382.9
	☐ Headache, Migraine 346.9	☐ Parkinsonism 332

☐ Peripheral Vascular Dis 443.9
☐ Pharyngitis 462.0
☐ Pneumonia, Bacterial 482.9
☐ Pneumonia, Viral 480.9
☐ Prostatitis, Chronic/Acute 601
☐ Rectal Bleeding 569.3
☐ Renal Failure, Chronic 585
☐ Rheumatoid Arthritis 714.0
☐ Sinusitis 461.9
☐ Supraventr. Tachycardia 427.0
☐ T.I.A. 435.9
☐ Tachycardia 426.89
☐ Tendinitis 726.90
☐ Tonsillitis 463
☐ Ulcer Duodenal 532.9
☐ Ulcer Gastric 531.9
☐ URI 465.9
☐ UTI 599.0
☐ Vaginitis 616.10
☐ Vertigo 780.4

DIAGNOSIS: (IF NOT CHECKED ABOVE)

REF. DR. & #

DOCTOR'S SIGNATURE / DATE	**NO SERVICES PURCHASED**	SERVICE PERFORMED	ACCEPT ASSIGNMENT	TODAY'S FEE	

INSTRUCTIONS TO PATIENT FOR FILING INSURANCE CLAIMS

1. MAIL THIS FORM DIRECTLY TO YOUR INSURANCE COMPANY.
   ATTACH YOUR OWN INSURANCE COMPANY'S FORM.

PLEASE REMEMBER THAT PAYMENT IS YOUR OBLIGATION, REGARDLESS OF INSURANCE OR OTHER THIRD PARTY INVOLVEMENT.

OFFICE ☐　YES ☐
E.R. ☐　NO ☐
HOME ☐

AMT. REC'D TODAY

TOTAL DUE

Name _____

Patient First Name	Patient Last Name		DATE OF ONSET FOR ILLNESS OR ACCIDENT
Responsible Party Last Name	Patient Last Name (If Different)	Date	/ /

CHANGE OF: ☐ NAME ☐ ADDRESS ☐ PHONE ☐ INSURANCE ☐ EMPLOYER

DIAGNOSIS:	CODE	DIAGNOSIS:	CODE	DIAGNOSIS:	CODE	DIAGNOSIS:	CODE	DIAGNOSIS:	CODE
__ Abdominal Pain	789.0	__ Chest Pain	786.50	__ Enteritis	008.0	__ Impetigo	684	__ Pneumonia	486
__ Abrasion	959.9	__ CHF	428.0	__ Esophagitis	530.1	__ Insomnia	780.51	__ Post Menopaus. Atr. Vag.	627.3
__ Abscess	682.9	__ Cholecystitis	575.1	__ Fatigue	780.7	__ Irritable Bowel Synd.	564.1	__ Pregnancy	V22
__ Acne	706.1	__ Cirrhosis	571.5	__ Flu Syndrome	487.1	__ Keratosis	701.1	__ Prostatis Hypertrophy	600
__ Alcoholism	303.9	__ Colitis	558.9	__ FUO	780.6	__ Labyrinthitis	386.3	__ Prostatitis	601.9
__ Allergic Reaction	995.3	__ Concussion	850.9	__ Furuncle	680.9	__ Laceration	882.0	__ Pyelonphritis	590.10
__ Allergic Rhinitis	477.9	__ Conjunctivitis	372.3	__ Gastritis	535.5	__ Laryngitis	464.0	__ Radiculitis	729.2
__ Amenorrhea	626.0	__ Constipation	564.9	__ Gastroenteritis	558.9	__ Low Back Pain	847.9	__ Renal Failure	586
__ Anemia	281.9	__ Costochondritis	733.6	__ GI Bleeding	578.9	__ Lumbar Disc Dis.	847.2	__ Rheum. Arthritis	714.0
__ Angina Pectoris	413.9	__ Contusion	924.9	__ Gingivitis	523.1	__ Lumbar Strain	846.7	__ Sebaceous Cyst	706.2
__ Anxiety State	300.00	__ COPD	496	__ Gout Unspecified	274.9	__ Menopausal Syndr.	672.2	__ Seborrhea	690
__ Appendicitis	541.	__ Corneal Abrasion	918.1	__ Headache, Migraine	346.9	__ Menorrhagia	626.2	__ Seizure Disorder	345.1
__ Arrhythmia	427.9	__ Cough	786.2	__ Headache, Tension	307.81	__ Mult. Contusions	924.0	__ Sinusitis	473.9
__ ASHD	414.0	__ CVA	431	__ Hematuria	599.7	__ Myocard. Inf	429.1	__ Sprain	848.9
__ Asthma	493.9	__ Cystitis	595.9	__ Hemorrhoids	455.6	__ Myositis	729.1	__ Suture Removal	V58.3
__ Atrial Fibrillation	427.31	__ Dementia	331.0	__ Hernia Hiatal	553.3	__ Nephrosclerosis	403.9	__ Tendonitis	726.90
__ Back Pain	724.2	__ Depression	296.2	__ Hernia Ventral	553.20	__ Nose Bleed	784.7	__ Thrombophleb	451.9
__ Breast Fibrocystic Dis.	610.1	__ Derangement Knee	717.9	__ Hernia, Inguinal	550.9	__ Obesity	278	__ Tonsilitis	463
__ Breast Tumor	239.3	__ Dermatitis	692.5	__ Herpes Simplex	054.9	__ Osteoarthritis	715.9	__ Urethritis	597.80
__ Bronchitis Nos.	493.9	__ Diabetes Mellitus	250.00	__ Herpes Zoster	053.9	__ Otitis Externa	380.12	__ URI	460
__ Bursitis	727.3	__ Diarrhea	558.9	__ Hypercholesteremia	272.0	__ Otitis Media	382.9	__ Vaginitis No. 5	616.1
__ CAD	746.85	__ Diverticulitis	562.11	__ Hyperlipidemia	272.4	__ Ovarian Cyst	620.2	__ Vaginitis Trich	131.01
__ Cellulitis		__ Duodenal Ulcer	532.1	__ Hypertension	401.9	__ Pancreatitis	577	__ Vaginitis Candida	112.1
__ Cerv. Disc. Disease	722.9	__ Dysfunct. Uterus Bid.	626.8	__ Hyperventilation	786.01	__ Paronychia, Finger	681.02	__ Vertigo	780.4
__ Cervical Strain Syndr.	723.8	__ Dysmenorrhes	625.3	__ Hypoestrogenism	256.3	__ Paronychia, Toe	681.11	__ Warts, Viral	078.1
__ Cervicitis Chronic	616.0	__ Electrolyte Imb.	276.9	__ Hypothyroidism	244.9	__ Pharyngitis	462		
__ CHD	414.9	__ Endometriosis	617.9	__ Impacted Cerumen	380.4	__ PID	614.9		

DIAGNOSIS: (IF NOT CHECKED ABOVE)

✓	DESCRIPTION	CODE/MD	DX	FEE	✓	DESCRIPTION	CODE/MD	DX	FEE	✓	DESCRIPTION	CODE/MD	DX	FEE
	OFFICE VISIT - ESTABLISHED PATIENT					**LABORATORY**					**DIAGNOSTIC PROCEDURES (Cont'd)**			
	Minimal Exam	99211				Venipuncture-DR.	36410				Spirometry	94010YB		
	Limited Exam	99212				Venipuncture	36415				Holter Recording	93224YB		
	Intermediate Exam	99213				Handling	99000				Sigmoidoscopy	45330		
	Extended Exam	99214				Throat Culture	87060				High Sigmoidoscopy	45360		
	Comprehensive Exam	99215				Monilia Culture	87086				Sigmoidoscopy w/ Biopsy	45331		
						Urinalysis	81000							
	OFFICE VISIT - NEW PATIENT					Urine Culture	87086							
	Limited Exam	99202									**PHYSICAL THERAPY**			
	Intermediate Exam	99203				**PROCEDURES**					Hydrocollator	97010		
	Extended Exam	99204				Arthrocentesis Small Joint	20600				Ultrasound	97128		
	Comprehensive Exam	99205				Arthrocentesis Interm. Joint	20605				PT Unlisted	97039		
	Accident Work-up	90020				Arthrocentesis Major Joint	20610							
						Trigger Point Injection	20550				**SUPPLIES**			
	INJECTIONS					Cryosurgery Cervix	57511				Surgical Tray A4550	99070		
	B12 J3420	90782				Face Cryosurgery	17000				Sterile Kit	84550		
	Cortisone J0810	90782				Not Face, 1st	17100							
	Flu	90724				Not Face, 2nd	17101				**MISCELLANEOUS**			
	Pneumovax	90732				Not Face 3 or More, Each	17102				Special Reports	99080		
	Tetanus Toxoid	90703				Ear Lavage	69210				Emergency O.V.	99058		
	DPT	90701									Review X-Ray Report	76140-26		
	Polio	90712												
	MMR	90707												
	HIB	90729												
	Estrogen J0970	90782				**DIAGNOSTIC PROCEDURES**								
	Lidocaine J2000	90782				Audiometry	92552							
	Skin Test (TB, Cocci, Histo)	86585				ECG	93000YB							
	Therapeutic Inj.	90782				ECG (Medicare)	93005							
	Drug:	Dose:												
	Antibiotic Inj.	90788												
	Drug:	Dose:												

REC'D BY:
☐ CASH
☐ CK. # _____
☐ CO-PAY
☐ MC/VISA

TOTAL FEE

AMT. REC'D

Authorization/Responsibility Agreement
I hereby authorize any insurance company to pay the proceeds of any benefits due me directly to: JAY RICHARD HODES, M.D. A copy of this can be considered as an original for insurance purposes.

Signed: _____ Date: _____

I hereby agree to pay my account as services are provided. If for any reason there is a balance owing on my account, I agree to pay promptly upon receipt of the monthly statement.

Signed: _____ Date: _____

I acknowledge and understand that I am responsible for all of the charges for all of the services rendered to me or any member of my family.
Although I have requested the doctor to bill my insurance company on my behalf, I clearly understand that it is still my responsibility to make sure the bill is paid in a reasonable time. If for any reason any portion of my bill is not paid by my insurance, I further agree to make arrangements for prompt payment of the bill.

Signed: _____ Date: _____

NEXT APPOINTMENT

MON	TUES	WED	THUR	FRI	SAT
2 WKS		1 M		2 M	
3 M		6 M		12 M	

DOCTOR'S SIGNATURE & DATE

ACHIEVING SKILL COMPETENCY

Reread the TPO for each procedure and then practice the skills listed below, following the procedure in your textbook.

Total Charges on Calculator—Procedure 4-1

Operate Copy Machine—Procedure 4-2

Operate Transcriber—Procedure 4-3

Operate Office Computer—rocedure 4-4

Open office—Procedure 4-5

Obtain preliminary patient information—Procedure 4-6

Close office—Procedure 4-7

After your instructor has returned your work to you, make all necessary corrections and place in a 3-ring notebook for future reference.

ASSIGNMENT SHEET

Chapter 5: INTERPERSONAL COMMUNICATIONS
Unit 1: VERBAL AND NONVERBAL MESSAGES

Review the objectives and text for each unit before completing the assignment sheet for that unit in this chapter. When all sheets for the chapter have been completed, remove them from this workbook and give them to the instructor for evaluation.

A. UNSCRAMBLE

1. _ _ _ _ _ _ _ _ _ _ _ _ _ _   RTMINTRSIEPE
2. _ _ _ _ _ _ _ _ _ _   TIAGBELNN
3. _ _ _ _ _ _ _   SDRTOIT
4. _ _ _ _ _ _ _ _ _ _   IUINONITT
5. _ _ _ _ _ _ _ _ _ _   OIPPETNREC
6. _ _ _ _ _ _ _ _ _ _ _   ICOGOUNNRSU
7. _ _ _ _ _ _ _ _ _ _ _ _   UOUSSRUCLLYP
8. _ _ _ _ _ _ _ _ _ _   NDTICARTCO
9. _ _ _ _ _ _ _ _ _ _ _ _   PIEMRIYLALC
10. _ _ _ _ _ _ _ _ _ _   CUETLTIARA
11. _ _ _ _ _ _ _ _ _ _ _ _ _   ENZCEOPCUTALI

B. LABELING: Add labels to each numbered section of this communication process model. Refer to Figure 5-1.

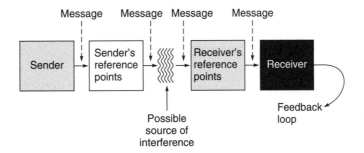

C. BRIEF ANSWER

1. Describe the basic pattern of communication. _____

_____

_____

2. Give examples of nonverbal communication. _____

_____

3. Explain how verbal and nonverbal communication can sometimes be misinterpreted. _____

_____

4. How can tone and speed of speech affect a message? _____

_____

5. Why is it important to wear appropriate dress, uniform, or business attire when working with patients? _____

_____

_____

_____

6. Explain what perception is. _____
_____

7. Why is it important to develop the skill of perception? _____
_____
_____

8. Why is silence such a powerful nonverbal message (communication)? _____
_____
_____

9. What benefit does the communication of touch provide to patients? _____
_____
_____

D. TRUE OR FALSE: Place a "T" for True or "F" for False. For any False answers you may have, number them below and explain why.

_____ 1. The medical assistant can be instrumental in providing comfort and compassion to patients in need.

_____ 2. A harmonious team effort makes for an efficient and pleasant work environment.

_____ 3. Becoming perceptive can only be attained by reading.

_____ 4. Your overall appearance sends out messages to anyone who looks at you.

_____ 5. Setting a good example is not a part of your responsibility in the care of others.

_____ 6. Your attitude has nothing to do with your overall appearance.

_____ 7. Gestures are body movements which can help the receiver understand the message being communicated.

_____ 8. Studies show that a caring touch of a patient can elicit better response in treatment.

_____ 9. It is possible to contradict a verbal message by an inappropriate facial expression.

_____ 10. Your attitude shows in your facial expression.

E. CRITICAL THINKING SITUATIONS: What would your response be in the following situations?

1. A 25-year-old female patient arrives a half hour early for her appointment. You notice that she is sitting off by herself and is sobbing. _____
_____

2. A middle-aged male patient has just finished a consultation with the doctor. The patient tells you that it is getting harder all the time taking care of his invalid father. _____
_____

3. You notice that a co-worker has made several charting errors in the past few days. It bothers you, for you are worried about quality patient care and the legal ramifications. _____
_____

4. Your physician-employer asks you to help an elderly patient overcome procrastination about taking his medication and eating regularly. _____
_____

5. A young mother of four (ranging in age from 6 months to 5 years) complains to you that she has no time for herself, is always exhausted, and is a nervous wreck. _____
_____
_____

F. CROSSWORD PUZZLE

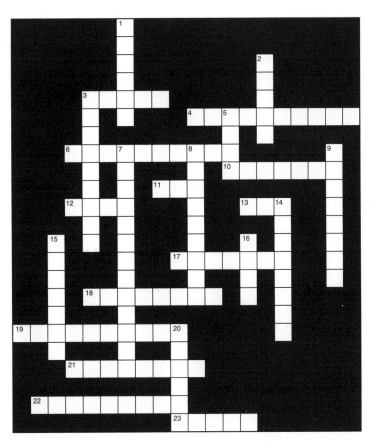

ACROSS

  3. How you project this is of utmost importance
  4. You must speak this way if you are to be understood
  6. Being aware of your own and others' feelings
 10. You should set a good _____
 11. Effective communication is an _____
 12. _____ work
 13. Conveys feelings of affection
 17. To twist or mess up
 18. Efficient use of time comes from _____
 19. Good rapport
 21. To send a message
 22. Unspoken
 23. Conveys a positive message

DOWN

  1. Spoken
  2. Gives patients a sense of security and caring
  3. To come between
  5. You should speak in a pleasant _____
  7. Exchange of information
  8. Perception
  9. Everyone has them
 14. Body movements that send messages
 15. What a team gives each other
 16. A strong communication (language)
 20. You must continually strive to master _____

Name _____

After your instructor has returned your work to you, make all necessary corrections and place in a 3-ring notebook for future reference.

ASSIGNMENT SHEET

Chapter 5: INTERPERSONAL COMMUNICATIONS
Unit 2: BEHAVIORAL ADJUSTMENTS

A. **MATCHING: Read the definition in Column II and then find the matching answer in Column I. Place the letter of the correct answer in the space provided.**

COLUMN I

_____ 1. Adjustment
_____ 2. Analytical
_____ 3. Ardently
_____ 4. Displacement
_____ 5. Intellectualization
_____ 6. Malinger
_____ 7. Projection
_____ 8. Rationalization
_____ 9. Repression
_____ 10. Stratagem
_____ 11. Sublimation
_____ 12. Unobtrusive

COLUMN II

a. To keep down or hold back
b. Devotedly
c. To pretend to be ill
d. To settle or bring into accord
e. Below the threshold of consciousness
f. Rationalism; reasoning without regard to feelings
g. A plan to deceive
h. Question/examine
i. Unconsciously blaming another for one's own inadequacies
j. Modest; unpretending
k. Transfer of feelings about another to an innocent person
l. Devising a socially acceptable explanation for inadequate behavior
m. Discord; confusion

B. **ANSWER THE FOLLOWING:**

1. List the commonly used defense mechanisms and give an example of each. _____

_____
_____
_____
_____
_____
_____
_____
_____
_____
_____
_____
_____
_____

2. What could happen to a person who habitually uses one or more of the commonly used defense mechanisms?

_____
_____
_____

3. Why is it necessary to know oneself before one can relate effectively with others? _____

_____
_____
_____
_____
_____

4. What are the problem-solving steps in this unit?

_____

_____

_____

_____

_____

5. Apply the problem-solving steps to a particular problem you may have. _____

_____

_____

_____

6. Explain the importance of one's mental and emotional status to overall health. _____

_____

_____

_____

C. FILL IN THE BLANK

1. Problem-solving skills can help one eliminate _____ .
2. How we view ourselves is our _____ .
3. Our response to others is dealt with by our _____ .
4. Unfortunately, many of us never come close to reaching our true _____ .
5. Making a list of our strengths and weaknesses is a good way to begin a _____ of ourselves.
6. Two good times to take a look at ourselves for evaluation and renew our goals and aspirations are _____ and _____ .
7. _____ is a complex process in which one has to be aware of all facets for complete information exchanges to occur.
8. The perceptive Medical Assistant should be able to decide what "_____" to ask a patient to determine whether the look on that patient's face matches the patient's demeanor.
9. The Medical Assistant must impart a genuine _____ for patient's well being.
10. Patients may open up about their problems or preoccupations if the Medical Assistant shows an _____ and takes the _____ with them that they need.

D. WORD SEARCH

1. **FIND THE FOLLOWING WORDS IN THE PUZZLE.**
2. **USE THE EVEN NUMBERED WORDS IN A SENTENCE.**

1. ACTS		11. ANXIETY
2. AVOID		12. RATIONALIZATION
3. DEFENSE MECHANISMS		13. CONCERN
4. SELF		14. BEHAVIOR
5. REGRESSION		15. PROBLEM
6. ACCEPT		16. DENIAL
7. MALINGER		17. PATIENTS
8. BLAME		18. EMOTIONS
9. KIND		19. CARE
10. INFLUENCE		20. EXPRESS

```
A N L V A Z E S P T V O F T K Q P R O E N
O B S O A C T S A C P S R T L Z M Y M R Y
D R W Z V T A L T S G W L P T O A A B A L
P Z E A O P N S E Q R O A E E S L Z Q C G
A Q R N I N T L Q S R Z P C L B I L R A B
N O V E D E F E N S E M E C H A N I S M S
T D D I O E P G T P G S M A D N G O T Z X
I N F L U E N C E D R A O D L M E B N W O
N I V A L B F I Y Z E D B H M E R L E B T
D K N X C W L T A A S L E F E L A A I L S
I S W A F B E O J L S M H T J B O M T F V
S Z R A T I O N A L I Z A T I O N Z A K A
O P R O X G Z C Q A O T V K B R P F P I L
P C O N C E R N L Z N H I A H P O E R N R
D A A X O W B J E K S N O S S E R P X E Q
Z M B E M O T I O N S A R S S R D M S C B
```

1. _____
2. _____
3. _____
4. _____
5. _____
6. _____
7. _____
8. _____
9. _____
10. _____

After your instructor has returned your work to you, make all necessary corrections and place in a 3-ring notebook for future reference.

ASSIGNMENT SHEET

Chapter 5: INTERPERSONAL COMMUNICATIONS
Unit 3: PATIENTS AND THEIR FAMILIES

A. MATCHING: Read the definition in Column II and then find the matching answer in Column I. Place the letter of the correct answer in the space provided.

COLUMN I

_____ 1. Marginal
_____ 2. Holistic
_____ 3. Terminal
_____ 4. Absurd
_____ 5. Incomprehensible
_____ 6. Nonchalant
_____ 7. Hostility
_____ 8. Inevitable
_____ 9. Devastate
_____ 10. Plight

COLUMN II

a. Cannot be understood
b. Showing no interest
c. A sad situation
d. Certain to happen
e. Overwhelm
f. Close to a limit
g. Pertaining to whole
h. Apprehension
i. Ridiculous
j. Antagonistic
k. Final

B. BRIEF ANSWER

1. Why is it important to develop good rapport with patients? _____
_____

2. How can the medical assistant safeguard the patient's right to confidentiality? _____
_____
_____

3. What are the patient's options in relation to the physician's treatment plan? _____
_____

4. Describe the stages which patients experience following the diagnosis of terminal illness. _____
_____
_____

5. What is the medical assistant's role in dealing with the terminally ill patient? _____
_____

6. What is the purpose of the living will (also referred to as Advance Directives)? _____
_____

7. What is the purpose of the hospice movement? _____
_____

8. List the services the hospice movement provides. _____
_____
_____

C. FILL IN THE BLANK

1. The first responsibility for the medical professional is to the _____ .

2. Facing unfamiliar surroundings and unfamiliar medical language adds to the patient's _____ .

3. Tact and good communication skills helps promote _____ with patients.

4. The patient's _____ must be obtained to release information about him/her to unauthorized persons.

5. The physician must be informed of a patient's _____ for it may have some bearing on the condition of the patient.

6. The medical assistant plays an integral part in _____ the physician's orders.

7. _____ is the key in helping patients accept and comply with treatment.

8. By being a good _____ , the medical assistant reinforces the physician's advice.

9. A copy of the living will is filed with the physician, the _____ , and the family of a terminally ill patient.

10. Patients and their families may need _____ guidance more at this time than ever before in their lives.

After your instructor has returned your work to you, make all necessary corrections and place in a 3-ring notebook for future reference.

ASSIGNMENT SHEET

Chapter 5: INTERPERSONAL COMMUNICATIONS
Unit 4: OFFICE INTERPERSONAL RELATIONSHIPS

A. UNSCRAMBLE

1. _ _ _ _ _   YETPT
2. _ _ _ _ _ _ _ _ _ _   LATNEAOIVU
3. _ _ _ _ _ _ _ _ _ _   RLXGNIPEPE
4. _ _ _ _ _   IRMTE
5. _ _ _ _ _ _ _ _ _ _ _   PDSECITRINO
6. _ _ _ _ _ _ _   ULISERE
7. _ _ _ _ _ _ _ _ _   VRJETENAUE

B. BRIEF ANSWER

1. What are the most important factors in the relationships between medical assistant, employers, and co-workers? _____
_____
_____

2. List positive factors of externship. _____
_____
_____

3. What are the reasons for staff meetings? _____
_____
_____

4. List some methods of intraoffice communication. _____
_____
_____

5. What is the purpose of the employee evaluation? _____
_____
_____
_____

C. MATCHING: Read the definition in Column II and then find the matching answer in Column I. Place the letter of the correct answer in the space provided.

COLUMN I

_____ 1. Annual evaluations
_____ 2. Positive attitude
_____ 3. Self-discipline
_____ 4. Medical assistant
_____ 5. Break-time
_____ 6. Cooperation
_____ 7. Intraoffice memo
_____ 8. Teamwork
_____ 9. Job descriptions
_____ 10. Good rapport
_____ 11. AAMA & ARMA

COLUMN II

a. Means of communicating important information to staff
b. Continuing education
c. Results in quality patient care
d. Promote efficiency
e. Necessary to accomplish objectives of physician and patient
f. Regular exercise
g. Creates pleasant work environment
h. Necessary in a professional setting
i. Essential in smooth office operation
j. Motivate employees and keep communication lines open
k. Must relate well to others
l. Essential to well-being

After your instructor has returned your work to you, make all necessary corrections and place in a 3-ring notebook for future reference.

ASSIGNMENT SHEET

Chapter 6: ORAL AND WRITTEN COMMUNICATIONS
Unit 1: TELEPHONE COMMUNICATIONS

Review the objectives and text for each unit before completing the assignment sheet for that unit in this chapter. When all sheets for the chapter have been completed, remove them from this workbook and give them to the instructor for evaluation.

A. COMPLETE THE FOLLOWING STATEMENTS.

1. Two essential items that should be next to each telephone in a medical facility are a *pad* and a *pen* .

2. The medical assistant who handles phone calls must be *courteous* , articulate, and a careful and *active listener.*

3. You should answer the phone in the medical facility as soon as possible or at least by the *3rd ring* .

4. The *rapport* established by the medical assistant who answers the phone will contribute to successful communication with patients.

5. The responsibility of responding to phone calls in a medical office takes a great deal of *maturity and patience* .

6. It is a sensible practice to have all _____ phone numbers listed by each phone in the office.

7. An established phone *triage manual* should be kept near the phone for reference so that each medical assistant who answers the phone will ask the same standard questions and give the same standard advice which the physician has pre-authorized.

8. All telephone messages that are urgent should be given _____ and handled as soon as possible.

9. When you hold the telephone receiver to your ear, it should be *2 to 3 inches* in front of your mouth so that the caller may clearly hear your voice.

10. You should be *honest* about your knowledge and experience with phone systems.

11. When answering a phone call of a patient, make sure you get the caller's *complete name / #* in case the call is an emergency and the call is interrupted.

12. Patients who phone for an appointment should be given a choice of *two* appointment times.

13. The appointment should be *confirmed* by reading the appointment time back to the patient after it has been recorded in the appointment book.

14. You should _____ file a report that the physician has not seen and initialed.

15. Only patient information that has been *authorized* by the patient in writing, with the patient's signature, may be given to another party.

16. If you have made an error on a patient's bill, be sure to *admit* it, *apologize* , and offer to send a *revised* statement.

17. When placing long distance phone calls, it is advisable to consult a telephone directory for a *time zone* so you can establish the appropriate time to call.

18. Never tell anyone over the phone (or in person) that you are *alone* as it may be an invitation for undesirable behavior.

19. If the physician requests that you monitor a phone call, it is important that the caller *agrees* to your listening and taking notes.

B. TRUE OR FALSE: PLACE A "T" FOR TRUE OR "F" FOR FALSE IN THE SPACE PROVIDED.

T   1. A pleasant voice and good listening skills are essential in telephone communications.

F   2. When a patient calls for information about their condition or for a lab report, it is not necessary to pull their chart.

T   3. All telephone calls, regardless of what you feel about their importance, should be documented.

F   4. The answering machine in the medical office should be turned on to leave a message to callers only on weekends when the physician is not in the office.

T   5. Telephone callers form a picture of you as they listen to your voice.

F   6. When you finish a conversation over the phone with a patient you should hang up first to let the patient know you are finished talking.

T   7. When an attorney phones for information about a patient, you must give them the necessary information immediately.

T   8. Always be sure to make a copy of any correspondence mailed out so you have a copy for the patient's chart.

T   9. The physician usually does not wish to speak to unidentified phone callers during busy office hours.

F   10. When answering the medical office phone, and the physician is not there, you should always know where to reach him/her.

T   11. You should never leave a patient on hold for more than 10 minutes.

F   12. You should screen and complete as many calls as possible before adding names to the physician's call back list.

C. ESSAY

1. List the common types of calls that are received in a medical office. Common types of Calls in the office are referrals, patients who call for apointments, prescriptions, or test results, Emergency calls, other physicians, hospitals, or laboratories, also personal calls/business calls.

2. Explain why a telephone triage manual should be kept by the phone to manage telephone calls in a medical facility. It should be kept by the phone for reference so that each assistant who answers the phone will ask the same standard questions/advice which the physician has pre-authorized.

3. List the important items of a telephone message. The important items of a phone message are the callers full name, spelled correctly, Brief note taking the nature of call, action required, Date, time of call, initial person recieving call, phone number of caller, including area code (if long distance.).

D. CROSSWORD PUZZLE: Solve the puzzle with the Words to Know and terms taken from this unit.

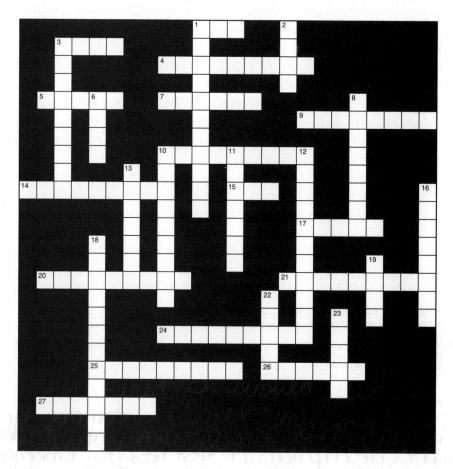

ACROSS

1. A number of sheets of paper fastened together
3. A given point of time
4. Relevant, applicable
5. To analyze by application of reagents-to prove knowledge
7. Induce to action
9. Mechanical device for recording sounds
10. An associate in an office, usually one of similar status
14. Person practicing medical profession
15. Writing instrument
17. A receptionist will answer telephone _____
20. Made known in words or action
21. Conventional rules for correct behavior
24. A preliminary or indicating procedure
25. A helper or co-worker in a specific occupation
26. Tool or plan
27. Pertaining to medicine

DOWN

1. The personal or individual quality that makes one person different from another
2. The sound of a bell
3. A book containing lists of names and address
6. A chance of a life _____
8. Place for healing
10. Verified; ratified
11. Sympathetically trying to identify one's feelings with those of another
12. Pronouncing clearly
13. Sixty in each hour
16. Type of work or commerce
18. Prove to be true; supported by facts
19. Depend; trust
22. Coming next after second in a series
23. Sound produced through mouth

DIRECTIONS: Read the following situations out loud in class and role play how you would handle. Answers will vary and your instructor may want to guide the situations.

TELEPHONE WORKSHEET #1: "I HAVE TO SEE THE DOCTOR-TODAY"

Doctor's Identity: (Use names of local physicians)

Solo or Group: Two-man partnership

Specialty: Family Practice

Time: 8:30 a.m.

Situation: Both physicians are on hospital rounds and are not expected until 10:00 a.m.
The appointment book is full.

Patient: (insert name of student or fictitious name), a patient since infancy

---

"I need an appointment today-right away. I'm leaving for college tomorrow and the doctor just has to see me. Just for a minute. I need a quick physical and a form filled out. It's nothing really."

"I can't register for class unless the doctor sees me. I just have to have an appointment. I know this is last minute-but just this once, please. Certainly, you understand, you have to.".

How did you handle this? First I would let the patient know that I will try my best to try to fit him into my busy schedule. I would get all call back information and tell him to hold so I can check my schedule. If I have a spot open I will let him know. If I dont I will simply explaine that I'm all booked, but if anyone cancels I will definitely call back.

TELEPHONE WORKSHEET #2: MOTHER WHO WANTS TO MAKE AN APPOINTMENT FOR HERSELF AND HER CHILD

Doctor's Identity:	(Use name of local physician)
Solo or Group:	Solo practice
Specialty:	OB-GYN
Time:	10:00 a.m.
Situation:	The physician is in an area where there are a number of pediatricians and he does not see pediatric patients.
Patient:	(fictitious name) Mrs. _____

Mrs. _____ is new in the area and got the doctor's name from calling the county medical society. She has a history of menstrual difficulty. She has no immediate problem, but wants to make an appointment with an OB-GYN physician in this new location in order to establish a "regular" doctor.

She tells the medical assistant that she wants to bring (fill in name of child) with her, and wants to make an appointment for _____ too, immediately following her appointment. _____ is her four year old daughter.

Mrs. _____ does not want to accept the fact that Dr. _____ will not see _____. She argues that she has to bring _____ with her, there is no one to take care of her, and this is not really an inconvenience to Dr. _____. It will just take a ten minute check for _____ , and Mrs. _____ is most willing to make an appointment two or three weeks in advance to meet the doctor's convenience.

How did you handle this?

TELEPHONE WORKSHEET #3: PATIENT INSISTS ON APPOINTMENT

Doctor's Identity: (Use names of local physicians)

Solo or Group: Two-man partnership

Specialty: Internal Medicine

Time: 3:30 p.m.

Situation: Dr. _____ is out of the office today.
Dr. _____ is in the examining room with a patient. The office is already behind schedule because Dr. _____ has had to work in a couple of emergency patients of Dr. _____.

Patient: (fictitious name) Mrs. _____ is a regular patient, that is, she has been to the office two or three times a year. The medical assistant knows her well enough to recognize the name and identify it with a 64-year-old widow living alone. Mrs. _____ has always been very nice, but is a little bit on the "dramatic" side.

- -

Mrs. _____ calls and says she is very ill and would like to see (Dr. who is out of the office) right away. She says she has had a headache since mid-morning and it is getting worse. She has had these headaches before, and Dr. _____ has always given her something to stop them, but she doesn't have any more of the little pills and she feels just awful. She knows she will be sick all night if something isn't done right away. Although she feels real bad she will get in a cab and come to the office right now.

She will see (Dr. in office) if necessary, but she prefers to see (Dr. who is out of the office) since he is her regular doctor. She thinks the doctor should see her now when she feels so bad. There is no use for the doctor to see her two or three days from now when she may be feeling all right - if she lives through the night.

She doesn't threaten or get abusive, but is really persistent and keeps repeating that she must see the doctor right now.

- -

How did you handle this? I will let her know the situation, and explain to her that the Dr. is not available, but this other doctor whom her primary doctor says under his supervision she should see until he is available. Or I could let her know I will contact the Dr. to see if he can prescribe the pills over the phone until he is able to see her.

TELEPHONE WORKSHEET #4: "WE'RE ON VACATION"

Doctor's Identity: (Use name of local physician)

Solo or Group: Solo practice

Specialty: Internist

Time: Late afternoon in July

Situation: The doctor is in and he is seeing his last scheduled patient for the day.

Patient: (fictitious name)

The caller simply identifies herself as Mrs. _____. She has a thick southern accent. The medical assistant does not know her.

The woman is sniffling and is saying, "My baby, my baby, _____ is so sick. Is the doctor there? I just know my baby needs help. Is the doctor there? I'm just visiting here, my husband left me in the hotel here and has been out fishing and camping for two days. The baby has a high fever and just keeps crying. I'm all alone, I don't know what to do."

How did you handle this? I would tell the Dr. my situation, and see if he is willing to wait and see her. If he is not available I would tell her the nearest hospetal to go to, and info. I would also tell her to go as soon as possible. I would take as much info as I can get.

TELEPHONE WORKSHEET #5: THE ANGRY AND ABUSIVE PATIENT

Doctor's Identity:	(Use name of local physician)
Solo or Group:	Solo practice
Specialty:	Family Practice
Time:	1:30 p.m.
Situation:	The appointment book is completely filled and the only time for a regular office visit is 2½ weeks ahead on Thursday at 2:00 p.m.
Patient:	(fictitious name) She has been in the office two or three times during the past year, and has always been rather quiet and reserved. Mrs. _____ has high blood pressure which is being handled very well with medication, but she is supposed to come in to the office every three or four months for a checkup. This office does not schedule appointments that far in advance. The doctor has simply said, "come back every two or three months." Mrs. _____ has never seemed unreasonable before, but today she is in a very bad mood.

- -

Mrs. _____ calls for an appointment and the medical assistant advises her that the first opening is 2½ weeks ahead. When the medical assistant gives her this information, her immediate and automatic response is that this is not at all convenient. She says that she planned to see the doctor in the next several days and that she has no idea where she will be in 2½ weeks. She thinks she might be taking a vacation trip somewhere, and she simply does not want to wait this long for an appointment.

As the conversation continues, Mrs. _____ gets more and more argumentative and points out that all she wants is a checkup which will take the doctor only a few minutes, and that if it was anything more than that she would probably be dead before the doctor could get around to seeing her. She argues that she isn't demanding to see the doctor immediately, that an appointment in the next three or four days will be satisfactory, but that waiting 2½ weeks for a simple checkup is not reasonable, etc., etc.

Finally, Mrs. _____ gets nasty. She says she wants to talk to the doctor. She wants to know just who is running the medical practice. She doesn't think the doctor really knows what is going on. She might even mention that she is running low on her pills and doesn't think that her medication will last for 2½ weeks more.

- -

How did you handle this? First I would try to calm the patient down. Let her know our situation. If she still needs it sooner, I will tell her if anyone cancels she is first on the list, and we will her know if anything comes up. If still not happy, I will let the Dr. speak with her, and let him know the circumstances.

TELEPHONE WORKSHEET #6: INSISTS ON TALKING TO THE DOCTOR

Doctor's Identity: (Use name of local physician)

Solo or Group: Solo practice

Specialty: Family Practice

Time: Early Monday morning

Situation: The doctor is in and in the examining room with a patient. The appointment schedule is already over-booked, and this is going to be another day when all of the patients have a long wait in the reception room and both the doctor and the medical assistant will be working overtime.

Patient: (fictitious name) An elderly widower, a regular patient who makes an appointment to see the doctor almost every month most of the time for imagined ills.

- -

Mr. _____ calls and says, "I need to talk with Dr. _____. I've had a splitting headache all weekend. I knew he would be out on the golf course or some such thing-so I waited until now to call. I just can't wait any longer. Put me through to him. I'll only take a minute."

The medical assistant replies that Dr. _____ is seeing a patient in the examining room and that he will call back. "That's what you always say" Mr. _____ replies, "if I was dying I would have to wait for a convenient time? All I want to do is talk to the doctor for just a minute."

The medical assistant repeats that the doctor is in the examining room and suggests a call-back.

Mr. _____, "I had to get out of bed to come to the phone, so I'll just hang on. That certainly isn't going to inconvenience him. You just tell him that I'm holding the phone. I don't like waiting-I waited all weekend and I don't want to be put off a moment longer than necessary. I pay my bills and I deserve to talk to the doctor when I need him."

- -

How did you handle this? I will let him know I am completely sorry, and that I will see to it that the Dr calls back A.S.A.P. Also I would tell him the wait will be long and it would jest be better if he waited for the Dr's call back.

TELEPHONE WORKSHEET #7: CALL TO NOTIFY PATIENT

Doctor's Identity: (Use names of local physicians)

Solo or Group: Partnership

Specialty: OB/GYN

Time: 1:00 p.m.

Situation: Both physicians have called in to say that they will be late in returning to the office. It seems all of the babies in town decided to be delivered today. Dr. _____ anticipating a Caesarean section, says he may not be in at all. Dr. _____ says that he will be at least one hour late, and maybe longer. Here office protocol is to notify patients, who have not as yet arrived, of the delay.

Patient: (fictitious name)

You call Mrs. _____ and tell her of the delay. She has an appointment for 3:00 p.m. and she made it some three weeks ago. She is upset-you can tell this from the tone of her voice.

The medical assistant knows from past experience that the best thing to do would be to cancel Mrs. _____ appointment and reschedule her. This can't be done, about the earliest time that Dr. _____ can see Mrs. _____ will be 5:00 to 5:30 p.m.

Mrs. _____ is not enthusiastic about either alternative.

How did you handle this?

TELEPHONE WORKSHEET #8: THE CASE OF THE HOLD BUTTON

Doctor's Identity:	(Use name of local physician, female)
Solo or Group:	Solo practice
Specialty:	General Surgery
Time:	10:00 a.m.
Situation:	Dr. _____ has advised the patient that if her incision continues to ooze, she is to call the doctor. The doctor has advised the medical assistant that if the patient calls, she will want to talk with her.
Patient:	(fictitious name)

Mrs. _____ calls; the doctor is in her consulting office and the medical assistant plans to transfer the call immediately to Dr. _____. Mrs. _____ is not upset, or doesn't seem to be, on the telephone. Dr. _____ is upset after talking with Mrs. _____ because she was having no trouble with her incision, all she needed was an appointment.

What did the medical assistant fail to do?

TELEPHONE WORKSHEET #9: THE PATIENT WHO HAS BEEN A NO-SHOW

Doctor's Identity: (Use name of local physician)

Solo or Group: Solo practice

Specialty: Family Practice

Time: 11:30 a.m.

Situation: The patient calls for an appointment. The patient had an appointment the previous week but didn't show and didn't call in. The patient simply says she was busy last Thursday and just couldn't make it. The appointment was only for a check-up, but she wants to make another appointment for now.

Patient: (fictitious name)

The medical assistant can make an appointment for approximately two weeks from today. Mrs. _____ is willing to accept that.

What does the medical assistant say in regard to the previous "no-show"?

ASSIGNMENT SHEET

Chapter 6: ORAL AND WRITTEN COMMUNICATIONS
Unit 3: WRITTEN COMMUNICATIONS

A. COMPLETION

1. List seven types of communication medical assistants may need to compose. _____
_____
_____
_____

2. Prepare an IOC to inform any six persons in your class about the following: Field trip to your local health department, one month from today at 9:00 a.m., returning by noon. Request verification of reading.

_____
_____
_____
_____
_____
_____
_____
_____
_____
_____

3. List six instances when form letters are appropriate. _____
_____
_____
_____

4. Using the following abbreviations, determine which type of correspondence is appropriate to the stated situation.
    Types: IOC, IN (informal note), Per Let (personal letter), Pro Let (professional letter), BL (business letter, IS (information sheet)
    _____ a. Sending information to a referred patient
    _____ b. Correspondence to colleagues on hospital board
    _____ c. Congratulations to a friend
    _____ d. Instructions for a diagnostic procedure
    _____ e. Request for membership information at a golf club
    _____ f. Request to accountant for mid-year status
    _____ g. Employee memo regarding change in office insurance benefits
    _____ h. Request for medical practice reciprocity in another state

5. Which words in the following lines are spelled correctly?

apostrophy	apostrofe	apostrophe
communication	comunication	communikation
congratulations	congradulations	congratulashuns
contraction	contrackion	contracshun
coresspondence	correspondence	correspondance
hiphen	hyfen	hyphen
mispelled	misspeled	misspelled
modafies	modifies	modifyes
stationery	stationairy	stationare

6. Following information in text on punctuation, capitalization, and mailable standards, type the three letters according to the instruction with each one; letterheads are provided. Final copy should meet mailable standards. _____

7. List the problem areas to watch when proofreading. _____

_____

_____

8. Type corrected letter #4 by interpreting proofreader's marks.

9. Given a dictating machine tape, produce a mailable letter according to Procedure 6-8, Type a Business Letter.

_____

10. Given a copy with errors, make corrections using eraser, correction paper and fluid and make typing error and correct with correction ribbon following Procedure 6-7, Make Corrections on Typewritten Copy.

LETTER #1

The first letter is to Robert Jones, M.D., 5000 N. High Street, Yourtown, US 43200. The name of the patient is Juan Gomez. Use full block style seen in Figure 6-20(b), proper capitalization, punctuation, and placement on the paper.

Dear dr jones

your patient juan gomez was first seen October 7, complaining of severe tinnitus in both ears.

On physical examination his hearing was 15/20 right ear 13/20 left ear audiogram was made which showed considerable loss of high tones Mr. gomez's complaints of tinnitus and decreased hearing are in accordance with the audiometric and clinical findings of beginning degeneration of his nerve of hearing. In all probability this condition has been caused by loud noises which he has encountered in his work.

despite treatment his hearing has not increased and tinnitus persists.

thank you for referring mr gomez.

very truly yours

LETTER #2

Type the second letter using modified block style seen in Figure 6-20(c). Use current date for the letter. Address the letter to John Jones, M.D. 3530 Main Street, Cold Springs, Kentucky, 41076. The name of the patient is Mrs. Patty Segal. The dictating physician is Samuel E. Matthews, M.D.

I saw _____ on _____ for x-ray examination.

AP and lateral roentgenograms of the cervical spine show an aberration of the normal cervical curve. The curve is convexed posteriorly at the level of the fifth, sixth, and seventh cervical vertebrae. Normally, the posterior curve should be concave. There are no significant hypertrophic changes, but there are minimal true arthritic changes involving the articular facets in the lower cervical region.

A roentgenogram of the right shoulder shows no evidence of intrinsic bone disease. There is no periarticular soft tissue calcification in the region of the bruise.

Thank you for your referral

Very truly yours,

LETTER #3

Type the following letter using modified block with indented paragraphs as seen in Figure 6-22(d). The letter is to Robert Jones, M.D., 5000 N. High Street, Yourtown, US 98765. The patient is Patricia Moriarty. The letter is from Kerry Smith, M.D.

Dear Dr. Jones:

I saw _____ in the office today. You will recall that she has suffered from menstrual discomfort and intermenstrual pain for the past 6 months.

On examination, the breasts are well developed and free of masses. On pelvic examination, the hymen is intact; and vaginal examination was not performed. On rectal examination, the uterus was anterior and freely movable. The right adnexa were normal. The left ovary was enlarged to the size of a walnut or slightly larger and was cystic. Compression of this ovary reproduced the patient's pain.

Patricia was asked to return in three weeks for re-examination to determine the need for treatment of ovarian enlargement.

Thank you for referring this patient.

Sincerely,

LETTER #1

SAMUEL E. MATTHEWS, M.D.

SUITE 120 100 E. MAIN STREET

YOURTOWN, US 98765-4321

LETTER #2

SAMUEL E. MATTHEWS, M.D.

SUITE 120 100 E. MAIN STREET

YOURTOWN, US 98765-4321

LETTER #3

KERRY SMITH, M.D.

101 LANE AVENUE

YOURTOWN, US 12345

LETTER #4
Letter to be corrected

Kerry Smith, M.D.
101 Lane Avenue
Yourtown, US 12345

Robrt Jones, M.D.
5000 N. High Street
Yourtown, US 98765

Dear Dr. Jones:

I saw Patricia Moriarty in the officetoday. You will recall that she has suffered from menstrual dis comfort and intermenstrual pain since July.

On examination, the breasts are well develloped and free of masses. on pelvic examination, the hymen is intact; and vaginal examination was not performed. On Rectal examination the uterus was anterior and freely movable. The right adnexa were normal. The left ovary was enlarged to the size of a walnut or slightly larger and was cystic Compression of this ovary reproduced the patient's pain. Patricia was asked to return in three weeks for re-examination to determine the need for treatment of ovarian enlargement.

Thank you for referring this patient.

Sincerely,

Kerry Smith, M.D.

LETTER #4

KERRY SMITH, M.D.

101 LANE AVENUE

YOURTOWN, US 12345

B. WORD PUZZLE

COMPLETE BLANKS USING DEFINITIONS BELOW.

1.   _ _ _ T _ _ _
2.   _ _ _ _ R _ _ _ _ _ _
3.   _ _ A _ _ _
4.   _ _ _ N _ _ _
5. _ _ _ _ _ S _ _
6.   C _ _ _ _ _ _ _
7   _ R _ _ _ _ _ _ _
8.   _ _ I _ _ _ _ _
9.   P _ _ _ _ _ _ _ _ _
10.   _ _ T _ _ _ _ _
11.   _ I _ _ _ _ _ _ _
12.   _ O _ _ _ _ _ _
13.   _ _ N _ _ _
14.   _ _ _ _ I _ _ _ _ _
15. _ _ _ _ _ S _
16.   T _ _ _ _ _ _ _ _

Definitions:

1. the part of a written or spoken statement that surrounds a particular word or passage and can clarify its meaning
2. a shortened word or words formed by omitting or combining some of the letters or sounds
3. a section of a sentence
4. a noun substitute
5. a mark or series of marks used in writing or printing to indicate an omission, especially of letters or words
6. a critical examination of a thing or situation
7. carefully read material for errors
8. an item suitable for mailing
9. an addition to a letter written after the writer's name
10. a mark imprinted on paper that is visible when it is held up to the light, usually a sign of quality
11. the name of a person as written by himself
12. to qualify or limit the meaning
13. to indicate, to mean
14. paper used for letters
15. to write, to form by combination of units or parts
16. a reference book containing words and their synonyms

ASSIGNMENT SHEET

Chapter 6: ORAL AND WRITTEN COMMUNICATIONS
Unit 4: RECEIVING AND SENDING OFFICE COMMUNICATIONS

A. BRIEF ANSWER

1. What supplies and equipment are needed to open the mail? _____

_____

2. What information may be different on the envelope than on the contents? _____

3. What incoming mail may be handled by the medical assistant alone? _____

_____

4. How should unwanted drug samples be disposed of? _____

5. Using the following information, address the envelope below so it can be read by the OCR and sorted by the BCS. Send to: Medical Records, University Hospital, 100 E. First Street, Ourtown, US, 12345-6789 (You may print your answer in lieu of typing). Use Elizabeth R. Evans, M.D., Suite 205 100 E. Main St., Yourtown, US 98765-4321 as the return address.

ELIZABETH R EVANS MD
SUITE 205 — 100 E MAIN ST
YOURTOWN US 98765-4321

MEDICAL RECORDS
UNIVERSITY HOSPITAL
100 EAST FIRST STREET
OURTOWN US 12345-6789

---

6. Below are some abbreviations pertaining to mail; give the words they stand for.
   A. USPS _____
   B. OCR _____
   C. BCS _____
   D. APT _____
   E. ATTN _____
   F. AVE _____
   G. BLVD _____
   H. HTS _____
   I. HOSP _____
   J. INST _____
   K. LN _____
   L. MGR _____

M. PKY _____

N. PL _____

O. PO _____

P. RR _____

7. What do the numbers in the following zip code 43221-4940 stand for?

4- _____

32- _____

21- _____

49- _____

40- _____

8. Name four things to remember in processing metered mail. _____

_____

_____

9. Mail is classified according to _____ , _____ and _____ .

10. Where can current postal information be obtained? _____

11. List the four classifications of mail. _____

12. In the following list, place a number 1 before first class mail, 2 before second, 3 before third or 4 before fourth class mail.

_____ 1. catalogs

_____ 2. payments from patients

_____ 3. bound printed matter

_____ 4. laboratory reports

_____ 5. newspapers

_____ 6. printed books

_____ 7. newsletters

_____ 8. books

_____ 9. handwritten or typed messages

_____ 10. payments from insurance companies

_____ 11. merchandise thru 15 ounces not required to be mailed first class

_____ 12. envelope with green diamond border

_____ 13. 16 mm or narrower films

_____ 14. periodicals issued at least quarterly

_____ 15. recordings

_____ 16. business mail up to 12 ounces

_____ 17. circulars

_____ 18. manuscripts

13. What special sending or receiving features are associated with the following types of mailings?

A. Priority- _____

B. Combination- _____

C. Express- _____

D. Special delivery- _____

E. Certificate of mailing- _____

F. Certified mail- _____

G. Registered- _____

B. MATCHING: Read the definition in Column II and then find the matching answer in Column I. Place the letter of the correct answer in the space provided.

COLUMN I

_____ 1. Fax
_____ 2. Pager
_____ 3. Voice mail
_____ 4. Cellular
_____ 5. Conference call
_____ 6. Teleconference
_____ 7. Telemedicine
_____ 8. E-mail
_____ 9. Internet

COLUMN II

a. Involves phones, cameras, and television
b. Portable telephone
c. Needs computer, electric address to receive messages
d. Requires appropriate software, a modem, and a search engine
e. Sends written material electronically over phone lines
f. Long distance physical assessment
g. Small receiver of electronic messages by phone signal
h. Multi-phone call
i. Receives messages into a "mailbox"

C. WORD PUZZLE

COMPLETE THE PUZZLE USING THE WORDS TO KNOW AND THE CLUES.

1. _ _ C _ _ _ _ _ _
2.   O _ _ _ _ _
3. _ _ _ _ M _ _ _
4.   _ _ M _ _ _ _
5.   _ U _ _ _ _ _ _ _ _
6.   _ _ N _ _ _ _ _ _ _
7. _ _ _ _ I _ _ _ _
8.   _ _ C _ _ _ _ _ _
9. _ _ _ _ _ A _ _ _
10.   _ _ _ _ T
11.   _ _ I _ _ _ _ _
12.   _ O _ _ _ _ _
13.   _ N _ _ _ _ _ _
14. _ _ _ _ S _ _ _ _ _

Clues

1. A copy
2. Where one works
3. Placed on mail
4. At home
5. Assures
6. To note
7. Testify in writing
8. Receiver
9. Uses heat
10. Number one
11. Overweight first class mail
12. Not domestic
13. Holds letter
14. Sent

Name _____

B. WORD SCRAMBLE: When you have unscrambled these terms, write a sentence with each word regarding the patient's medical record.

1. _ _ _ _ _ _ _ _   DIFIGNSN
2. _ _ _ _ _ _ _ _   PSEFICCI
3. _ _ _ _ _ _   RDOCRE
4. _ _ _ _ _ _ _ _ _ _   CEJEVTIBSU
5. _ _ _ _ _ _ _ _   SPGESRRO
6. _ _ _ _ _ _ _   ACEDITT
7. _ _ _ _ _ _ _ _ _ _ _ _ _ _ _   NFOICTTYLIDAEIN
8. _ _ _ _ _ _ _ _ _ _ _ _   TANECIVOONNL
9. _ _ _ _ _ _ _ _ _   CEBTJIOVE
10. _ _ _ _ _ _ _ _ _ _   MDDCEUONTE
11. _ _ _ _ _ _ _   RTSHYIO
12. _ _ _ _ _ _ _ _ _ _   ENIOMRIPSS

B. USE THESE LINED SPACES TO WRITE YOUR SENTENCES:

1. _____
2. _____
3. _____
4. _____
5. _____
6. _____
7. _____
8. _____
9. _____
10. _____
11. _____
12. _____

C. TRUE OR FALSE: Place a "T" for True or "F" for False in the space provided.

T   1. The confidentiality of the patients' medical records must be maintained by careful management as they are used.

F   2. Only parts of the patient's record are necessary when the patient wishes the physician to testify in an injury case.

T   3. The patient must always sign an authorization form before any information may be released.

F   4. All patient information contained in the medical record is considered as subjective information.

T   5. Progress notes should be arranged in chronological order with the most recent date on top.

T   6. The date and time should be recorded on the page for progress notes each time the patient is seen.

F   7. Using correction fluid is recommended to completely eliminate an error made on a patient's record.

T   8. Using black ink on the patient's record will make good copies whenever necessary.

T   9. An error found on a typewritten report regarding a patient should be corrected the same way as a handwritten error, by drawing a single line through it with the correction above or next to it.

T   10. The POMR record begins with the standard data base.

After your instructor has returned your work to you, make all necessary corrections and place it in a 3-ring notebook for future reference.

ASSIGNMENT SHEET

Chapter 7: RECORDS MANAGEMENT
Unit 2: FILING

A. BRIEF ANSWER

1. What is meant by indexing? *It requires you to make a decision as to the name subject, or other caption under which you will file the material.*

2. Name and define the four basic filing methods.
   a. *inspect each report or piece of correspondence to see if released for filing*
   b. *indexing (decicison as to name, subject, or caption.*
   c. *coding done by marking the index caption on file*
   d. *sort the materia. sort in alphabetical order*

3. Name and define the five steps in filing.
   a. *inspect - make sure it is available for filing.*
   b. *index - giving the pt a subject.*
   c. *code - to find a paticular chart*
   d. *sort - distribute mail*
   e. *store - all important info.*

4. Describe the proper method of placing material in a file folder. _____
   _____
   _____

5. Describe the most efficient method of removing and replacing patient files. · _____
   _____
   _____
   _____

6. List the storage media used for "paperless" filing systems. _____
   _____
   _____

B. INDEXING PRACTICE

1. Index each name below on a 3x5 card or paper cut to that size. Start each name ½ inch from the top and ½ inch in from the left margin. Arrange the cards in alphabetical order.

   a. Curtis Koch *20*
   b. Dianne Hanning *18*
   c. Dezzie Harris *19*
   d. Connie Graves *16*
   e. Anna Epstein *15*
   f. Melvin Edwards *14*
   g. Charles L. Davis *11*
   h. Gertrude Carter *9*
   i. Barbara Cahill *7*
   j. Earl Block *6*
   k. Robert Blair *4*
   l. C.L. Benson *5*
   m. L.K. Ander *1*
   n. Elmo Applegate *3*
   o. Nathan Appleby *2*
   p. Bruce Carr *8*
   q. Sandra Dyer *13*
   r. Pauline Hall *17*
   s. P.A. Dennis *12*
   t. Dave Daniels *10*

2. Index each name below on a 3x5 card or paper cut to that size. Start each name ½ inch from the top and ½ inch in from the left margin. Arrange the cards in alphabetical order.

a. Edgar Underwood
b. Richard Poff
c. Thomas Meyer
d. Felix Lee
e. Helen Thornton
f. Hubert Landers
g. Ann Stone
h. Mary June Quinn
i. Peter Nye
j. G. Saunders

k. Glen Ochs
l. Clyde Rambo
m. Russel Owens
n. Thomas Jefferson
o. June Guthrie
p. Theresa Frost
q. Kenneth Ford
r. Vivian Booth
s. Jimmy Block
t. Stephen Bergstrom

3. Code the names listed below by underlining the first unit and place 2, 3, 4 above other units in correct filing order. Then arrange the names in correct alphabetic and indexing order on the form provided.

Ex: Lïsa / Ãnn / Hale

a. Steve Van Meter
b. Victor Li-Lelaez
c. Min Kwang-Shik
d. Joan Vanmatre
e. Judy Kavang
f. Esther Corbie-Bender
g. Marila Corbitt
h. Asad Al-Alowi
i. Louise Gage
j. Frances Buntyn
k. Letticia Galindo
l. Don Durflinger
m. Anna Gunton

n. Louie Gage
o. Alfred D'Ambrosio
p. A. M. FitzHugh
q. Kelly LaBarba
r. Sylvia D'Ambrogi
s. Bill Fitz
t. Bryan LaBeff
u. C. W. McBrayer
v. Dr. Larry Mathis
w. Mrs. M.W. Smith (Mary)
x. Rev. Joan Sanders
y. Mrs. Carol Long (Mrs. William)

WORKSHEET FOR FILING ASSIGNMENTS

1st unit	2nd Unit	3rd Unit	4th Unit
a.			
b.			
c.			
d.			
e.			
f.			
g.			
h.			
i.			
j.			
k.			
l.			
m.			
n.			
o.			
p.			
q.			
r.			
s.			
t.			
u.			
v.			
w.			
x.			
y.			

4. Code the names listed below by underlining the first unit and place 2, 3, 4 above other units in correct filing order. Then arrange the names in correct alphabetic and indexing order on the form provided.

Ex: Abbott-Coltman. / Inc.

   a. Neu-Mor Corp.
   b. Mt. Vernon Mobile Homes
   c. Richard's Antiques
   d. Robt. Moriconi, (Jr.)
   e. Japan Air Lines
   f. Aus- Tex Garden Supply
   g. A. Ingram
   h. Northwest Airlines
   i. Bill New Law Office
   j. San Antonio Tours, Inc.
   k. So-Lo Diet Center
   l. M N Insurance Agency
   m. McFarland Down Town Motor Co.
   n. Vivian Richards, M.D.
   o. St. Paul Printing Co.

WORKSHEET FOR FILING ASSIGNMENTS

1st unit	2nd Unit	3rd Unit	4th Unit
a.			
b.			
c.			
d.			
e.			
f.			
g.			
h.			
i.			
j.			
k.			
l.			
m.			
n.			
o.			

5. Use the 25 cards prepared in question 3. Write the following registry numbers in the upper right-hand corner of the cards. Arrange the cards in numerical order and list the 25 names in the order in which they now appear.

a. _____   j. _____   r. _____
b. _____   k. _____   s. _____
c. _____   l. _____   t. _____
d. _____   m. _____   u. _____
e. _____   n. _____   v. _____
f. _____   o. _____   w. _____
g. _____   p. _____   x. _____
h. _____   q. _____   y. _____
i. _____

Van Meter 19-2-10   Kavang 10-11-65   Gage, Louise 12-70-45
Li-Lelaez 22-12-65   Corbie-Bender 50-30-25   Buntyn 60-20-15
Kwang-Shik 13-11-65   Corbitt 13-30-25   Galindo 12-70-45
Vanmatre 10-22-10   Al-Alowi 10-10-15   Durflinger 40-40-25
Gunton 10-70-45   D'Ambrogi 19-40-25   Mathis 40-12-75
Gage, Louise 12-70-45   Fitz 20-60-35   Smith 13-23-95
D'Ambrosio 10-10-25   LaBeff 20-12-65   Sanders 18-10-95
FitzHugh 10-13-35   McBrayer 30-23-75   Long 13-30-65
LaBarba 11-12-65

C. WORD SEARCH: FIND THE FOLLOWING WORDS IN THE PUZZLE.

1. ACCUMULATED
2. ALPHABETICAL
3. CODING
4. DATA
5. EXPEDITE
6. FILING
7. GEOGRAPHIC
8. ILLUMINATING
9. INDEXING
10. INSPECT
11. NUMERICAL
12. SEQUENCE
13. SORT
14. STORE
15. SUBSEQUENT
16. SUPPLEMENTED
17. SYSTEMATICALLY
18. UNIT
19. UNPRODUCTIVE

```
P O I U L K J H M N B V O I U Y L L A C I T A M E T S Y S
Q W E R F D S A Z X C V K J H N B U N P R O D U C T I V E
H J K F G H D F H S T O R E S D A W Q E T R E F O C N M Q
B V C X Z G F D S O M D E T A L U M U C C A I U D O S N U
L K J M N B T Y U R I O T M N B H G F A P O I U I K P L E
S U B S E Q U E N T X P I W A B M Y I P O U J H N B E M N
L O J Y F E D S W G Z Q D B Y N T M I T T R E W G D C X C
O P U I T Y T R E N A S E W E R I P F I L I N G Y N T G E
L K J M N B H G F I P L P D E X N V B O M I Y R E D D L K
A S D W E Q R T B X N H X I L L U M I N A T I N G C A B N
P O K I J M N B F E D T E H G F D S A Q W E R T Y O T L K
F D S A E R T W C D B N M J H L A C I T E B A H P L A K J
L O I K J M N H Y N P O M N U M E R I C A L J N B M L O P
E R W D S F B V C I M J H K I U O C I H P A R G O E G I N
P O I N T S U P P L E M E N T E D P O K E R D C S Q N T L
```

ACHIEVING SKILL COMPETENCY

Reread the TPO for each procedure and then practice the skills listed below, following the procedure in your textbook.

File Folders or Cards Alphabetically-Procedure 7-1

File Folders Numerically-Procedure 7-2

Pull File Folders from Numerical File-Procedure 7-4

When you have mastered the performances of a skill, sign your name on the appropriate evaluation sheet and give it to your instructor to indicate you are prepared to perform the procedure for evaluation.

After your instructor has returned your work to you, make all necessary corrections and place in a 3-ring notebook for future reference.

ASSIGNMENT SHEET

Chapter 8: COLLECTING FEES
Unit 1: MEDICAL CARE EXPENSES

   Review the objectives and text for each unit before completing the assignment sheet for that unit in this chapter. When all sheets for the chapter have been completed, remove them from this workbook and give them to the instructor for evaluation.

A. ESSAY

1. What are the factors to consider to determine fees for patient care?

_____
_____
_____

2. When insurance companies and government agencies establish a fee profile for physicians, how does it affect payment for patients?

_____
_____
_____

3. Explain what you should do if an indigent patient wants an appointment in your facility and your physician cannot accept another indigent patient at this time.

_____
_____
_____
_____

4. List the information that should be obtained on the personal data sheet of each patient.

_____
_____
_____
_____
_____
_____
_____
_____
_____
_____
_____

5. What is professional courtesy?

_____
_____
_____

B. TRUE OR FALSE: Place a "T" for True or "F" for False in the space provided.

_____ 1. Physicians are the ones who discuss fees with patients.

_____ 2. Insurance companies and government agencies establish a fee profile for physicians based on charges averaged over a period of time.

_____ 3. Physicians should never be told when a patient is unhappy with the cost of treatment.

_____ 4. Indigent patients should receive the same care as paying patients.

_____ 5. Two copies of the reduced fee agreement, with the words without prejudice stated, should be witnessed as they are signed for those with limited income.

_____ 6. Payment should never be accepted from those who should receive professional courtesy.

_____ 7. Each time the patient comes in for an appointment, you should verify the personal data sheet information.

_____ 8. The personal data sheet should ask for additional insurance coverage.

_____ 9. It is not necessary for the records release form to have a witness sign it.

_____ 10. On the third party liability statement the name of the patient and the name of the responsible party are always one and the same person.

C. WORD PUZZLE: Provide another word using the words listed below that means the same (or is similar in meaning) to fill in the blank spaces:

1. complicated   1. _ _ _ _ _ _ _ _ _ _

2. poor   2. _ _ _ _ _ _ _ _

3. inexpensive   3. _ _ _ _ _ _ _

4. succeeding   4. _ _ _ _ _ _ _ _ _ _

5. confirm   5. _ _ _ _ _ _

After your instructor has returned your work to you, make all necessary corrections and place in a 3-ring notebook for future reference.

ASSIGNMENT SHEET

Chapter 8: COLLECTING FEES
Unit 2: CREDIT ARRANGEMENTS

A. ESSAY

1. Explain when you should discuss payment planning and health insurance coverage with patients and give examples.

   _____
   _____
   _____
   _____

2. What is specified in the Truth in Lending Act?

   _____
   _____

3. How are physicians required under the AMA Code of Ethics to allow patients to use credit cards for services?

   _____
   _____

4. Why are credit card payments advantageous if there is a 1 to 3% assessment charged to the physician?

   _____
   _____

5. What is the purpose of the Bureau of Medical Economics?

   _____

6. If a request is received from a credit bureau regarding a patient, what information are you to disclose in your answer?

   _____
   _____

B. WORD SEARCH: Find the following words in the puzzle.

```
I A D V A N C E A C T
A D D I S C L O S E H
D E L I N Q U E N T C
V C L O E T H I C S O
T R U T H   C A R D S
I N S T A L L M E N T
C P A Y M E N T D E S
I A F I N A N C I N G
L T E S T I M A T E F
O I N C H A R G E S A
S U B S T A N T I A L
```

1. CARDS
2. INSTALLMENT
3. CHARGES
4. FINANCING
5. ETHICS
6. COSTS
7. DISCLOSE
8. PAYMENT
9. TRUTH
10. ESTIMATE
11. DELINQUENT
12. ADVANCE
13. ACT
14. CREDIT
15. SOLICIT
16. SUBSTANTIAL

C. TRUE OR FALSE: Place a "T" for True or "F" for False in the space provided.

_____ 1. A cost estimate sheet for surgery should include cost of the surgery and the approximate cost of the anesthesia, consultants, and hospital costs.

_____ 2. The Truth in Lending Act is enforced by the International Trade Commission.

_____ 3. Physicians may increase charges for services to patients who wish to use credit cards for medical services.

_____ 4. It is not only lawful but a good practice to disclose information to referring offices regarding paying habits of patients.

_____ 5. The Truth in Lending form must be signed by the patient in your presence.

After your instructor has returned your work to you, make all necessary corrections and place in a 3-ring notebook for future reference.

ASSIGNMENT SHEET

Chapter 8: COLLECTING FEES
Unit 3: BOOKKEEPING PROCEDURES

MIXED QUIZ

1. Use the following information to fill in a daily log for each of the three days indicated. Be careful to calculate charges when more than one is listed and put only total in charge column. Be sure to itemize in column listing description. Be careful to list payments in payment column and break down each in either cash or check payment column. _____

December 27, 19____

      Juan Gomez - paid $17.00 ck

      Sue Schmidt - O.C. limited $27.00; Inj. B 12 $15.00

      Susan Segal - O.C. New intermediate $48.00

      Sue Schmidt - paid $62.00 ck

      Carol Sue Kostrevski - O.C. Comprehensive $70.00; paid $50.00 cash

      LaChar Holley - (NP) Comprehensive $85.00

January 5, 19____

      Geoff Segal - paid $48.00 cash for Susan

      Juan Gomez - Extended exam $46.00

      June Kostrevski - Allergy testing $100.00

      Carol Sue Kostrevski - Inj. Penicillin $12.00

      Joan Moriarty - O.C. Intermediate $30.00; x-ray left knee $76.00; paid $50.00 ck

      Carol Schmidt - O.C. Extended $46.00

      Boris Kostrevski - Paid $150.00 ck

January 8, 19____

      Boris Kostrevski - CPE comprehensive New $85.00; chest x-ray $79.00;

            EKG $50.00; Lab Physical Profile $113.00;

            Draw blood $5.00; Urinalysis $10.00

      Patrick Moriarty - O.C. Intermediate $30.00; paid $38.00 ck

      Tina Schmidt - cast removal $35.00

      Juan Gomez- O.C. Limited $27.00

      Geoff Segal - N.C.

      June Kostrevski - Ck. Aetna Ins. $100.00

      LaChar Holley - Hospital 12/29 thru 1/6

           Initial visit $85.00

           6 days at $25.00

           Total charges $235.00

      Boris Kostrevski - Medicare pd. Ck $40.00

      Juan Gomez - Medical pd. ck $12.50

DATE	NAME	DESCRIPTION	CHARGES	CREDITS		CASH	CHK
				PAYMENTS	ADJ.		

| DATE | NAME | DESCRIPTION | CHARGES | √ | CREDITS | | CASH | CHK |
					PAYMENTS	ADJ.		

| DATE | NAME | DESCRIPTION | CHARGES | √ | CREDITS | | CASH | CHK |
					PAYMENTS	ADJ.		

2. Prepare ledger cards for the patients listed below. The additional names are of family members who would be listed on the separate account cards. After the account cards are prepared, post the three daily log days to the account cards. Be sure to itemize all charges under description column. Your instructor may provide you with account cards or you may use the blank cards printed in this workbook for completion of this assignment. If you use separate cards, they should always be in alphabetical order. _____

Boris Kostrevski - Mrs. June; Carol Sue
1493 S. James Road
(Your city and ZIP code)
$55.00 Balance brought forward

Patrick Moriarty - Mrs. Joan
397 North Tony Road
(Your city and ZIP code)
$38.00 Balance brought forward

George Schmidt - Mrs. Sue; Tina; Carol Susan
2349 E. Remington Road
(Your city and ZIP code)
$75.00 Balance brought forward

Juan Gomez
293 West High Street
(Your city and ZIP code)
$25.00 Balance brought forward

Patty and Geoff Segal - Susan
410 North Tony Road
(Your city and ZIP code)

LaChar Holley
4567 Charcoal Lane
(Your city and ZIP code)

If you would like more practice experience in completion of day sheets and account cards, your instructor has additional assignments in the Instructor's Guide.

Samuel E Matthews, M D
Suite 120
100 E Main Street
Yourtown US 98765-4321
(654) 789-0123

Gomez, Juan
293 West High Street
Anywhere, USA 00000

DATE	DESCRIPTION	CHARGE	CREDITS		CURRENT BALANCE
			PAYMENTS	ADL.	
	BALANCE FORWARD				

PLEASE PAY LAST AMOUNT IN THIS COLUMN

276L

Samuel E Matthews, M D
Suite 120
100 E Main Street
Yourtown US 98765-4321
(654) 789-0123

Segal, Patty
410 North Tony Road
Anywhere, USA 00000

DATE	DESCRIPTION	CHARGE	CREDITS		CURRENT BALANCE
			PAYMENTS	ADL.	
	BALANCE FORWARD				

PLEASE PAY LAST AMOUNT IN THIS COLUMN

276L

Statement 1

Samuel E Matthews, M D
Suite 120
100 E Main Street
Yourtown US 98765-4321
(654) 789-0123

Holley, LaChar
4567 Charcoal Lane
Anywhere, USA 00000

DATE	DESCRIPTION	CHARGE	CREDITS PAYMENTS	CREDITS ADJ.	CURRENT BALANCE
	BALANCE FORWARD →				

PLEASE PAY LAST AMOUNT IN THIS COLUMN ←

276L

Statement 2

Samuel E Matthews, M D
Suite 120
100 E Main Street
Yourtown US 98765-4321
(654) 789-0123

Moriarty, Joan
397 Tony Road
Anywhere, USA 00000

DATE	DESCRIPTION	CHARGE	CREDITS PAYMENTS	CREDITS ADJ.	CURRENT BALANCE
	BALANCE FORWARD →				

PLEASE PAY LAST AMOUNT IN THIS COLUMN ←

276L

Statement 1

Samuel E Matthews, M D
Suite 120
100 E Main Street
Yourtown US 98765-4321
(654) 789-0123

Kostrevski, Carol Sue
1493 S. James Road
Anywhere, USA 00000

| DATE | | DESCRIPTION | CHARGE | CREDITS | | CURRENT |
				PAYMENTS	ADL.	BALANCE
		BALANCE FORWARD				

PLEASE PAY LAST AMOUNT IN THIS COLUMN ◄

276L

Statement 2

Samuel E Matthews, M D
Suite 120
100 E Main Street
Yourtown US 98765-4321
(654) 789-0123

Moriarty, Patrick
397 North Tony Road
Anywhere, USA 00000

| DATE | | DESCRIPTION | CHARGE | CREDITS | | CURRENT |
				PAYMENTS	ADL.	BALANCE
		BALANCE FORWARD				

PLEASE PAY LAST AMOUNT IN THIS COLUMN ◄

276L

Form 1 (Top)

Samuel E Matthews, M D
Suite 120
100 E Main Street
Yourtown US 98765-4321
(654) 789-0123

Kostrevski, June
1493 S. James Road
Anywhere, USA 00000

| DATE | DESCRIPTION | CHARGE | CREDITS | | CURRENT |
			PAYMENTS	ADL.	BALANCE
	BALANCE FORWARD				

PLEASE PAY LAST AMOUNT IN THIS COLUMN

276L

Form 2 (Bottom)

Samuel E Matthews, M D
Suite 120
100 E Main Street
Yourtown US 98765-4321
(654) 789-0123

Kostrevski, Boris
1493 S. James Road
Anywhere, USA 00000

| DATE | DESCRIPTION | CHARGE | CREDITS | | CURRENT |
			PAYMENTS	ADL.	BALANCE
	BALANCE FORWARD				

PLEASE PAY LAST AMOUNT IN THIS COLUMN

276L

Samuel E Matthews, M D
Suite 120
100 E Main Street
Yourtown US 98765-4321
(654) 789-0123

Schmidt, Sue
2349 E. Remington Road
Anywhere, USA 00000

| DATE | DESCRIPTION | CHARGE | CREDITS | | CURRENT |
			PAYMENTS	ADL.	BALANCE
	BALANCE FORWARD →				

PLEASE PAY LAST AMOUNT IN THIS COLUMN ←

276L

Samuel E Matthews, M D
Suite 120
100 E Main Street
Yourtown US 98765-4321
(654) 789-0123

Schmidt, George
2349 E. Remington Road
Anywhere, USA 00000

| DATE | DESCRIPTION | CHARGE | CREDITS | | CURRENT |
			PAYMENTS	ADL.	BALANCE
	BALANCE FORWARD →				

PLEASE PAY LAST AMOUNT IN THIS COLUMN ←

276L

Samuel E Matthews, M D
Suite 120
100 E Main Street
Yourtown US 98765-4321
(654) 789-0123

Schmidt, Carol Susan
2349 E. Remington Road
Anywhere, USA 00000

DATE	DESCRIPTION	CHARGE	CREDITS PAYMENTS	ADL	CURRENT BALANCE
	BALANCE FORWARD				

PLEASE PAY LAST AMOUNT IN THIS COLUMN ←

276L

Samuel E Matthews, M D
Suite 120
100 E Main Street
Yourtown US 98765-4321
(654) 789-0123

Schmidt, Tina
2349 E. Remington Road
Anywhere, USA 00000

DATE	DESCRIPTION	CHARGE	CREDITS PAYMENTS	ADL	CURRENT BALANCE
	BALANCE FORWARD				

PLEASE PAY LAST AMOUNT IN THIS COLUMN ←

276L

Form 1

Samuel E Matthews, M D
Suite 120
100 E Main Street
Yourtown US 98765-4321
(654) 789-0123

Segal, Geoff
410 North Tony Road
Anywhere, USA 00000

DATE	DESCRIPTION	CHARGE	CREDITS PAYMENTS	ADJ.	CURRENT BALANCE
	BALANCE FORWARD				

PLEASE PAY LAST AMOUNT IN THIS COLUMN

276L

Form 2

Samuel E Matthews, M D
Suite 120
100 E Main Street
Yourtown US 98765-4321
(654) 789-0123

Segal, Susan
410 North Tony Road
Anywhere, USA 00000

DATE	DESCRIPTION	CHARGE	CREDITS PAYMENTS	ADJ.	CURRENT BALANCE
	BALANCE FORWARD				

PLEASE PAY LAST AMOUNT IN THIS COLUMN

276L

3. Use half sheets of paper and type the letterhead from Figure 8-7. Type itemized statements from the five families who still owe money. _____

_____

4. Describe the exceptions to the usual billing procedures. _____

_____

_____

_____

_____

5. Describe the advantages of a one-write bookkeeping system. _____

_____

_____

_____

_____

6. Define bookkeeper. _____

7. Define chemotherapy. _____

_____

8. Define posted. _____

9. Define proprietorship. _____

10. Define journalizing. _____

11. Define trial balance. _____

12. Define bankruptcy. _____

_____

13. Define petition. _____

_____

After your instructor has returned your work to you, make all necessary corrections and place in a 3-ring notebook for future reference.

ASSIGNMENT SHEET

Chapter 8: COLLECTING FEES
Unit 4: COMPUTER BILLING

1. Describe advantages of computerized billing. _____
   _____
   _____
   _____
   _____

2. Describe different ways to locate an account in a computer system. _____
   _____

3. Describe an account history. _____

4. List reasons why billing statements would/should be withheld. _____
   _____
   _____

5. Define account history. _____

6. Define alpha search. _____
   _____
   _____

After your instructor has returned your work to you, make all necessary corrections and place in a 3-ring notebook for future reference.

ASSIGNMENT SHEET

Chapter 8: COLLECTING FEES
Unit 5: COLLECTING OVERDUE PAYMENTS

1. Define aging of accounts. _____
   _____

2. How long are accounts ordinarily carried before being referred to a collection agency? _____
   _____

3. Should accounts automatically be referred to collection after the prescribed period of time? Why? _____
   _____

4. List the advantages of the use of telephone calls for account collection. _____
   _____

5. List conditions necessary when using the telephone for account collection.

   _____
   _____
   _____
   _____
   _____
   _____
   _____
   _____
   _____
   _____

6. Compose and type collection letters for the accounts of LaChar Holley, Juan Gomez, George Schmidt, and Boris Kostrevski. Use the examples in Figure 8-11 as a guide. If you use dates, be sure they are ones which are compatible with the account cards you are using for a reference. Use a different form for each letter.

   _____

7. Define the statute of limitations. _____
   _____
   _____

SAMUEL E. MATTHEWS, MD
SUITE 120
100 E. MAIN STREET
YOURTOWN, US 98765-4321
(654) 789-0123

SAMUEL E. MATTHEWS, MD
SUITE 120
100 E. MAIN STREET
YOURTOWN, US 98765-4321
(654) 789-0123

SAMUEL E. MATTHEWS, MD
SUITE 120
100 E. MAIN STREET
YOURTOWN, US 98765-4321
(654) 789-0123

SAMUEL E. MATTHEWS, MD
SUITE 120
100 E. MAIN STREET
YOURTOWN, US 98765-4321
(654) 789-0123

ACHIEVING SKILL COMPETENCY

Reread the TPO for each procedure and then practice the skills listed below, following the procedure in your textbook.

Prepare Patient Ledger Card-Procedure 8-1

Record Charges and Credits-Procedure 8-2

Type Itemized Statement-Procedure 8-3

When you feel you have mastered the performance of the skill, sign your name on the appropriate evaluation sheet and give it to your instructor to indicate you are prepared to perform the procedure for evaluation.

After your instructor has returned your work to you, make all necessary corrections and place in a 3-ring notebook for future reference.

ASSIGNMENT SHEET

Chapter 9: HEALTH CARE COVERAGE
Unit 1: FUNDAMENTALS OF MANAGED CARE

Review the objectives and text for each unit before completing the assignment sheet for that unit in this chapter. When all sheets for the chapter have been completed, remove them from this workbook and give them to the instructor for evaluation.

A. BRIEF ANSWER

1. What type of medical insurance has created competition in the insurance industry? _____

_____

2. Why are HMOs so popular? _____

_____

3. Where did the phrase "managed care" originate? _____

_____

4. What is generally the cost of health care to employees whose employer offers an HMO as part of an employee's benefit package? _____

_____

5. Describe managed care today. _____

_____

_____

6. What is the initial purpose of the HMO? _____

_____

7. What are the two major types of health insurance? _____

_____

8. In regard to health insurance coverage, how can the medical assistant be helpful to patients? _____

_____

_____

_____

9. Where can patients find the names of physicians who are participating members of their HMO? _____

_____

10. Describe a helpful practice which should be performed at the beginning of each office visit regarding the patient's insurance card. _____

_____

_____

11. Explain the Birthday Rule in regard to insurance coverage. _____

_____

_____

12. What is critical to assure successful reimbursement for medical services rendered to patients? _____

_____

_____

_____

13. List the subject areas that are necessary for the medical assistant to process medical claims forms. And why?

_____

_____

_____

B. MATCHING: Read the definition in Column II and then find the matching answer in Column I. Place the letter of the correct answer in the space provided.

COLUMN I

_____ 1. attending physician
_____ 2. signed authorization
_____ 3. advance directives
_____ 4. admitting physician
_____ 5. capitation
_____ 6. balance billing
_____ 7. assignment of benefits
_____ 8. accounts receivable
_____ 9. Claim

COLUMN II

a. fixed amount paid to doctor per month
b. physician who admits patient to hospital
c. total charges that have not been paid
d. patient authorizes payment directly to the physician
e. physician who cares for patient in hospital
f. authorization to release medical information
g. also known as a Living Will
h. charges insurance did not pay
i. request for insurance company payment

C. FILL IN THE BLANK

1. _____ was established to aid personnel and dependents of the armed services with medical expenses.

2. _____ was established for disabled veterans, their spouses and dependents to aid with medical expenses.

3. A predetermined amount that the insured must pay before the insurance company pays is called the _____ .

4. A printed description of the benefits provided by the insurer to the beneficiary is known as the _____ .

5. _____ is the term given to the primary care physician for coordinating the patient's care to specialists, hospital admissions, and so on.

6. A specific amount which the insured must pay toward the charge for professional services rendered is called _____

7. The _____ is the one who writes his/her signature on the back of a check that is made out to him/her.

8. A list of approved professional services for which the insurance company will pay with the maximum fee paid for each service is called a _____ .

9. A _____ is a printed form that has patient information and a listing of the services and code numbers with the total charges.

10. A program that provides complete health care for children and encourages early detection of health problems is known as _____ .

11. _____ is an organized system of medical team members into groups to provide quality and cost-effective care that encompasses both the delivery of health care and the payment of services

D. WORD SEARCH: Find the terms from their meanings listed below, plus the words in italics within the meanings (abbreviations may be used):

1. Standard claims *form* of the *Health* Care Finance Administration to submit for *third* party payment.

_____

2. A joint funding program by federal/state governments (not in Arizona) for those on public assistance for medical *care*. _____

3. Private *insurance* to supplement Medicare benefits for non-covered services. _____

4. A *group* of physicians who continue to practice independently in their own offices. _____

5. Coding system used to *document* diseases, injuries, illnesses, and modalities. _____

_____

6. Non-profit organization created to improve patient care *quality* and health plan performance. _____

_____

7. Another name for *encounter* form. _____

8. Transferring words into numbers to facilitate use of *computers* in claims processing. _____

9. Moneys paid for an insurance *contract.* _____

10. *Fee* schedule based on relative value of resources that physicians spend to provide services to Medicare patients. _____

11. The person who has been insured; insurance *policy* holder. _____

12. Prior authorization must be obtained before the patient is admitted to the hospital or some specified outpatient or in-office *procedures.* _____

```
V  A  L  U  E  R  M  I  N  S  U  R  A  N  C  E
E  R  A  C  I  D  E  M  N  C  Z  A  U  C  O  D
R  A  M  I  F  I  D  A  C  O  A  T  I  E  N  T
B  O  C  A  R  E  I  D  Q  D  H  E  A  L  T  H
R  W  O  R  A  H  C  F  A  I  5  0  0  L  R  D
V  S  M  M  C  H  A  J  P  N  S  W  X  L  A  T
S  U  P  E  R  B  I  L  L  G  Y  B  P  F  C  J
P  B  U  D  I  C  D  9  C  M  F  O  R  M  T  Q
O  S  T  I  F  E  N  C  O  U  N  T  E  R  E  U
L  C  E  F  E  E  G  P  R  T  F  A  M  I  P  A
I  R  R  I  P  A  R  T  Y  S  X  D  I  K  U  L
C  I  S  L  N  C  O  G  J  X  K  O  U  Z  M  I
Y  B  M  L  B  T  U  X  D  O  C  U  M  E  N  T
M  E  D  I  G  A  P  R  O  C  E  D  U  R  E  Y
P  R  E  C  E  R  T  I  F  I  C  A  T  I  O  N
```

E. TRUE OR FALSE: Place a "T" for True or "F" for False in the space provided.

_____ 1. An indemnity plan is a company that bills the physician for medical services.

_____ 2. The Medicare fee schedule is a list of approved professional services that Medicare will pay listing the maximum fee it pays for each service.

_____ 3. A preexisting condition is a condition that existed before the insured's policy was issued.

_____ 4. A contract is an agreement between two or more parties for certain services or obligations to be discussed.

_____ 5. For patients who are minors or who are incompetent, a guardian must sign for any release of information and for any services to be completed.

_____ 6. Utilization management refers to a panel that keeps track of what services were ordered and check if their medical care was completed.

_____ 7. The usual fee is the charge that physicians make for services for their private patients.

_____ 8. A skilled nursing facility is a medical facility licensed to primarily provide skilled nursing care to patients ordered by Workers' Compensation.

After your instructor has returned your work to you, make all necessary corrections and place in a 3-ring notebook for future reference.

ASSIGNMENT SHEET

Chapter 9: HEALTH CARE COVERAGE
Unit 2: HEALTH CARE PLANS

A. BRIEF ANSWER

1. What is significant regarding premiums and benefits of private commercial insurance companies?
   _____

2. Why was Blue Cross health insurance originally set up?
   _____

3. What coverage does Blue Cross now include besides hospital expenses?
   _____

4. Name the additional plans Blue Cross and Blue Shield offer today.
   _____

5. What do indemnity plans require of the patient regarding payments?
   _____

6. What is the usual co-payment required of patients who have an HMO plan?
   _____

7. List the available types of HMOs and briefly describe each of them.
   _____
   _____
   _____
   _____
   _____

8. What are the responsibilities of the NCQA?
   _____

B. COMPLETION: Place a "P" before private insurance plans listed below and a "G" before the government health insurance plans:

_____ 1. Foundations for medical care

_____ 2. Medicare

_____ 3. Blue Shield

_____ 4. Champus

_____ 5. Workers' compensation

_____ 6. Blue Cross

_____ 7. Easter Seal Rehabilitation Centers

_____ 8. Medicaid

_____ 9. Commercial health insurance

_____ 10. Health Maintenance Organizations

C. FILL IN THE BLANK

1. To qualify as a/an _____, an organization must present proof of its ability to provide comprehensive health care.

2. One of the four levels of NCQA accreditation is full accreditation given for _____ indicating excellent performance.

3. The primary care physician is also referred to as _____ .

4. HMOs mail _____ to the provider's office to keep the office apprised of policy changes between representatives' visits.

5. Besides the four principal types of state benefits, Workers' Compensation also includes _____ _____ for severely disabled employees.

6. Patients who have had an industrial injury should have a _____ for that injury and a separate account card.

7. One common reason for delay in payment of claims is that they are _____ .

8. The physician and the staff should always provide quality care to all patients regardless of their _____ status.

9. Medicare B is the coverage that pays for _____ .

10. Physicians who choose not to be a participating provider must collect _____ _____ for the services rendered.

11. If the physician provides a non-covered service for a Medicare patient, an _____ must be signed by the patient.

12. There is a special _____ on the HCFA-1500 form which allows the claims processor to assign a unique identification number to the claim during microfilming.

13. In processing Medicare forms, use ICDA codes for _____ , CPT codes for _____ , and HCPCS codes for _____ .

D. TRUE OR FALSE: Place a "T" for True or "F" for False in the space provided.

_____ 1. CHAMPUS covers all military personnel.

_____ 2. Medicare encourages all providers to file claims electronically.

_____ 3. The NPI (National Provider Identification) is used in blocks 24k and 33 of the HCFA-1500 to identify the location of the service.

_____ 4. Ideally, all insurance forms should be signed and dated by the patient.

_____ 5. The only time a patient's signature is not necessary is when you have been given verbal permission from that patient to release information.

_____ 6. Claims will be returned to the provider if the NPI number is missing from the HCFA form.

_____ 7. Medicare Part B patients usually are responsible for the first $100 of covered services.

_____ 8. For Medicaid patients, a general rule is that prior authorization is necessary to provide medical treatment except in an emergency.

_____ 9. Workers' Compensation requires that patients have reevaluations at intervals with their physician who must promptly give a supplemental report regarding the patient's condition.

After your instructor has returned your work to you, make all necessary corrections and place in a 3-ring notebook for future reference.

ASSIGNMENT SHEET

Chapter 9: HEALTH CARE COVERAGE
Unit 3: PREPARING CLAIMS

MIXED QUIZ

1. What does the phrase "third party reimbursement" mean? _____
_____

2. Why were claim forms developed? _____
_____

3. When did the first attempt at classifying the causes of deaths occur? _____

4. What significant event occurred in 1938? _____
_____
_____

5. Fill in the blanks:

Coding is in reality, the _____ of _____ and/or _____

of _____ or _____ into _____ to _____

_____ , which can be _____ into _____ and

_____ .

6. List three reasons why coding is beneficial.

1. _____
_____

2. _____

3. _____
_____

7. What change occurred with the Catastrophic Coverage Act of 1988? _____
_____

8. What does sequencing mean? _____

9. What is the main rule to remember when coding and what does it mean? _____
_____

10. Look at a copy of the approved HCFA 1500 insurance form; where would you enter the following information?

_____ A. Health care coverage being billed

_____ B. Patient's name

_____ C. Insured's name

_____ D. Patient's condition is result of their employment

_____ E. Name of insured's employer

_____ F. Indicate there is another health plan

_____ G. Have patient sign

_____ H. Dates patient unable to work

_____ I. Diagnosis codes

_____ J. Procedure codes

_____ K. Physician's tax ID number

_____ L. Assignment acceptance

_____ M. Physician's signature

11. Complete five insurance forms using the following information: Code 11, office, for places of service: (24B) The physician is Samuel E. Matthews, MD, Suite 120, 100 E. Main Street, Yourtown, US 98765-4321. His SS# is 987654321. Phone 654-789-0123. PIN 7654321. The patients all live in Yourtown, US.

a. Juan Gomez, 293 West High Street, 98765

Medicare. Phone 263-5538. BD 2/17/21. Male. SS# 291166966-A. Patient is insured person. Other insurance BC, BS #2911669660; signature on file. Abdominal pain and Diabetes Mellitus. (Consult this unit for code numbers. Consult code book for code numbers needed for procedures.) Seen in office.

5/18/__	Office visit, intermediate	30.00
	Test feces for blood	15.00
	Automated hemogram	10.00
	Blood Drawing	5.00

b. LaChar Holley, 4567 Charcoal Lane 98765

Travelers Insurance. Phone 122-7768. BD 10/7/60. Female, SS# 505209821. Patient is insured person. No other insurance. Not related to employment or accident. Signature on file. Arthritis, acute and back pain. Seen in office.

6/15/__	Office visit, intermediate	30.00
	X-ray lumbar spine, AP & lateral	118.00
	Blood Drawing	5.00
	Automated hemogram	10.00

c. Tina Schmidt, daughter. BD 12/27/90. Phone 891-7145. Insured George Schmidt, 1249 E. Remington Road, 98769. Self-employed. BC and BS Insurance. SS# of insured 888207777. BD 10/6/49. No other insurance. Phone 441-0050. Signature on file. Impetigo. Seen in office.

| 6/20/__ | Office visit, limited | 27.00 |

d. Joan Moriarty, wife. BD 12/19/62. Insured Patrick Moriarty, 397-½ North Tony Road 98768. Self employed. Metropolitan-Insurance. SS# of insured 887105566. BD 11/14/60. Phone 431-6943. No other insurance. Signature on file. Cervicitis, Cystitis, acute and edema. Patient seen in office.

9/20/__	Office visit, extended	46.00
	Catheterization, urethra	20.00
	Endometrial Biopsy	125.00
	Urinalysis	10.00

e. Boris Kostrevski, 1493 S. James Road 98765. Medicare and Aetna Insurance. SS# of insured 505208800-A. BD 7/14/22. Phone 298-6483. Signature on file. Diabetes Mellitus, coronary atherosclerosis. Seen in office.

6/20/__	Office visit, intermediate	30.00
	Assay blood fluid, glucose	10.00
	Blood drawing	5.00

Name _____

APPROVED OMB-0938-0008

PICA

HEALTH INSURANCE CLAIM FORM

PICA

1. MEDICARE MEDICAID CHAMPUS CHAMPVA GROUP HEALTH PLAN FECA BLK LUNG OTHER

☐ (Medicare #) ☐ (Medicaid #) ☐ (Sponsor's SSN) ☐ (VA File #) ☐ (SSN or ID) ☐ (SSN) ☐ (ID)

1a. INSURED'S I.D. NUMBER   (FOR PROGRAM IN ITEM 1)

2. PATIENT'S NAME (Last Name, First Name, Middle Initial)

3. PATIENT'S BIRTH DATE   SEX
MM   DD   YY   M ☐   F ☐

4. INSURED'S NAME (Last Name, Firts Name, Middle Initial)

5. PATIENT'S ADDRESS (No., Street)

6. PATIENT RELATIONSHIP TO INSURED
☐ Self ☐ Spouse ☐ Child ☐ Other

7. INSURED'S ADDRESS (No., Street)

CITY   STATE

8. PATIENT STATUS
☐ Single ☐ Married ☐ Other

CITY   STATE

ZIP CODE   TELEPHONE (Include Area Code)
(   )

Employed ☐   Full-Time ☐   Part-Time ☐
                Student   Student

ZIP CODE   TELEPHONE (Include Area Code)
(   )

9. OTHER INSURED'S NAME (Last Name, First Name, Middle Initial)

10. IS PATIENT'S CONDITION RELATED TO:

11. INSURED'S POLICY GROUP OR FECA NUMBER

a. OTHER INSURED'S POLICY OR GROUP NUMBER

a. EMPLOYMENT? (CURRENT OR PREVIOUS)
☐ YES ☐ NO

a. INSURED'S DATE OF BIRTH   SEX
MM   DD   YY   M ☐   F ☐

b. OTHER INSURED'S DATE OF BIRTH   SEX
MM   DD   YY   M ☐   F ☐

b. AUTO ACCIDENT?   PLACE (State)
☐ YES ☐ NO

b. EMPLOYER'S NAME OR SCHOOL NAME

c. EMPLOYER'S NAME OR SCHOOL NAME

c. OTHER ACCIDENT?
☐ YES ☐ NO

c. INSURANCE PLAN NAME OR PROGRAM NAME

d. INSURANCE PLAN NAME OR PROGRAM NAME

d. RESERVED FOR LOCAL USE

d. IS THERE ANOTHER HEALTH BENEFIT PLAN?
☐ YES ☐ NO If yes, return to and complete item 9 a-d.

READ BACK OF FORM BEFORE COMPLETING & SIGNING THIS FORM.

12. PATIENT'S OR AUTHORIZED PERSON'S SIGNATURE I authorize the release of any medical or other information necessary to process this claim. I also request payment of government benefits either to myself or to the party who accepts assignments below.

13. INSURED'S OR AUTHORIZED PERSON'S SIGNATURE I authorize payment of medical benefits to the undersigned physician or supplier for services described below.

SIGNED_____   DATE_____

SIGNED_____

14. DATE OF CURRENT:
MM   DD   YY
ILLNESS (First sympton) OR INJURY (Accident) OR PREGNANCY (LMP)

15. IF PATIENT HAS HAD SAME OR SIMILAR ILLNESS. GIVE FIRST DATE   MM   DD   YY

16. DATES PATIENT UNABLE TO WORK IN CURRENT OCCUPATION
MM   DD   YY   MM   DD   YY
FROM   TO

17. NAME OR REFERRING PHYSICIAN OR OTHER SOURCE

17a. I.D. NUMBER OF REFERRING PHYSICIAN

18. HOSPITALIZATION DATES RELATED TO CURRENT SERVICES
MM   DD   YY   MM   DD   YY
FROM   TO

19. RESERVED FOR LOCAL USE

20. OUTSIDE LAB?
☐ YES ☐ NO $ CHARGES

21. DIAGNOSIS OR NATURE OF ILLNESS OR INJURY. (RELATE ITEMS 1,2,3 OR 4 TO ITEM 24E BY LINE)

1. I_____.___   3. I_____.___

2. I_____.___   4. I_____.___

22. MEDICAID RESUBMISSION
CODE   ORIGINAL REF. NO.

23. PRIOR AUTHORIZATION NUMBER

24.	A					B	C	D		E	F	G	H	I	J	K
	DATE(S) OF SERVICE					Place of Service	Type of Service	PROCEDURES, SERVICES, OR SUPPLIES (Explain Unusual Circumstances)		DIAGNOSIS CODE	$ CHARGES	DAYS OR UNITS	EPSDT Family Plan	EMG	COB	RESERVED FOR LOCAL USE
	From			To				CPT/HCPCS	MODIFIER							
	MM	DD	YY	MM	DD	YY											
1																	
2																	
3																	
4																	
5																	
6																	

25. FEDERAL TAX I.D. NUMBER   SSN ☐ EIN ☐

26. PATIENT'S ACCOUNT NO.

27. ACCEPT ASSIGNMENT? (For govt. claims, see back)
☐ YES ☐ NO

28. TOTAL CHARGE
$

29. AMOUNT PAID
$

30. BALANCE DUE
$

31. SIGNATURE OF PHYSICIAN OR SUPPLIER INCLUDING DEGREES OR CREDENTIALS (I certify that the statements on the reverse apply to this bill and are made a part thereof.)

32. NAME AND ADDRESS OF FACULTY WHERE SERVICES WERE RENDERED (If other than home or office)

33. PHYSICIAN'S, SUPPLIER'S BILLING NAME, ADDRESS, ZIP CODE & PHONE#

SIGNED _____   DATE _____

PIN #   GRP #

(APPROVED BY AMA COUNCIL ON MEDICAL SERVICE 8/88)   *PLEASE PRINT OR TYPE*

FORM HCFA-1500 (U2) (12-90)
FORM OWCP -1500   FORM RRB-1500

CARRIE

PATIENT AND INSURED INFORMATION

PHYSICIAN OR SUPPLIER INFORMATION

APPROVED OMB-0938-0008

← CARRIER →

HEALTH INSURANCE CLAIM FORM

PICA   PICA

PLEASE DO NOT STAPLE IN THIS AREA

1. MEDICARE MEDICAID CHAMPUS CHAMPVA GROUP HEALTH PLAN FECA BLK LUNG OTHER

☐ (Medicare #) ☐ (Medicaid #) ☐ (Sponsor's SSN) ☐ (VA File #) ☐ (SSN or ID) ☐ (SSN) ☐ (ID)

1a. INSURED'S I.D. NUMBER (FOR PROGRAM IN ITEM 1)

2. PATIENT'S NAME (Last Name, First Name, Middle Initial)

3. PATIENT'S BIRTH DATE SEX
MM DD YY M ☐ F ☐

4. INSURED'S NAME (Last Name, Firts Name, Middle Initial)

5. PATIENT'S ADDRESS (No., Street)

6. PATIENT RELATIONSHIP TO INSURED
☐ Self ☐ Spouse ☐ Child ☐ Other

7. INSURED'S ADDRESS (No., Street)

CITY   STATE

8. PATIENT STATUS
☐ Single ☐ Married ☐ Other

CITY   STATE

ZIP CODE TELEPHONE (Include Area Code)
( )

Employed ☐ Full-Time Student ☐ Part-Time Student ☐

ZIP CODE TELEPHONE (Include Area Code)
( )

9. OTHER INSURED'S NAME (Last Name, First Name, Middle Initial)

10. IS PATIENT'S CONDITION RELATED TO:

11. INSURED'S POLICY GROUP OR FECA NUMBER

a. OTHER INSURED'S POLICY OR GROUP NUMBER

a. EMPLOYMENT? (CURRENT OR PREVIOUS)
☐ YES ☐ NO

a. INSURED'S DATE OF BIRTH SEX
MM ¦ DD ¦ YY M ☐ F ☐

b. OTHER INSURED'S DATE OF BIRTH SEX
MM ¦ DD ¦ YY M ☐ F ☐

b. AUTO ACCIDENT? PLACE (State)
☐ YES ☐ NO

b. EMPLOYER'S NAME OR SCHOOL NAME

c. EMPLOYER'S NAME OR SCHOOL NAME

c. OTHER ACCIDENT?
☐ YES ☐ NO

c. INSURANCE PLAN NAME OR PROGRAM NAME

d. INSURANCE PLAN NAME OR PROGRAM NAME

d. RESERVED FOR LOCAL USE

d. IS THERE ANOTHER HEALTH BENEFIT PLAN?
☐ YES ☐ NO If yes, return to and complete item 9 a-d.

READ BACK OF FORM BEFORE COMPLETING & SIGNING THIS FORM.

12. PATIENT'S OR AUTHORIZED PERSON'S SIGNATURE I authorize the release of any medical or other information necessary to process this claim. I also request payment of government benefits either to myself or to the party who accepts assignments below.

13. INSURED'S OR AUTHORIZED PERSON'S SIGNATURE I authorize payment of medical benefits to the undersigned physician or supplier for services described below.

SIGNED_____ DATE_____

SIGNED_____

← PATIENT AND INSURED INFORMATION →

14. DATE OF CURRENT: ILLNESS (First symptom) OR
MM ¦ DD ¦ YY INJURY (Accident) OR
PREGNANCY (LMP)

15. IF PATIENT HAS HAD SAME OR SIMILAR ILLNESS. GIVE FIRST DATE MM ¦ DD ¦ YY

16. DATES PATIENT UNABLE TO WORK IN CURRENT OCCUPATION
MM ¦ DD ¦ YY MM ¦ DD ¦ YY
FROM TO

17. NAME OR REFERRING PHYSICIAN OR OTHER SOURCE

17a. I.D. NUMBER OF REFERRING PHYSICIAN

18. HOSPITALIZATION DATES RELATED TO CURRENT SERVICES
MM ¦ DD ¦ YY MM ¦ DD ¦ YY
FROM TO

19. RESERVED FOR LOCAL USE

20. OUTSIDE LAB? $ CHARGES
☐ YES ☐ NO

21. DIAGNOSIS OR NATURE OF ILLNESS OR INJURY. (RELATE ITEMS 1,2,3 OR 4 TO ITEM 24E BY LINE)

1. I_____.___ 3. I_____.___

2. I_____.___ 4. I_____.___

22. MEDICAID RESUBMISSION CODE ORIGINAL REF. NO.

23. PRIOR AUTHORIZATION NUMBER

24. A		B	C	D		E	F	G	H	I	J	K
DATE(S) OF SERVICE		Place of Service	Type of Service	PROCEDURES, SERVICES, OR SUPPLIES (Explain Unusual Circumstances)		DIAGNOSIS CODE	$ CHARGES	DAYS OR UNITS	EPSDT Family Plan	EMG	COB	RESERVED FOR LOCAL USE
From MM DD YY	To MM DD YY			CPT/HCPCS	MODIFIER							
1												
2												
3												
4												
5												
6												

25. FEDERAL TAX I.D. NUMBER SSN ☐ EIN ☐

26. PATIENT'S ACCOUNT NO.

27. ACCEPT ASSIGNMENT? (For govt. claims, see back)
☐ YES ☐ NO

28. TOTAL CHARGE $

29. AMOUNT PAID $

30. BALANCE DUE $

31. SIGNATURE OF PHYSICIAN OR SUPPLIER INCLUDING DEGREES OR CREDENTIALS (I certify that the statements on the reverse apply to this bill and are made a part thereof.)

32. NAME AND ADDRESS OF FACULTY WHERE SERVICES WERE RENDERED (If other than home or office)

33. PHYSICIAN'S, SUPPLIER'S BILLING NAME, ADDRESS, ZIP CODE & PHONE#

SIGNED _____ DATE _____

PIN # GRP #

← PHYSICIAN OR SUPPLIER INFORMATION →

(APPROVED BY AMA COUNCIL ON MEDICAL SERVICE 8/88) ***PLEASE PRINT OR TYPE*** FORM HCFA-1500 (U2) (12-90)
FORM OWCP -1500 FORM RRB-1500

PLEASE
DO NOT
STAPLE
IN THIS
AREA

PICA

APPROVED OMB-0938-0008

HEALTH INSURANCE CLAIM FORM

PICA

CARRIE ▼ ▲ PATIENT AND INSURED INFORMATION

1. MEDICARE   MEDICAID   CHAMPUS   CHAMPVA   GROUP   FECA   OTHER
   ☐ (Medicare #) ☐ (Medicaid #) ☐ (Sponsor's SSN) ☐ (VA File #) HEALTH PLAN BLK LUNG
   ☐ (SSN or ID) ☐ (SSN) ☐ (ID)

1a. INSURED'S I.D. NUMBER   (FOR PROGRAM IN ITEM 1)

2. PATIENT'S NAME (Last Name, First Name, Middle Initial)

3. PATIENT'S BIRTH DATE   SEX
   MM │ DD │ YY   M ☐ F ☐

4. INSURED'S NAME (Last Name, Firts Name, Middle Initial)

5. PATIENT'S ADDRESS (No., Street)

6. PATIENT RELATIONSHIP TO INSURED
   ☐ Self ☐ Spouse ☐ Child ☐ Other

7. INSURED'S ADDRESS (No., Street)

CITY   STATE

8. PATIENT STATUS
   ☐ Single   ☐ Married   ☐ Other

CITY   STATE

ZIP CODE   TELEPHONE (Include Area Code)
                (   )

   Employed ☐ Full-Time ☐ Part-Time ☐
             Student   Student

ZIP CODE   TELEPHONE (Include Area Code)
                  (   )

9. OTHER INSURED'S NAME (Last Name, First Name, Middle Initial)

10. IS PATIENT'S CONDITION RELATED TO:

11. INSURED'S POLICY GROUP OR FECA NUMBER

a. OTHER INSURED'S POLICY OR GROUP NUMBER

a. EMPLOYMENT? (CURRENT OR PREVIOUS)
   ☐ YES   ☐ NO

a. INSURED'S DATE OF BIRTH   SEX
   MM │ DD │ YY   M ☐ F ☐

b. OTHER INSURED'S DATE OF BIRTH   SEX
   MM │ DD │ YY   M ☐ F ☐

b. AUTO ACCIDENT?   PLACE (State)
   ☐ YES   ☐ NO

b. EMPLOYER'S NAME OR SCHOOL NAME

c. EMPLOYER'S NAME OR SCHOOL NAME

c. OTHER ACCIDENT?
   ☐ YES   ☐ NO

c. INSURANCE PLAN NAME OR PROGRAM NAME

d. INSURANCE PLAN NAME OR PROGRAM NAME

d. RESERVED FOR LOCAL USE

d. IS THERE ANOTHER HEALTH BENEFIT PLAN?
   ☐ YES   ☐ NO If yes, return to and complete item 9 a-d.

READ BACK OF FORM BEFORE COMPLETING & SIGNING THIS FORM.

12. PATIENT'S OR AUTHORIZED PERSON'S SIGNATURE I authorize the release of any medical or other information necessary to process this claim. I also request payment of government benefits either to myself or to the party who accepts assignments below.

13. INSURED'S OR AUTHORIZED PERSON'S SIGNATURE I authorize payment of medical benefits to the undersigned physician or supplier for services described below.

SIGNED_____ DATE_____

SIGNED_____

14. DATE OF CURRENT:
    MM │ DD │ YY
    ◄ ILLNESS (First sympton) OR
      INJURY (Accident) OR
      PREGNANCY (LMP)

15. IF PATIENT HAS HAD SAME OR SIMILAR ILLNESS.
    GIVE FIRST DATE   MM │ DD │ YY

16. DATES PATIENT UNABLE TO WORK IN CURRENT OCCUPATION
    MM │ DD │ YY   MM │ DD │ YY
    FROM   TO

17. NAME OR REFERRING PHYSICIAN OR OTHER SOURCE

17a. I.D. NUMBER OF REFERRING PHYSICIAN

18. HOSPITALIZATION DATES RELATED TO CURRENT SERVICES
    MM │ DD │ YY   MM │ DD │ YY
    FROM   TO

19. RESERVED FOR LOCAL USE

20. OUTSIDE LAB?
    ☐ YES ☐ NO $ CHARGES

21. DIAGNOSIS OR NATURE OF ILLNESS OR INJURY. (RELATE ITEMS 1,2,3 OR 4 TO ITEM 24E BY LINE)

1. l_____.___   3. l_____.___

2. l_____.___   4. l_____.___

22. MEDICAID RESUBMISSION
    CODE   ORIGINAL REF. NO.

23. PRIOR AUTHORIZATION NUMBER

24.	A		B	C	D		E	F	G	H	I	J	K
	DATE(S) OF SERVICE		Place of Service	Type of Service	PROCEDURES, SERVICES, OR SUPPLIES (Explain Unusual Circumstances)		DIAGNOSIS CODE	$ CHARGES	DAYS OR UNITS	EPSDT Family Plan	EMG	COB	RESERVED FOR LOCAL USE
	From MM DD YY	To MM DD YY			CPT/HCPCS	MODIFIER							
1													
2													
3													
4													
5													
6													

25. FEDERAL TAX I.D. NUMBER   SSN EIN
    ☐ ☐

26. PATIENT'S ACCOUNT NO.

27. ACCEPT ASSIGNMENT?
    (For govt. claims, see back)
    ☐ YES ☐ NO

28. TOTAL CHARGE
    $ │

29. AMOUNT PAID
    $ │

30. BALANCE DUE
    $ │

31. SIGNATURE OF PHYSICIAN OR SUPPLIER INCLUDING DEGREES OR CREDENTIALS
    (I certify that the statements on the reverse apply to this bill and are made a part thereof.)

32. NAME AND ADDRESS OF FACULTY WHERE SERVICES WERE RENDERED (If other than home or office)

33. PHYSICIAN'S, SUPPLIER'S BILLING NAME, ADDRESS, ZIP CODE & PHONE#

SIGNED _____ DATE _____

(APPROVED BY AMA COUNCIL ON MEDICAL SERVICE 8/88)

PLEASE PRINT OR TYPE

PIN #   GRP #

FORM HCFA-1500 (U2) (12-90)
FORM OWCP -1500   FORM RRB-1500

PHYSICIAN OR SUPPLIER INFORMATION

PLEASE
NOT
STAPLE
IN THIS
AREA

APPROVED OMB-0938-0008

PICA

HEALTH INSURANCE CLAIM FORM

PICA

1. MEDICARE MEDICAID CHAMPUS CHAMPVA GROUP FECA OTHER
HEALTH PLAN BLK LUNG
☐(Medicare #) ☐(Medicaid #) ☐(Sponsor's SSN) ☐(VA File #) ☐(SSN or ID) ☐(SSN) ☐(ID)

1a. INSURED'S I.D. NUMBER (FOR PROGRAM IN ITEM 1)

2. PATIENT'S NAME (Last Name, First Name, Middle Initial)

3. PATIENT'S BIRTH DATE SEX
MM ┆ DD ┆ YY
M☐ F☐

4. INSURED'S NAME (Last Name, Firts Name, Middle Initial)

5. PATIENT'S ADDRESS (No., Street)

6. PATIENT RELATIONSHIP TO INSURED
☐ Self ☐Spouse ☐Child ☐Other

7. INSURED'S ADDRESS (No., Street)

CITY STATE

8. PATIENT STATUS
☐ Single ☐ Married ☐Other

CITY STATE

ZIP CODE TELEPHONE (Include Area Code)
( )

Employed ☐ Full-Time ☐Part-Time
Student Student

ZIP CODE TELEPHONE (Include Area Code)
( )

9. OTHER INSURED'S NAME (Last Name, First Name, Middle Initial)

10. IS PATIENT'S CONDITION RELATED TO:

11. INSURED'S POLICY GROUP OR FECA NUMBER

a. OTHER INSURED'S POLICY OR GROUP NUMBER

a. EMPLOYMENT? (CURRENT OR PREVIOUS)
☐ YES ☐ NO

a. INSURED'S DATE OF BIRTH SEX
MM ┆ DD ┆ YY
M☐ F☐

b. OTHER INSURED'S DATE OF BIRTH SEX
MM ┆ DD ┆ YY
M☐ F☐

b. AUTO ACCIDENT? PLACE (State)
☐ YES ☐ NO

b. EMPLOYER'S NAME OR SCHOOL NAME

c. EMPLOYER'S NAME OR SCHOOL NAME

c. OTHER ACCIDENT?
☐ YES ☐ NO

c. INSURANCE PLAN NAME OR PROGRAM NAME

d. INSURANCE PLAN NAME OR PROGRAM NAME

d. RESERVED FOR LOCAL USE

d. IS THERE ANOTHER HEALTH BENEFIT PLAN?
☐ YES ☐ NO If yes, return to and complete item 9 a-d.

READ BACK OF FORM BEFORE COMPLETING & SIGNING THIS FORM.
12.PATIENT'S OR AUTHORIZED PERSON'S SIGNATURE I authorize the release of any medical or other information necessary to process this claim. I also request payment of government benefits either to myself or to the party who accepts assignments below.

SIGNED_____ DATE_____

13. INSURED'S OR AUTHORIZED PERSON'S SIGNATURE I authorize payment of medical benefits to the undersigned physician or supplier for services described below.

SIGNED_____

14. DATE OF CURRENT: ILLNESS (First sympton) OR
MM ┆ DD ┆ YY INJURY (Accident)OR
PREGNANCY (LMP)

15. IF PATIENT HAS HAD SAME OR SIMILAR ILLNESS.
GIVE FIRST DATE MM ┆ DD ┆ YY

16. DATES PATIENT UNABLE TO WORK IN CURRENT OCCUPATION
MM ┆ DD ┆ YY MM ┆ DD ┆ YY
FROM ┆ ┆ TO ┆ ┆

17.NAME OR REFERRING PHYSICIAN OR OTHER SOURCE

17a. I.D. NUMBER OF REFERRING PHYSICIAN

18. HOSPITALIZATION DATES RELATED TO CURRENT SERVICES
MM ┆ DD ┆ YY MM ┆ DD ┆ YY
FROM ┆ ┆ TO ┆ ┆

19.RESERVED FOR LOCAL USE

20. OUTSIDE LAB? $ CHARGES
☐YES ☐NO

21.DIAGNOSIS OR NATURE OF ILLNESS OR INJURY. (RELATE ITEMS 1,2,3 OR 4 TO ITEM 24E BY LINE)

1.I____.___

3. I____.___

2.I____.___

4. I____.___

22. MEDICAID RESUBMISSION
CODE ORIGINAL REF. NO.

23. PRIOR AUTHORIZATION NUMBER

24.	A				B	C	D		E	F	G	H	I	J	K
	DATE(S) OF SERVICE				Place of Service	Type of Service	PROCEDURES, SERVICES, OR SUPPLIES (Explain Unusual Circumstances)		DIAGNOSIS CODE	$ CHARGES	DAYS OR UNITS	EPSDT Family Plan	EMG	COB	RESERVED FOR LOCAL USE
	From		To				CPT/HCPCS	MODIFIER							
	MM	DD YY	MM	DD YY											
1															
2															
3															
4															
5															
6															

25.FEDERAL TAX I.D. NUMBER SSN EIN
☐ ☐

26. PATIENT'S ACCOUNT NO.

27.ACCEPT ASSIGNMENT?
(For govt. claims, see back)
☐YES ☐NO

28. TOTAL CHARGE
$

29. AMOUNT PAID
$

30. BALANCE DUE
$

31. SIGNATURE OF PHYSICIAN OR SUPPLIER
INCLUDING DEGREES OR CREDENTIALS
(I certify that the statements on the reverse apply to this bill and are made a part thereof.)

SIGNED _____ DATE _____

32. NAME AND ADDRESS OF FACULTY WHERE SERVICES WERE RENDERED (If other than home or office)

33. PHYSICIAN'S, SUPPLIER'S BILLING NAME, ADDRESS, ZIP CODE & PHONE#

PIN # GRP #

(APPROVED BY AMA COUNCIL ON MEDICAL SERVICE 8/88)

PLEASE PRINT OR TYPE

FORM HCFA-1500 (U2) (12-90)
FORM OWCP -1500 FORM RRB-1500

CARRIER

PATIENT AND INSURED INFORMATION

PHYSICIAN OR SUPPLIER INFORMATION

121

Name _____

APPROVED OMB-0938-0008

PICA

HEALTH INSURANCE CLAIM FORM

PICA

1. MEDICARE ☐ (Medicare #) MEDICAID ☐ (Medicaid #) CHAMPUS ☐ (Sponsor's SSN) CHAMPVA ☐ (VA File #) GROUP HEALTH PLAN ☐ (SSN or ID) FECA BLK LUNG ☐ (SSN) OTHER ☐ (ID)

1a. INSURED'S I.D. NUMBER   (FOR PROGRAM IN ITEM 1)

2. PATIENT'S NAME (Last Name, First Name, Middle Initial)

3. PATIENT'S BIRTH DATE   SEX
MM | DD | YY   M ☐ F ☐

4. INSURED'S NAME (Last Name, Firts Name, Middle Initial)

5. PATIENT'S ADDRESS (No., Street)

6. PATIENT RELATIONSHIP TO INSURED
Self ☐ Spouse ☐ Child ☐ Other ☐

7. INSURED'S ADDRESS (No., Street)

CITY   STATE

8. PATIENT STATUS
Single ☐ Married ☐ Other ☐

CITY   STATE

ZIP CODE   TELEPHONE (Include Area Code)
(   )

Employed ☐ Full-Time Student ☐ Part-Time Student ☐

ZIP CODE   TELEPHONE (Include Area Code)
(   )

9. OTHER INSURED'S NAME (Last Name, First Name, Middle Initial)

10. IS PATIENT'S CONDITION RELATED TO:

11. INSURED'S POLICY GROUP OR FECA NUMBER

a. OTHER INSURED'S POLICY OR GROUP NUMBER

a. EMPLOYMENT? (CURRENT OR PREVIOUS)
☐ YES ☐ NO

a. INSURED'S DATE OF BIRTH   SEX
MM | DD | YY   M ☐ F ☐

b. OTHER INSURED'S DATE OF BIRTH   SEX
MM | DD | YY   M ☐ F ☐

b. AUTO ACCIDENT?   PLACE (State)
☐ YES ☐ NO

b. EMPLOYER'S NAME OR SCHOOL NAME

c. EMPLOYER'S NAME OR SCHOOL NAME

c. OTHER ACCIDENT?
☐ YES ☐ NO

c. INSURANCE PLAN NAME OR PROGRAM NAME

d. INSURANCE PLAN NAME OR PROGRAM NAME

d. RESERVED FOR LOCAL USE

d. IS THERE ANOTHER HEALTH BENEFIT PLAN?
☐ YES ☐ NO If yes, return to and complete item 9 a-d.

READ BACK OF FORM BEFORE COMPLETING & SIGNING THIS FORM.
12. PATIENT'S OR AUTHORIZED PERSON'S SIGNATURE I authorize the release of any medical or other information necessary to process this claim. I also request payment of government benefits either to myself or to the party who accepts assignments below.

13. INSURED'S OR AUTHORIZED PERSON'S SIGNATURE I authorize payment of medical benefits to the undersigned physician or supplier for services described below.

SIGNED_____ DATE_____

SIGNED_____

14. DATE OF CURRENT:
MM | DD | YY
ILLNESS (First sympton) OR INJURY (Accident) OR PREGNANCY (LMP)

15. IF PATIENT HAS HAD SAME OR SIMILAR ILLNESS.
GIVE FIRST DATE MM | DD | YY

16. DATES PATIENT UNABLE TO WORK IN CURRENT OCCUPATION
FROM MM | DD | YY TO MM | DD | YY

17. NAME OR REFERRING PHYSICIAN OR OTHER SOURCE

17a. I.D. NUMBER OF REFERRING PHYSICIAN

18. HOSPITALIZATION DATES RELATED TO CURRENT SERVICES
FROM MM | DD | YY TO MM | DD | YY

19. RESERVED FOR LOCAL USE

20. OUTSIDE LAB?
☐ YES ☐ NO $ CHARGES

21. DIAGNOSIS OR NATURE OF ILLNESS OR INJURY. (RELATE ITEMS 1,2,3 OR 4 TO ITEM 24E BY LINE)

1. |_____.____   3. |_____.____

2. |_____.____   4. |_____.____

22. MEDICAID RESUBMISSION
CODE   ORIGINAL REF. NO.

23. PRIOR AUTHORIZATION NUMBER

24.	A		B	C	D		E	F	G	H	I	J	K
	DATE(S) OF SERVICE		Place of Service	Type of Service	PROCEDURES, SERVICES, OR SUPPLIES (Explain Unusual Circumstances)		DIAGNOSIS CODE	$ CHARGES	DAYS OR UNITS	EPSDT Family Plan	EMG	COB	RESERVED FOR LOCAL USE
	From MM DD YY	To MM DD YY			CPT/HCPCS	MODIFIER							
1													
2													
3													
4													
5													
6													

25. FEDERAL TAX I.D. NUMBER   SSN ☐ EIN ☐

26. PATIENT'S ACCOUNT NO.

27. ACCEPT ASSIGNMENT?
(For govt. claims, see back)
☐ YES ☐ NO

28. TOTAL CHARGE
$

29. AMOUNT PAID
$

30. BALANCE DUE
$

31. SIGNATURE OF PHYSICIAN OR SUPPLIER INCLUDING DEGREES OR CREDENTIALS
(I certify that the statements on the reverse apply to this bill and are made a part thereof.)

32. NAME AND ADDRESS OF FACULTY WHERE SERVICES WERE RENDERED (If other than home or office)

33. PHYSICIAN'S, SUPPLIER'S BILLING NAME, ADDRESS, ZIP CODE & PHONE#

SIGNED _____ DATE _____

PIN #   GRP #

(APPROVED BY AMA COUNCIL ON MEDICAL SERVICE 8/88)   *PLEASE PRINT OR TYPE*

FORM HCFA-1500 (U2) (12-90)
FORM OWCP -1500   FORM RRB-1500

ACHIEVING SKILL COMPETENCY

Reread the TPO for the procedure and then practice the skill listed below, following the procedure in your textbook.

Complete a Claim Form-Procedure 9-1

When you have mastered the performance of the skill, sign your name on the appropriate evaluation sheet and give it to your instructor to indicate you are prepared to perform the procedure for evaluation.

SUGGESTED ACTIVITIES

After your instructor has returned your work to you, make all necessary corrections and place in a 3-ring notebook for future reference.

ASSIGNMENT SHEET

Chapter 10: MEDICAL OFFICE MANAGEMENT
Unit 1: THE LANGUAGE OF BANKING

Review the objectives and text for each unit before completing the assignment sheet for that unit in this chapter. When all sheets for the chapter have been completed, remove them from this workbook and give them to the instructor for evaluation.

MIXED QUIZ

1. Matching: Read the definition in Column I and then find the matching answer in Column II. Place the letter of the correct answer in the space provided.

COLUMN I

_____ 1. Agent
_____ 2. Bankbook
_____ 3. Bank statement
_____ 4. Cashier's check
_____ 5. Check register
_____ 6. Certified check
_____ 7. Checking account
_____ 8. Currency
_____ 9. Deposit
_____ 10. Deposit record
_____ 11. Deposit slip

COLUMN II

a. Record of deposit given to customer by bank
b. A person authorized to act for another
c. A bank account against which checks are written
d. Record of deposits, withdrawals, and interest earned
e. An itemized list of cash and checks deposited
f. Check stub
g. Purchaser pays full amount of check issued by bank
h. Paper money issued by government
I. A record sent to customer showing all banking activity for a set period of time
j. Money being placed in a bank account
k. Bank stamps customer's own check and holds funds aside to cover check

2. Matching: Read the definition in Column I and then find the matching answer in Column II. Place the letter of the correct answer in the space provided.

COLUMN I

_____ 1. Endorsement
_____ 2. Endorser
_____ 3. Insufficient funds
_____ 4. Limited check
_____ 5. Maker
_____ 6. Money order
_____ 7. Note
_____ 8. Payee
_____ 9. Payer
_____ 10. Postdated check

COLUMN II

a. Negotiable instrument purchased for a fee to be used instead of a check
b. Check made out for a future date
c. Person to whom check is written
d. Payee's signature on back of check
e. A bank term used to indicate that writer of check did not have enough money in account to cover check
f. Person who signs check
g. Legal evidence of debt
h. Same as payee on check
i. Check which will be void if written over designated amount or kept beyond time limit of when it should be cashed
j. Individual who signs a check

3. Matching: Read the definition in Column I and then find the matching answer in Column II. Place the letter of the correct answer in the space provided.

COLUMN I

_____ 1. Power of attorney
_____ 2. Savings account
_____ 3. Service charge
_____ 4. Stale check
_____ 5. Stop payment
_____ 6. Teller
_____ 7. Traveler's check
_____ 8. Voucher check
_____ 9. Warrant
_____ 10. Withdrawal

COLUMN II

a. Bank employee who is main contact between customer and bank
b. Fees charged by bank for services rendered
c. Removal of funds from depositor's account
d. Method by which maker of check may change his mind about making payment
e. Check with detachable form used to state purpose for which check was written
f. A bank account upon which depositor earns interest
g. Evidence of a debt due but is not negotiable
h. Special check issued by bank in exchange for cash that must be signed when purchased and again when used
i. A check presented for payment after date specified when would be honored
j. A legal procedure that authorizes one person to act as agent for another

4. Explain the bank code on a check.
   a. What is an ABA number? _____
   b. Who originated the number concept? _____
   c. What is its purpose? _____
   _____

5. Define the term MICR. _____
   a. Explain what each series of numbers means
      1. _____
      2. _____
      3. _____
   b. What does a bank add to the check? _____
   c. Why is MICR used? _____
   _____

6. Identify the ABA and MICR codes on the check.

JAMES C. MORRISON   101
1765 SHERIDAN DRIVE
YOUR CITY, STATE, 12345   _____ , 19 ____   00–6789/0000

PAY TO THE
ORDER OF _____ | $ _____

_____ DOLLARS

DELUXE CHECK PRINTERS
YOUR CITY, U.S.A. 12345

MEMO _____

⑈:00006 7894⑈: 12345678;'   0101 ;0000039158;

   a. _____
   b. _____
   c. _____
   d. _____
   e. _____

7. Explain the difference between overdraft and overdrawn. _____
   _____
   _____
   _____

8. A. List five pieces of information the bank requires to stop payment on a check.
   1. _____
   2. _____
   3. _____
   4. _____
   5. _____
   B. For what reasons may payment be stopped?
   1. _____
   2. _____

9. Define the term "postdated check" and explain what you must do with such a check. _____
   _____
   _____
   _____

10. What is an electronic fund transfer system? _____
    _____
    _____

11. Describe the one-write check writing system. _____
    _____
    _____

12. What would you do in the event a bank deposit is not credited? _____
    _____
    _____

After your instructor has returned your work to you, make all necessary corrections and place in a 3-ring notebook for future reference.

ASSIGNMENT SHEET

Chapter 10: MEDICAL OFFICE MANAGEMENT
Unit 2: CURRENCY, CHECKS, AND PETTY CASH

MIXED QUIZ

1. Explain why comparing shipments to packing lists or invoices is important. _____
   _____
   _____
   _____

2. Using the following information, complete four checks to suppliers of goods and services. Use the current date and sign the checks with the physician's name with your name below the line. Complete the stub end, subtracting each subsequent check. (Two extra checks are provided in case you make an error.)
   a. Physician's Supply, Inc. $125.50
   b. Clinical Laboratory Services $987.45
   c. Brown Office Equipment $535.99
   d. Jones Building Maintenance $1,248.75

1490	BAL. BRO'T FOR'D				ELIZABETH R. EVANS, M.D.	1490
	19___		DEPOSITS		SUITE 205 100 E. MAIN ST. YOURTOWN, US 98765-4321	___ 19 ___ 25-64/440
TO ___					PAY TO THE ORDER OF ___ $ ___	
FOR ___					___ DOLLARS	
	TOTAL				THE NEVER FAIL BANK ANYWHERE, U.S.A 00000	7-88-25
	THIS CHECK				FOR ___	
	BALANCE				|:00006 7894|: 12345678;' 01490 ;0000039158;	

1491	BAL. BRO'T FOR'D				ELIZABETH R. EVANS, M.D.	1491
	19___		DEPOSITS		SUITE 205 100 E. MAIN ST. YOURTOWN, US 98765-4321	___ 19 ___ 25-64/440
TO ___					PAY TO THE ORDER OF ___ $ ___	
FOR ___					___ DOLLARS	
	TOTAL				THE NEVER FAIL BANK ANYWHERE, U.S.A 00000	7-88-25
	THIS CHECK				FOR ___	
	BALANCE				|:00006 7894|: 12345678;' 01491 ;0000039158;	

1492	BAL. BRO'T FOR'D				ELIZABETH R. EVANS, M.D.	1492
	19___		DEPOSITS		SUITE 205 100 E. MAIN ST. YOURTOWN, US 98765-4321	___ 19 ___ 25-64/440
TO ___					PAY TO THE ORDER OF ___ $ ___	
FOR ___					___ DOLLARS	
	TOTAL				THE NEVER FAIL BANK ANYWHERE, U.S.A 00000	7-88-25
	THIS CHECK				FOR ___	
	BALANCE				|:00006 7894|: 12345678;' 01492 ;0000039158;	

1493	BAL. BRO'T FOR'D				ELIZABETH R. EVANS, M.D.	1493
	19___		DEPOSITS		SUITE 205 100 E. MAIN ST. YOURTOWN, US 98765-4321	___ 19 ___ 25-64/440
TO ___					PAY TO THE ORDER OF ___ $ ___	
FOR ___					___ DOLLARS	
	TOTAL				THE NEVER FAIL BANK ANYWHERE, U.S.A 00000	7-88-25
	THIS CHECK				FOR ___	
	BALANCE				|:00006 7894|: 12345678;' 01493 ;0000039158;	

1494	BAL. BRO'T FOR'D				ELIZABETH R. EVANS, M.D.	1494
	19___		DEPOSITS		SUITE 205 100 E. MAIN ST. YOURTOWN, US 98765-4321	___ 19 ___ 25-64/440
TO ___					PAY TO THE ORDER OF ___ $ ___	
FOR ___					___ DOLLARS	
	TOTAL				THE NEVER FAIL BANK ANYWHERE, U.S.A 00000	7-88-25
	THIS CHECK				FOR ___	
	BALANCE				|:00006 7894|: 12345678;' 01494 ;0000039158;	

1495	BAL. BRO'T FOR'D				ELIZABETH R. EVANS, M.D.	1495
	19___		DEPOSITS		SUITE 205 100 E. MAIN ST. YOURTOWN, US 98765-4321	___ 19 ___ 25-64/440
TO ___					PAY TO THE ORDER OF ___ $ ___	
FOR ___					___ DOLLARS	
	TOTAL				THE NEVER FAIL BANK ANYWHERE, U.S.A 00000	7-88-25
	THIS CHECK				FOR ___	
	BALANCE				|:00006 7894|: 12345678;' 01495 ;0000039158;	

3. Why should you refuse a third party check? _____

4. Why should you not accept a check for more than the amount due? _____
_____

5. Why may a check marked "payment in full" be a problem? _____
_____

6. Name the two kinds of endorsements, explaining the meaning of each one.
   a. _____
   b. _____

7. How do you process a check when the name of the payee is misspelled? _____
_____

8. Where should a check be endorsed? _____

9. Prepare a bank deposit using the following list of cash and check payments.

   Currency/coin: $35.50, $40.00, $50.75, $25.00, $15.75

   Checks: Holley, check #134 - $40.00
                     Segal, check #285 - $25.00
                     Gomez, check #596 - $55.00
                     Schmidt, check #436 - $32.00
                     Moriarty, check #1073 - $38.00
                     Kostrevski, check #735 - $47.00
                     Kendrix, check #489 - $150.00
                     Cartloano, check #634 - $45.00

   Money Orders: Chin, $45.00; Jackson, $55.00

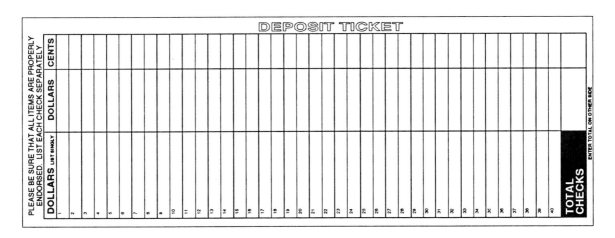

10. What must you do if a mail deposit is lost? _____

_____

11. Use the following figures to reconcile the bank account on the form provided. You may assume the opening balance agrees with the previous statement.

STATEMENT OF ACCOUNT

THE NEVER FAIL BANK • ANYWHERE, USA 00000

For the Month of _____, _____(Year)

Checks written during the month

#101	25.00	111	500.00	122	35.00
102	600.00	112	18.22	123	95.94
103	75.00	113	133.28	124	19.00
104	37.54	114	57.50	125	75.00
105	30.00	115	38.60	126	400.00
106	95.94	116	500.00	127	78.37
107	73.87	117	785.00	128	95.94
108	44.00	118	28.37	129	200.00
109	130.00	119	60.00	130	33.60
110	95.94	120	36.30	131	1200.00
		121	115.45	132	100.00

Checkbook balance end of last month - $3173.71

Deposit mailed but not appearing on statement $191.00

Checks Paid Out		Deposits	Balance
Balance Brought Forward			1840.57
25.00	95.94	500.00	1815.57
600.00	44.00	750.00	1715.57
30.00	500.00	350.00	2339.63
73.87	38.60	700.00	2441.76
95.94	115.45	335.00	2394.32
57.50	95.94	500.00	2133.22
28.37	75.00	440.50	2604.85
60.00	78.37	180.00	2985.35
36.30	33.60	175.00	3013.60
35.00	130.00	520.00	3057.66
19.00	18.22	522.50	3483.66
400.00	500.00	720.00	3431.85
200.00	95.94	600.00	3918.25
100.00	133.28	662.00	4414.98
	3.27 SC		5076.98

No. Checks = 28

No. Deposits = 14

Service Charge = 3.27

Ending Balance 5076.98

RECONCILE THE BANK STATEMENT

Bank Statement Balance   _____
Outstanding checks

    _____
    _____
    _____
    _____

Total _____
Subtract total outstanding checks   _____
Adjusted balance   _____
Add deposits not credited   _____
Corrected Bank Statement Balance   _____
Checkbook balance   _____
Subtract bank charges   _____
Corrected Checkbook Balance   _____

12. For what purpose is a petty cash fund used? _____
_____

13. Fill in the spaces with the Words to Know plus other appropriate words.

    1.   __ E __ __ __ __ __ __
    2.   __ __ __ __ N __ __ __ __
    3.   __ __ __ __ D __ __ __ __ __
    4.   __ O __ __
    5.   __ __ __ R __ __ __ __
    6.   __ __ __ S __ __ __ __
    7   __ E __ __ __ __ __
    8.   __ __ __ M __ __ __ __
    9.   __ __ __ __ __ E __
    10.   __ __ __ N __ __ __ __ __ __ __ __
    11. __ __ __ __ __ __ __ __ __ T __ __ __

CLUES
    1. All consumed, none left
    2. Make agree
    3. Payee other than patient
    4. Cancel, make invalid
    5. Cash
    6. A record
    7. To place in an account
    8. A sum paid toward a balance
    9. A paper designating payment
    10. Action occurring
    11. Power given, permission granted

After your instructor has returned your work to you, make all necessary corrections and place in a 3-ring notebook for future reference.

ASSIGNMENT SHEET

Chapter 10: MEDICAL OFFICE MANAGEMENT
Unit 3: SALARY, BENEFITS, AND TAX RECORDS

MIXED QUIZ

1. Fill in the blanks to complete the following sentences:
   All employees in a physician's office must have a _____ . Forms to apply for the number can be obtained from local _____ , _____ , and _____ . Each employee must also complete an _____ indicating the number of exemptions claimed. In addition, recent federal legislation requires the completion of an _____ _____ . This form is issued by the _____ . Its purpose is to ensure all persons employed are either _____ , or _____ _____ . In addition to these federal requirements, forms must also be processed for _____ and _____tax records.

2. What information should be listed on payroll record keeping forms?

   a. _____
   b. _____
   c. _____
   d. _____
   e. _____
   f. _____
   g. _____
   h. _____
   i. _____
   j. _____
   k. _____
   l. _____
   m. _____

3. a. What determines the amount of federal tax withheld?

   1. _____
   2. _____
   3. _____
   4. _____

   b. How are state and local taxes determined? _____

   c. What is net pay? _____

4. What is the physician's responsibility in relation to state and federal regulations?

   a. _____
   b. _____
   c. _____
   d. _____

5. List six examples of fringe benefits.

   a. _____
   b. _____
   c. _____
   d. _____
   e. _____
   f. _____
   g. _____

6. What does the term "vested" mean? _____

_____

7. Underline the correctly spelled term in each line.

accountent	accontant	accountant
disability	disibility	disebility
longevity	lonjevity	longitevy
egemption	exeption	exemption
deducktions	deductions	deductshuns

8. Using the information below, fill in the spaces from the Words to Know and other appropriate words.

1.   _ _ _ <u>U</u> _ _ _ _ _ _
2.   _ _ _ _ _ <u>N</u> _ _ _ _
3.   _ <u>E</u> _ _ _ _ _ _
4.   <u>U N E M P L O Y M E N T</u>
5.   _ _ _ _ <u>P</u> _ _ _ _
6.   _ _ _ _ _ _ <u>L</u> _ _ _
7   _ _ <u>O</u> _ _
8.   _ _ _ _ _ _ _ _ <u>Y</u>
9.   _ <u>M</u> _ _ _ _ _ _
10.   _ <u>E</u> _ _ _ _
11.   <u>N</u> _ _
12.   _ _ _ _ _ <u>T</u> _ _ _ _ _ _ _

CLUES
1. Eligible credits to reduce tax
2. One who examines fiscal matters
3. Additional to salary
4. Without work
5. To excuse
6. Lack of ability
7. Total earnings
8. Length of time
9. One hired for a job
10. Eligible to receive
11. Remaining
12. Participation in distribution of earnings

After your instructor has returned your work to you, make all necessary corrections and place in a 3-ring notebook for future reference.

ASSIGNMENT SHEET

Chapter 10: MEDICAL OFFICE MANAGEMENT
Unit 4: GENERAL MANAGEMENT DUTIES

MIXED QUIZ

1. Why is it necessary to maintain a sense of fiscal status? _____

   _____

2. What kinds of information are supplied to the practice monthly by an accountant?

   a. _____

   b. _____

   c. _____

3. What are three consequences of a missed appointment?

   a. _____

   b. _____

   c. _____

4. What kind of information should be indicated on an inventory card?

   a. _____

   b. _____

   c. _____

   d. _____

5. When might a patient's account be overpaid? _____

   What must you check before refunding any amount? _____

6. All items must be stored properly. Identify the following correct storage places.

   a. Medications in _____

   b. Narcotics in _____

   c. Some laboratory supplies in _____

   d. Supplies _____

7. List an office manager's responsibility to the support staff.

   a. _____

   b. _____

   c. _____

   d. _____

   e. _____

   f. _____

   g. _____

8. List five office manager's responsibilities to the physicians.

   a. _____

   b. _____

   c. _____

   _____

   d. _____

   e. _____

9. Find and circle the following 18 words in the puzzle below.

```
A P R E M I U M S D B C D
M E E S F G E D H E M A I
A C I T F I X R J L A C N
N A M A I N T E N A N C E
A L B T S C E C K G U O G
G I U U C O N O L A A U L
E B R S A M S R M T L N I
M R S N L E I D O I P T G
E A E Q R S V S T O U V E
N T M W X R E F U N D Y N
T I E X P E D I T U R E T
Z O N I N V E N T O R Y A
B N T C P O L I C Y D E F
```

1. ACCOUNT	10. MANAGEMENT
2. CALIBRATION	11. MANUAL
3. DELEGATION	12. NEGLIGENT
4. EXPENDITURE	13. POLICY
5. EXTENSIVE	14. PREMIUMS
6. FISCAL	15. RECORDS
7. INCOME	16. REFUND
8. INVENTORY	17. REIMBURSEMENT
9. MAINTENANCE	18. STATUS

ACHIEVING SKILL COMPETENCY

Reread the TPO for each procedure and practice the skills listed below, following the procedures in your textbook.

Write a Check-Procedure 10-1

Prepare a Deposit Slip-Procedure 10-2

Reconcile a Bank Statement-Procedure 10-3

When you feel you have mastered the performance of the skill, sign your name on the appropriate evaluation sheet and give it to your instructor to indicate you are prepared to perform the procedure for evaluation.

After your instructor has returned your work to you, make all necessary corrections and place in a 3-ring notebook for future reference.

ASSIGNMENT SHEET

SECTION III: STRUCTURE AND FUNCTION OF THE BODY

Chapter 11: ANATOMY AND PHYSIOLOGY OF THE HUMAN BODY

Review the objectives and text for each unit before completing the assignment sheet for that unit in this chapter. When all sheets for each unit have been completed, remove them from this workbook and give them to the instructor for evaluation.

UNIT 1: ANATOMICAL DESCRIPTORS AND FUNDAMENTAL BODY STRUCTURES

A. MIXED QUIZ

1. Define anatomy. _____
2. Name and define the two subdivisions of anatomy. _____
   _____
3. Define physiology. _____
4. Describe the meaning of the phrase *anatomical position*. _____
   _____
   _____

5. Fill in the blanks.
   In anatomical position, the patient's right side is across from your _____ side. References made to something toward the midline is said to be _____; if it is away from the midline it is _____. Arms and legs are known as _____. The front of the body is called the _____ or _____ section. The back section is called the _____ or _____ side. The body has two main cavities. The anterior cavity is further divided into an upper _____ and a lower _____ cavity. The posterior body section has a _____ cavity and a _____ cavity.

6. List the organs within each body cavity.
   a. Thoracic: _____
   b. Abdominal: _____
   c. Pelvic: _____
   d. Cranial: _____
   e. Spinal: _____

7. Identify the directional reference terms on the illustrations of anatomical position.

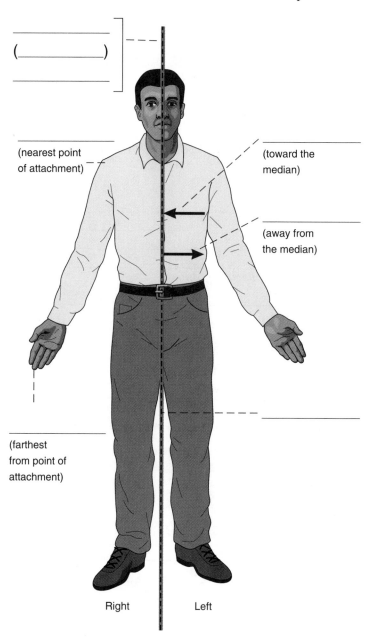

(_____)

(_____)

_____
(nearest point
of attachment)

_____
(toward the
median)

_____
(away from
the median)

_____
(farthest
from point of
attachment)

_____

Right   Left

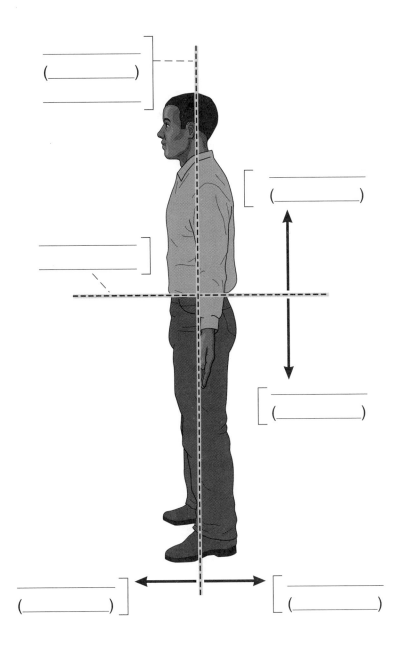

(_____)

_____

[_____]
(_____)

_____
_____

[_____]
(_____)

_____
(_____)

[_____]
(_____)

8. Identify the eight body cavities on the following illustration.

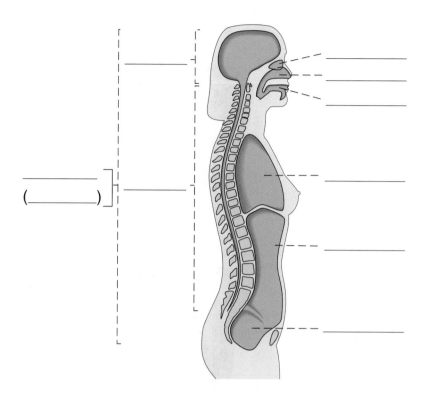

9. Identify the thoracic and abdominal organs.

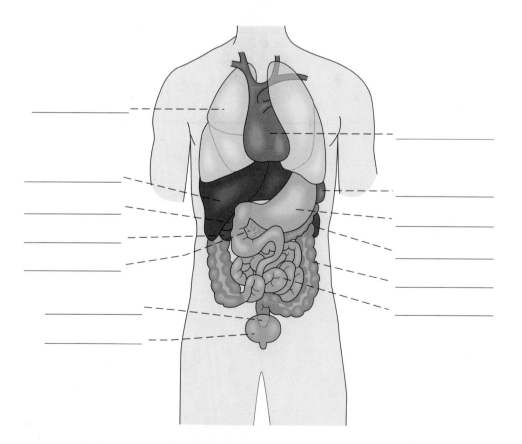

10. The abdomen can be divided into four sections for reference purposes. Name the sections.

   a. _____
   b. _____
   c. _____
   d. _____

11. Identify the nine anatomical divisions and one reference point of the abdomen on the following illustration.

12. List the structures of a cell.

   a. _____
   b. _____
   c. _____
   d. _____
   e. _____
   f. _____
   g. _____
   h. _____
   i. _____
   j. _____

13. List three things which may cause a mutation to occur. _____
   _____

14. Name three types of inheritance patterns and tell how they affect an individual's inherited traits.

   _____
   _____
   _____
   _____

15. List the six processes by which materials pass through cell membranes.

   1. _____
   2. _____
   3. _____
   4. _____
   5. _____
   6. _____

16. Complete the following sentences.

The osmotic characteristics of solutions are classified by their effect on _____ . If the solution is the same osmotic pressure as blood serum, it is known as an _____ solution. When osmolality is lower, the solution is called _____ if it is higher, it is called _____ . A salt solution with the same salt content as that of a red blood cell is called _____ .

17. Match the following acid or base with its possible location; enter the appropriate letter in the space before the acid or base.

_____ Acetic acid   a. Found in batteries

_____ Boric acid   b. Household liquid cleaners

_____ Hydrochloric acid   c. Lye

_____ Sulfuric acid   d. Found in vinegar

_____ Ammonium hydroxide   e. Found in the stomach

_____ Magnesium hydroxide   f. Weak eyewash

_____ Sodium hydroxide   g. Milk of Magnesia

18. Indicate whether the following pH value is acidic or alkaline and what body fluid has a similar value.

pH Value	Acidic/Alkaline	Body Fluid
a. 8.0		
b. 7.4		
c. 6.0		
d. 7.3		
e. 1.5		

19. The following genetic conditions have visible abnormal characteristics which make them readily recognized. Match the condition to its visible sign by placing the number of the sign in the space before the condition.

_____ Cleft lip   1. male with long legs with short obese trunk

_____ Cleft palate   2. malformation of one or both feet

_____ Down syndrome   3. verticle split in upper lip

_____ Spina Bifida   4. female with webbing of the neck

_____ Klinefelter's syndrome   5. opening in the top of mouth

_____ Talipes   6. small head and slanting eyes

_____ Turner's syndrome   7. a malformation of the back

20. What is the name of the project that is sequencing genes? _____

21. Explain the term DNA fingerprinting and how can it be used? _____

_____

_____

22. List the four types of tissues. Identify three places in the body where the tissue can be found.

a. _____

  1. _____

  2. _____

  3. _____

b. _____

  1. _____

  2. _____

  3. _____

c. _____

  1. _____

  2. _____

  3. _____

d. _____
   1. _____
   2. _____
   3. _____

23. List the ten systems of the body.

   1. _____
   2. _____
   3. _____
   4. _____
   5. _____
   6. _____
   7. _____
   8. _____
   9. _____
   10. _____

24. Word Search: There are 31 words hidden in the puzzle. Can you find them?

anatomy	epithelial	organ
anterior	feet	pelvic
cavity	gene	PKU
cleft	genetic	posterior
connective	iliac	skin
cranial	lateral	smooth
DNA	lip	spina
dorsal	lumbar	tissue
down	midline	ventral
edema	muscle	
epigastric	nerve	

```
S P I N A G E N E T I C W P
S P L N C L E F T D O W N C
P K U I A F E N M T I C T V
S P I E P I T H E L I A L E
S P A N T E R I O R G A N K
S M I N A G P N S T I C E P
S U I N A G E E S I C R O
S S V E N T R A L T U C V S
S C I N A G O N I V F E E T
S L R N E D E M A L I C T E
S E I A A G E N Y T I C T R
S C O N N E C T I V E A T I
S P I E P I G A S T R I C O
S P D O R S A L U M B A R R
S L A T E R A L S M O O T H
S M I D L I N E C A V I T Y
```

25. Match the following term (Column I) with a meaning (Column II). Place the correct number in the space provided.

COLUMN1

_____ a. Cardiac
_____ b. Cranial
_____ c. Cytoplasm
_____ d. Diaphragm
_____ e. Dorsal
_____ f. Epigastric
_____ g. Homeostasis
_____ h. Hypochondriac
_____ i. Inguinal
_____ j. Lateral
_____ k. Medial
_____ l. Myelin
_____ m. Neuron
_____ n. Proximal
_____ o. Smooth
_____ p. Striated
_____ q. Thoracic
_____ r. Tissue
_____ s. Umbilical
_____ t. Ventral
_____ u. Mutation
_____ v. Chromosome
_____ w. X-linked gene
_____ y. PKU
_____ z. Down syndrome

COLUMN II

1. Groin area
2. A nerve cell
3. A covering on a nerve
4. Heart tissue
5. Toward the midline
6. Change in the genetic code
7. Part of extremity nearest the body
8. Cavity which holds the brain
9. Lack of liver enzyme to act upon phenylalanine
10. Muscle tissue in organs
11. Abdominal area around navel
12. Stores hereditary material of the cell
13. Constructed of like cells
14. Skeletal muscle tissue
15. A genetic condition due to improper chromosome 21 division
16. Cellular fluid
17. Part of extremity farthest away from body
18. State of normal functioning
19. Muscle that divides anterior cavity
20. Away from the midline
21. Carried by X chromosome
22. The anterior section
23. Abdominal area above umbilical
24. Chest area
25. The posterior section
26. The abdominal area below the umbilical
27. The cell nucleus
28. Swelling in the tissues
29. Abdominal area below ribs

B. CRITICAL THINKING SITUATIONS. WHAT WOULD YOU SAY? WHAT WOULD YOU DO?

1. Your friend Nancy Martin, shares with you that she is trying to become pregnant. You know whe is 37 years old and has a younger brother with Down's Syndrome. _____

_____

_____

2. A neighbor confides in you that her 15-year-old son has not shown any signs of sexual maturity, even though he is very tall. You know he has also had some difficulty with school. _____

_____

_____

_____

After your instructor has returned your work to you, make all necessary corrections and place in a 3-ring notebook for future reference.

ASSIGNMENT SHEET

Chapter 11
Unit 2: THE NERVOUS SYSTEM

A. MIXED QUIZ

1. List the two main divisions of the nervous system.
    a. _____
    b. _____

2. What is a synapse?
    _____

3. Identify two types of peripheral nerves.
    a. _____
    b. _____

4. List the two types of spinal nerves and describe their functions.
    a. _____
    b. _____

5. Fill in the blanks to describe simple and complex reflex actions.
    Simple reflex actions involve an impulse traveling along a nerve to the _____ and
    _____ . A common test used to illustrate this action is called the _____ .
    Complex reflex actions involve an impulse traveling from its source through _____ to the
    _____ and up to the _____ . The message is interpreted and the
    _____ carry the response message back to the _____ and out the
    appropriate nerve.

6. What is the purpose or function of the autonomic nervous system? _____
    _____

7. Name the two divisions of the autonomic system, explaining their actions.
    a. _____
    b. _____

8. List the five divisions of the brain and identify what function each division provides.
    a. _____
       _____
    b. _____
    c. _____
    d. _____
    e. _____

9. List the lobes of the cerebrum and their associated functions.
    a. _____
       _____
    b. _____
    c. _____
       _____
    d. _____

10. List the two structures between the cerebrum and the midbrain, describing their functions.
    a. _____
       1. _____
    b. _____
       1. _____
       2. _____
       3. _____
       4. _____
       5. _____

6. _____

7. _____

8. _____

11. List the three meninges, describing their location and function as given in the text.

    a. _____

    b. _____

    c. _____

12. What are the spaces called between the a) dura mater and the arachnoid and b) the arachnoid and the pia?

    a. _____

    b. _____

13. Name the fluid within the cavities of the CNS and describe its function. _____

_____

14. Match the following diagnostic tests with their purpose. Place the number of the purpose (Column II) in the space before the test name, (Column I).

COLUMN1

_____ a. Arteriography

_____ b. Brain scan

_____ c. Glasgow Coma Scale

_____ d. CAT scan

_____ e. E.E.G.

_____ f. Electromyography

_____ g. Lumbar puncture

_____ h. Myelography

_____ i. Skull X ray

_____ j. Position Emission Tomography

COLUMN II

1. Detects abnormal electrical impulses in the brain

2. To detect tumors, bleeding, clots, brain size, and edema

3. Measure cerebrospinal fluid pressure or obtain a sample of fluid

4. Images enhanced with color

5. To detect cranial fractures or dense cerebral areas

6. Instill a dye or air to show irregularities in the CNS

7. Detects cerebral hemorrhage, aneurysm, or CVA

8. To detect neuromuscular disorders or nerve damage

9. Radioisotopes measured to detect abnormal masses or blood vessel lesions

10. To describe the level of consciousness

15. From the list below, enter the number of the disease or disorder to match the symptoms given.

a. _____ : Sudden acute onset of fever, headache, and vomiting which progresses to a stiff neck and back, drowsiness, and eventual coma.

b. _____ : Blurred or double vision with sensations of tingling or numbness; periods of attacks and remission characterized by tremor, muscular weakness, paralysis, etc.

c. _____ : Severe muscle rigidity, drooling, tremor, and a characteristic bent forward position when walking.

d. _____ : Temporary double vision, slurred speech, dizziness, staggering, and falling.

e. _____ : Loss of sensation with paralysis of one side of the body.

f. _____ : Sharp, piercing pain in the back of the thigh extending down the side of the leg

g. _____ : Weakness and paralysis on one side of the face causing drooping mouth, drooling, and inability to close the affected eye.

h. _____ : Fluid-filled vesicles on the skin associated with fever, severe deep pain, itching, and abnormal skin sensations.

i. _____ : Seizures of varying duration, possible loss of consciousness, loss of body function control, and convulsions.

j. _____ : Abnormally large head, distended scalp veins, shiny scalp skin, irritability, vomiting.

k. _____ : Hyperactive tendon reflexes, underdeveloped affected extremities, muscular contractions; may also have seizures, mental retardation, and impaired speech.

l. _____ : High fever, chills, headache, positive Brudzinski and Kernig signs.

m. _____ : Severe pain along the course of a nerve anywhere in the body.

n. _____ : Excruciating facial pain upon stimulation of a trigger zone.

o. _____ : Paralysis with loss of sensation and reflexes in lower extremities.

p. _____ : Muscular weakness and atrophy. Problems with speech, chewing, and swallowing. Respirations may be affected; choking, and drooling.

q. _____ : Prodromal symptoms of fatigue, visual disturbances, tingling of face and lips, sensitivity to light, nausea and vomiting.

r. _____ : Incomplete closure of one or more vertebra, bladder and bowel control problems, hydrocephalus, weakness or paralysis of legs, often mental retardation.

s. _____ : Vomiting, lethargy, liver dysfunction, hyperventilation, delirium and coma, with eventual respiratory arrest.

1. Amyotrophic Lateral Sclerosis
2. Bell's Palsy
3. Cerebral Palsy
4. Encephalitis
5. Epilepsy
7. Herpes Zoster
6. Hemiplegia
8. Hydrocephalus
9. Meningitis
10. Migraine headache

11. Multiple Sclerosis
12. Neuralgia
13. Paraplegia
14. Parkinson's Disease
15. Reye's Syndrome
16. Sciatica
17. Spina Bifida
18. Transient Ischemic Attack
19. Trigeminal Neuralgia

16. Complete the following puzzle.

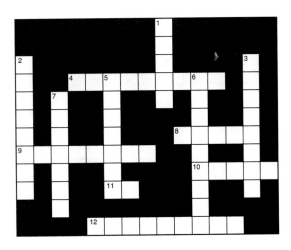

ACROSS
4. Posterior lobe of cerebrum
8. Nerve which causes action or movement
9. Contains sensory nerve cell bodies
10. Nerve of vision
11. Abbreviation for multiple sclerosis
12. Cavity within the brain

DOWN
1. Portion of CNS in cranium
2. Membrane covering CNS
3. Small brain part at top of brain stem
5. The skull
6. Part of peripheral nervous system
7. Portion of cerebrum behind forehead

B. CRITICAL THINKING SITUATIONS: WHAT WOULD YOU SAY? WHAT WOULD YOU DO?

1. Mr. Burns recently suffered a CVA which caused damage to the right side of his brain. He has difficulty with his left leg and has numbness in his left arm and hand. He cannot understand why his left side is affected.

_____

_____

2. Yesterday your nephew was injured severely in a motorcycle accident. Your brother is very concerned because his son has no apparent sensations or control of his body from the waist down. Can you give him any encouragement? _____

_____

_____

3. A patient phones the office complaining of painful blisters on the right side of his chest. He wants the doctor to call the pharmacy to order something to put on them. _____

_____

_____

_____

_____

4. A female patient calls late Saturday morning complaining of severe throbbing headache with nausea and sensitivity to light. It has been going for for the past 12 hours and she's afraid she is having a stroke. She is very frightened. _____

_____

_____

_____

5. A male patient tells you that on two separate occasions he has had "spells" of double vision, dizziness, and a tendency to lose his balance and fall. He says it only lasts about a half day so it's probably just old age and he's not going to bother the doctor about it. _____

_____

After your instructor has returned your work to you, make all necessary corrections and place in a 3-ring notebook for future reference.

4. List six functions of the skeletal system.

a. _____

b. _____

c. _____

d. _____

e. _____

f. _____

5. Describe the spinal column. _____

_____

6. Label the following illustration of the vertebral column.

Cervical

Coccyx

Lumbar

Sacrum

Thoracic

7. Fill in the blanks.

The rib cage consists of _____ pairs of ribs which attach by _____ to the _____ anteriorly and to the _____ posteriorly. The top _____ pairs are attached both anteriorly and posteriorly. The bottom _____ pairs are attached only to the _____ and are therefore called _____. The rib cage is also classified as having _____ and _____ ribs. This division considers the first _____ pairs to be _____ ribs because _____. The last _____ pairs are called _____ ribs because _____. The primary function of the rib cage is to protect the _____ and _____.

163

8. Label the illustration of the rib cage with the following terms:
   Clavicle
   Costal Cartilage
   False Ribs
   Floating Ribs
   Manubrium
   Spinal Column
   Sternum
   True Ribs
   Xiphoid Process

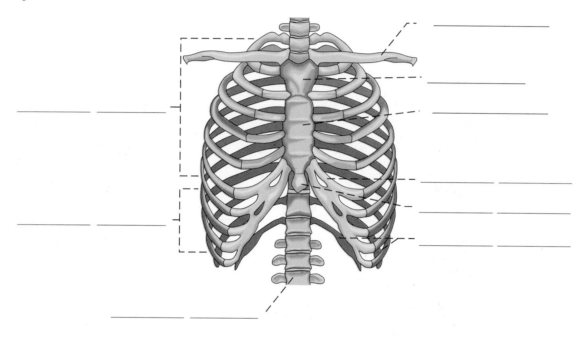

9. How is a long bone constructed? _____
   _____
   _____

10. How do long bones grow? _____
   _____

11. Identify three kinds of synovial joints, giving an example of each.
   a. _____
   b. _____
   c. _____

12. List the seven types of fractures, describing the characteristics of each type.
   a. _____
   b. _____
   c. _____
   d. _____
   e. _____
   f. _____
   g. _____

13. Identify each type of fracture illustrated below.

    a. _____

    b. _____

    c. _____

    d. _____

    e. _____

    f. _____

    g. _____

    h. _____

Transverse

Oblique

(A)   (B)   (C)   (D)   (E)   (F)

(G)   (H)

14. Describe the initial and follow-up treatment of fractures. _____

_____

_____

_____

_____

15. How does bone heal? _____

_____

_____

_____

16. What is a fat embolus and how does it occur? _____

_____

_____

17. What conditions might result in the need for an amputation?

    a. _____   c. _____

    b. _____   d. _____

18. Explain the condition known as phantom limb. _____

_____

19. Match the disease or disorder to the appropriate symptom. Enter the number from Column II in the space provided in Column I.

COLUMN I

_____   a. Osteoarthritis

_____   b. Rheumatoid arthritis

_____   c. Bursitis

_____   d. Congenital hip dysplagia

_____   e. Dislocation

_____   f. Epicondylitis

_____   g. Gout

_____   h. Hallux valgus

_____   i. Herniated disk

_____   j. Kyphosis

_____   k. Osteoporosis

_____   l. Scoliosis

_____   m. Sprain

_____   n. Carpal tunnel syndrome

_____   o. Bunion

_____   p. Lordosis

_____   q. Subluxation

COLUMN II

1. Painful displacement of the bones of the joint, usually fingers, shoulder, knees; often resulting in joint fracture

2. A metabolic disease resulting in severe joint pain due to deposits of urates

3. A lateral spinal curvature, usually thoracic, resulting from spinal column rotation

4. Porous, brittle bones, prone to fracture, caused by metabolic disorder, found primarily in postmenopausal women

5. Progressive deterioration of joint cartilage, usually hip and knee, joint pain, stiffness, grating and joint fluid

6. The dislocation of a child's hip joint at birth

7. A bowing of the back, usually at the thoracic level

8. Inflammation of forearm extensor tendon at its attachment on the humerus; more painful with twisting of forearm

9. Chronic inflammatory disease occurring intermittently; damages synovial membrane causing edema and congestion, bone atrophy, deformities

10. Causes severe low back pain, radiating deep into buttocks and down back of the leg

11. A tear of the ligaments of a joint resulting in pain, swelling, and local bleeding

12. Painful inflammation of the joint sac usually at the knee, elbow or shoulder

13. Lateral deviation of the great toe with enlarged first metatarsal and the formation of a bunion

14. Partial or incomplete dislocation of the articulating surfaces of bones at a joint causing deformity, pain, and extremity length change

15. An inflamed barsa of the great toe filled with fluid and covered with a callus

16. Decreased sensitivity in the first two fingers and thumb, often with atrophy of the thumb muscle on the palm side

17. Abnormal anterior convex curvature of the lumbar spine

20. Complete the following puzzle.

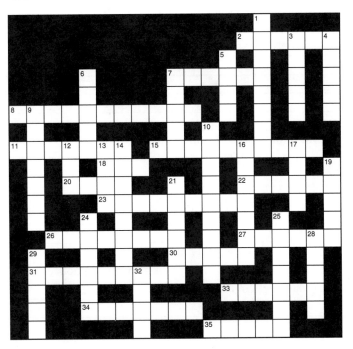

ACROSS

2. Uncomplicated
7. Leg bone
8. Sensation after amputation
11. Floating mass in blood vessel
15. Incomplete fracture
18. Last known address (abbr.)
20. Calcified cartilage
22. Stretch ligaments
23. To straighten a fracture
26. Break
27. Fills long bones
30. Harvests
31. Bones of the hands and feet
33. Bone in the forearm
34. Bone in the rib cage
35. Pelvic bone

DOWN

1. Attaches bone to bone at joints
3. A student
4. Joint between the humerus and the ulna and radius
5. Make well
6. Lethal
7. Thigh bone
9. Upper arm bone
10. Bones of spine
12. Circular object
13. Bone of forearm
14. Bony framework
16. The body _____
17. Outer garment
19. To furnish with a permanent source of income
21. Goes into
24. Bulgy deposit around a new fracture
25. The skull
28. Grossly overweight
29. Backbone
32. Female child

B. CRITICAL THINKING SITUATIONS: WHAT WOULD YOU SAY? WHAT WOULD YOU DO?

1. Mrs. Martin calls the office wondering if she should bring in her son. He fell off his bicycle and hurt his arm. He can move all his fingers but his arm hurts and there is a swollen area just above the wrist. _____

   _____

   _____

   _____

   _____

2. Mrs. Stone called the office for information. Mr. Stone suffered a broken leg yesterday at work. She is concerned because he is perspiring, is pale, has a moderate fever, and his heart rate and breathing is faster than normal. _____

   _____

   _____

3. Your friend Sally has been working on an assembly line attaching upholstery to automobile seats. She said that she is losing the strength in her hands. When you look at them you notice she is unable to make a fist and she says that she has pain and numbness in her thumb and first two fingers. _____

   _____

   _____

   _____

4. Your child has a friend spend the night. They are playing twister in their pajamas. You notice when the friend bends over that there is a hump at her mid-back area. _____

   _____

   _____

5. Your neighbor calls because an ankle he sprained yesterday is a lot more swollen today and is more painful. He had put a heating pad around it like his friend said. _____

   _____

   _____

After your instructor has returned your work to you, make all necessary corrections and place in a 3-ring notebook for future reference.

ASSIGNMENT SHEET

Chapter 11
Unit 6: THE MUSCULAR SYSTEM

A. MIXED QUIZ

1. What is a motor unit? _____

    _____

2. Why does muscular activity produce heat in the body? _____

    _____

    _____

3. List six functions of skeletal muscles.

    a. _____

    b. _____

    c. _____

    d. _____

    e. _____

    f. _____

4. List the three types of muscular tissue and describe the characteristics of each type, where located in the body, and the type of function performed.

TYPE	CHARACTERISTICS	LOCATION	FUNCTION
a. _____ _____	_____ _____	_____ _____	_____ _____
b. _____ _____ _____ _____	_____ _____ _____ _____	_____ _____ _____ _____	_____ _____ _____ _____
c. _____ _____ _____	_____ _____ _____	_____ _____ _____	_____ _____ _____

5. What is the purpose of a muscle team? Locate one example. _____

    _____

6. What does the term "muscle tone" mean? _____

7. Label the six illustrations below to indicate direction of movement in the muscle teams.

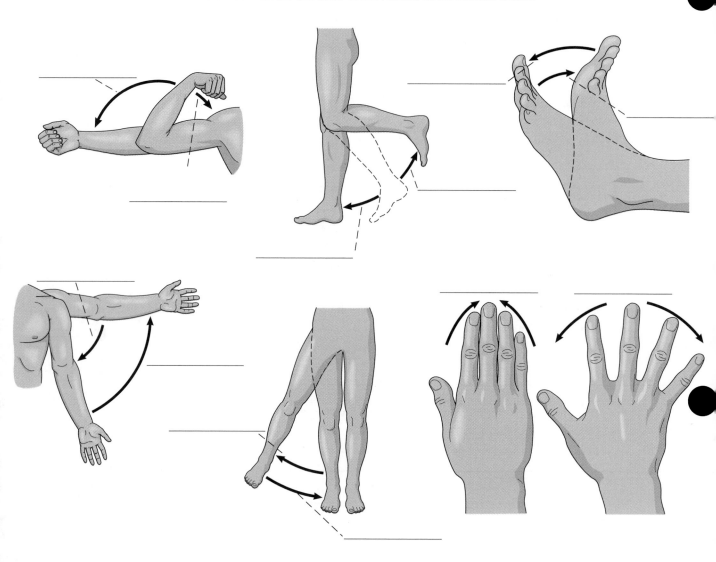

8. Describe the structure and function of a tendon, locating the body's strongest example. _____
_____

9. Explain the meaning of the terms "origin" and "insertion." _____
_____

10. Describe a muscle sheath and bursa; explain their functions. _____
_____

11. Identify the muscles of respiration and explain their action. _____
_____
_____
_____

12. Label the following major anterior body muscles on the illustration.

Biceps Brachi
Deltoid
External Oblique
Intercostals
Masseter
Orbicularis Oculi
Orbicularis Oris

Pectoralis Major
Quadriceps Femoris
Rectus Abdominis
Sartorius
Tibialis Anterior
Vastus Lateralis

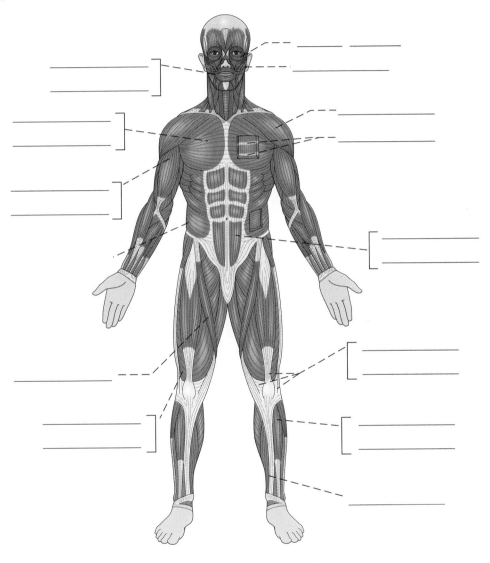

13. Label the following major posterior body muscles on the illustration.

Achilles Tendon
Biceps Femoris
Deltoid
Gastrocnemius
Gluteus Maximus
Gluteus Medius
Hamstring Group

Latissimus Dorsi
Occipitalis
Semi-Membranous
Semi-Tendinosus
Sternocleidomastoid
Trapazius
Triceps Brachii

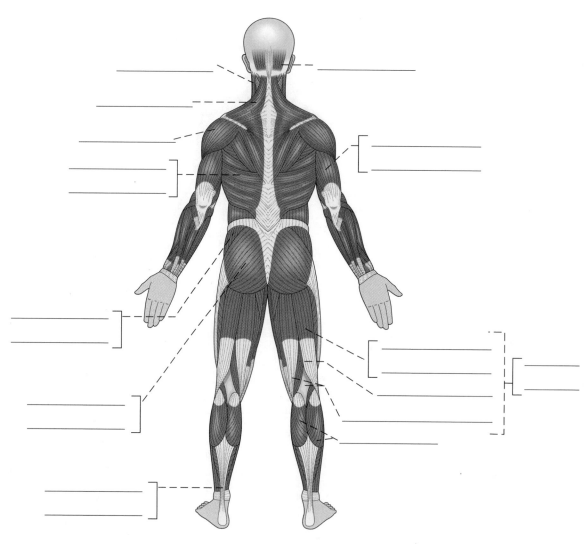

14. Explain peristaltic action. _____
_____
_____

15. Describe the structure and function of a sphincter. _____
_____
_____

16. Describe the following disorders or diseases of the muscular system.
   a. Bursitis _____
   b. Tendonitis _____
   c. Epicondylitis _____
   d. Fibromyalgia syndrome _____
   e. Muscular dystrophy _____
   f. Torticollis _____
   _____

17. Match the term in Column I with its numbered definition in Column II.

COLUMN I   COLUMN II
   _____ a. Abduction   1. Spasmotic contractions of the diaphragm
   _____ b. Adduction   2. Excessive stress on a skeletal muscle
   _____ c. Anchor   3. A donut-shaped muscle
   _____ d. Atrophy   4. A progressive wasting of muscle tissue from lack of use
   _____ e. Contracture   5. A tough membrane sheath attachment
   _____ f. Dystrophy   6. To move an extremity away from the body's center
   _____ g. Fascia   7. The origin of a muscle
   _____ h. Hiccough   8. Permanent shortening of flexor muscles with bent joints
   _____ i. Spasm   9. Congenital progressive skeletal muscle wasting
   _____ j. Strain   10. A state of partial muscle contraction
                                  11. To move an extremity toward the body's center
                                  12. A painful contracted muscle that will not relax

18. Using the Words to Know for this unit, complete the following puzzle.

    _ _ M _ _ _ _ _ _   (muscle group)
    _ _ _ _ _ U _ _ _ _ _   (muscle attachment)
    S Y S T E M   (group of organs)
    _ _ _ C _ _ _ _ _ _ _ _ _ _ _ (combination of two systems)
    _ _ _ _ _ _ _ _ U _   (back muscle)
    _ _ _ _ _ _ _ L _ _ _   (smooth muscle action)
    _ _ _ _ _ A _ _ _ _   (a permanent condition)
    _ _ _ _ _ R _ _ _   (named for occupation)

19. Each line contains four different spellings of a word. Underline the correctly spelled word.
   a. distrophy   dystrophy   distraphy   dystraphy
   b. pecktoralis   pecktorales   pectorales   pectoralis
   c. extensor   extenser   egtenser   egtensor
   d. gastructnemius   gastrocnemius   gastrocnemious   gastructnemious
   e. hiccoff   hiccupp   hiccough   hicough
   f. intercostal   intracostal   intracoastal   intercoastal
   g. spincter   spinctor   sphinctor   sphincter
   h. tortacollis   tortacolis   torticollis   torticolis
   i. fibramyositis   fibromyositis   fibromyasitis   fibermyositis

20. Find the 25 words hidden in the puzzle.

abduct	dystrophy	smooth
adduct	extensor	spasm
anchor	fascia	strain
atrophy	flexor	team
bend	insertion	tendon
bicep	muscle	tone
bursa	origin	tricep
cardiac	relax	
cramp	sheath	

```
C  J  I  A  T  R  O  P  H  Y  F  H
B  A  B  D  U  C  T  R  M  C  A  E
I  P  F  L  E  X  O  R  I  M  S  X
C  N  C  A  R  D  I  A  C  G  C  T
E  T  S  H  E  A  T  H  O  Q  I  E
P  E  M  E  C  V  T  O  N  E  A  N
S  A  O  C  R  A  M  P  I  U  W  S
T  M  O  B  O  T  A  B  I  D  Q  O
R  U  T  K  E  O  I  N  U  L  W  R
A  S  H  Q  X  N  O  O  C  R  W  X
I  C  P  T  E  N  D  O  N  H  S  P
N  L  U  A  D  D  U  C  T  W  O  A
P  E  D  Y  S  T  R  O  P  H  Y  R
R  E  L  A  X  M  T  R  I  C  E  P
```

B. CRITICAL THINKING QUESTIONS: WHAT WOULD YOU SAY - WHAT WOULD YOU DO?

1. A male patient is being treated for tendonitis of the elbow. He calls to complain that for the last two days he has experienced more pain than he did when he first came in for treatment. He has been using heat to the area as he was told. _____

_____

_____

_____

_____

After your instructor has returned your work to you, make all necessary corrections and place in a 3-ring notebook for future reference.

ASSIGNMENT SHEET

Chapter 11
Unit 7: THE RESPIRATORY SYSTEM

A. MIXED QUIZ

1. Where is oxygen produced and how important is it to the human body? _____
_____

2. What occurs to cause a breath to be taken? _____
_____

3. Trace the pathway of oxygen to an internal cell. _____
_____
_____
_____
_____

4. Describe the structure and function of each of the following parts of the respiratory system.

   a. Nose:_____
   _____

   b. Pharynx:_____

   c. Epiglottis:_____
   _____

   d. Larynx:_____
   _____
   _____

   e. Trachea:_____
   _____

   f. Bronchi:_____

   g. Bronchioles:_____
   _____

   h. Alveolus:_____
   _____
   _____

5. How is voice sound produced? _____
_____

6. Explain the difference between external and internal respiration. _____
_____
_____

7. What is surfactant and how does it affect inflation of the lungs? _____
_____
_____
_____

8. What are the six symptoms of hyaline membrane disease?

a. _____

b. _____

c. _____

d. _____

e. _____

f. _____

9. List five instances when a breathing pattern is altered normally.

a. _____

b. _____

c. _____

d. _____

e. _____

10. Describe the pleural coverings of the lungs and explain their purpose. _____

_____

_____

_____

_____

_____

11. Match the disorders or diseases in Column I with their major symptoms (Column II).

COLUMN I

_____ a. Allergic rhinitis
_____ b. Asthma
_____ c. Atelectasis
_____ d. Bronchitis
_____ e. COPD
_____ f. Emphysema
_____ g. Epistaxis
_____ h. Histoplasmosis
_____ i. Hyaline membrane disease
_____ j. Influenza
_____ k. Laryngectomy
_____ l. Legionnaires' disease
_____ m. Paroxysmal nocturnal dyspnea
_____ n. Pleural effusion
_____ o. Pleurisy
_____ p. Pneumoniosis
_____ q. Pneumonia
_____ r. Pneumothorax
_____ s. Pulmonary edema
_____ t. Pulmonary embolism
_____ u. SIDS
_____ v. Tuberculosis
_____ w. URI

COLUMN II

1. A progressive, complex disease with marked dyspnea, productive cough, frequent respiratory infections, barrel chest, respiratory failure
2. A nose bleed
3. Cold-like symptoms at first, progressing to involve liver, spleen and lymph glands. Productive cough, dyspnea, weakness
4. Acute, contagious disease with chills, fever, headache, muscular aches, non-productive cough
5. Sharp, stabbing pain with lung respirations, some dyspnea, usually one-sided
6. Surgical removal of the larynx
7. Fluid collection within lung tissue associated with heart disease; causes dyspnea, orthopnea, frothy bloody sputum
8. Dyspnea, chest pain, rapid heart, productive cough, low-grade fever; caused by blood vessel obstruction
9. Reaction to airborne allergens causing sneezing, profuse watery nasal discharge, and nasal congestion
10. Prolonged apnea in infants, irregular heart rate, severe lack of oxygen
11. Nodular lesions and patchy infiltration of lung tissue causing fatigue, weakness, lack of appetite, weight loss, night sweats
12. An infectious, acute, or chronically developed disease causing wheezing, dyspnea, productive cough
13. Sore throat, nasal congestion, headache, burning, watery eyes, fever, non-productive cough
14. Diarrhea, lack of appetite, headache, chills, fever that persists, weakness, grayish sputum
15. Bronchospasms; an allergic disorder causing wheezing, dyspnea, sputum production
16. Affects infants causing respiratory distress, rapid and shallow breathing, retracted sternum, flared nostrils, grunting
17. Acute infection causing coughing, sputum, chills, fever, pleural chest pain; impairs exchange of oxygen and carbon dioxide
18. Inability to exchange oxygen and carbon dioxide causing chronic cough, pursed lips breathing, cyanosis, weight loss
19. Sudden sharp pain, unequal chest wall expansion, may be chest wound, may be weak rapid pulse, dyspnea, lung collapse
20. Environmental disease causing dyspnea, lack of oxygen, bronchial congestion
21. Dyspnea due to collapse of the alveoli
22. Awaken from sleep with feeling of suffocation
23. Hypoxia due to the presence of excess fluid in the pleural space

12. Label the following illustration of the lungs below.

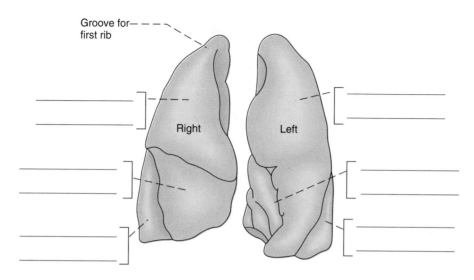

Groove for——first rib

Right   Left

13. Match the diagnostic examinations from Column I with their purpose from Column II.

COLUMN I

_____ a. Bronchoscopy
_____ b. Chest X ray
_____ c. Lung scan
_____ d. Sputum analysis
_____ e. Thoracentesis
_____ f. Arterial blood gases
_____ g. Lung perfusion scan
_____ h. Lung ventilation scan
_____ i. Pulmonary angiography

COLUMN II

1. To evaluate pulmonary emboli
2. To withdraw fluid from the pleural space
3. To determine basic condition of the lungs or identify a disease process
4. To observe the trachea and bronchial tree, obtain a sample, or remove a foreign body
5. To diagnose infectious organisms or cancer cells
6. Aid in diagnosing pulmonary emboli and evaluate pulmonary circulation in certain heart conditions before surgery.
7. To measure the partial pressures of O_2 and CO_2 in the lungs by determining the pH of the blood.
8. To provide a visual image of pulmonary blood flow to diagnose blood vessel obstruction.
9. To determine the distribution pattern of an inhaled gas to identify obstructed airways.

14. Unscramble the following Words to Know.

a. _ _ _ _ _ _ _   ELIVALO
b. _ _ _ _ _ _ _ _   IHISTRIN
c. _ _ _ _ _ _   ALXNYR
d. _ _ _ _ _ _ _ _ _ _   ITEGPLOTSI
e. _ _ _ _ _ _ _ _ _ _   OHRIELBONC
f. _ _ _ _ _ _ _ _ _   MSHEPEYAM
g. _ _ _ _ _ _ _ _   SYNCOASI
h. _ _ _ _ _ _ _   RATAHEC
i. _ _ _ _ _ _ _ _ _   UNOLYPRAM
j. _ _ _ _ _ _ _ _ _   EYPILSUR
k. _ _ _ _ _ _   HAMTAS
l. _ _ _ _ _ _ _   EYPSADN
m. _ _ _ _ _ _ _ _ _ _   PROHNAEOT
n. _ _ _ _ _ _ _ _ _   ENPIMUANO
o. _ _ _ _ _ _ _ _ _ _ _ RIYPSORTARE
p. _ _ _ _ _ _ _ _ _   SUCCHGIHO
q. _ _ _ _ _ _ _   AIPYOHX
r. _ _ _ _ _ _   ENXGOY

B. CRITICAL THINKING SITUATIONS: WHAT WOULD YOU SAY? WHAT WOULD YOU DO?

1. A young mother calls the office crying because her small child is having temper tantrums and is holding his breath. She is afraid he is going to quit breathing and die. _____

_____

_____

_____

2. An elderly patient calls with complaints of high fever, muscle aches, a headache, and chills. He says he feels like he has the "flu" but he had a flu shot about 9 months ago at the end of last year's season. _____

_____

_____

_____

_____

_____

3. A male patient is having a difficult time adjusting to his laryngectomy. He is very depressed because he cannot talk and even his food doesn't seem to taste the same. He is very self conscious about his appearance and does not want anyone to see him. _____

_____

_____

_____

_____

_____

4. A co-worker has just returned from sick leave due to tuberculosis. She appears well and looks much better than when she was diagnosed. She has been on medication for the past 6 weeks. You overhear other co-workers say they are not going to get too close to her and make remarks about her being back to work that are very unkind. _____

_____

_____

After your instructor has returned your work to you, make all necessary corrections and place in a 3-ring notebook for future reference.

ASSIGNMENT SHEET

Chapter 11
Unit 8: THE CIRCULATORY SYSTEM

A. MIXED QUIZ

1. List the four major parts of the circulatory system.

   a. _____

   b. _____

   c. _____

   d. _____

2. Identify the following structures of the heart on the illustration below: apex, right atrium (auricle), left atrium (auricle), right ventricle, left ventricle, aortic arch, right coronary artery and vein, left coronary artery and vein, right pulmonary artery, left pulmonary artery, superior vena cava

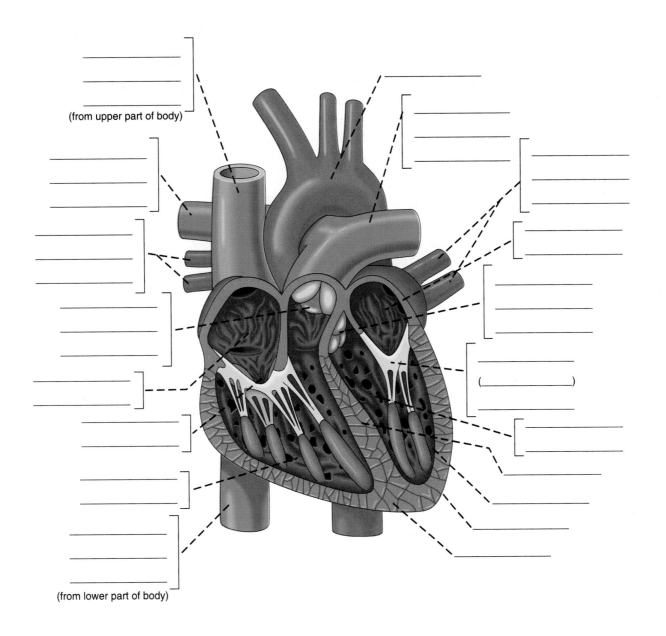

(from upper part of body)

(from lower part of body)

4. What is the difference between pulmonary and systemic circulation? _____
_____
_____

5. Describe the heart sounds and what heart action causes the sound. Identify where the sounds may be auscultated.

Sound	Caused by	Where auscultated
a)		
b)		

6. Describe the location and action of the pacemaker.
_____
_____
_____

7. Explain how the action of the pacemaker is related to the symptoms of heart block and fibrillation. ____
_____
_____
_____
_____

8. What causes arrhythmia? _____
_____

9. Describe the characteristics of bigeminal and trigeminal rhythm. _____
_____

10. What purpose does an artificial pacemaker serve and how does it function? _____
_____
_____

11. Explain how the rate of the heartbeat is controlled. _____
_____
_____
_____

12. List the five types of blood vessels, explaining the structure and purpose of each type.

TYPE	STRUCTURE	FUNCTION
a. _____		
b. _____		
c. _____		
d. _____		
e. _____		

13. How does a capillary bed function? _____
_____
_____

14. Trace the pathway of blood through pulmonary and systemic circulation beginning at the vena cava, going to a capillary of the body and returning to the atrium of the heart. Name the structures of the heart and lungs, and the major vessels. _____
_____
_____
_____
_____

15. From where does the blood in the portal circulation come, where does it go and why? _____
_____
_____

16. Fill in the blanks. (Begin with "Lymph vessels")
The lymphatic system consists of lymph vessels which are located throughout the body. Lymph capillaries _____ and other substances and return them to the circulatory system. The system is a _____ system; there are no vessels bringing _____ to the _____ . The capillaries join to become _____ which in turn become larger vessels called _____ . The lymphatics eventually form two main _____ , a _____ duct and a _____ duct. _____ are located along lymph vessels at various places in the body. During an infection, the nodes become _____ and _____ because of the collection of lymphocytes.

17. List four actions of the spleen.
a. _____
b. _____
c. _____
d. _____

18. Name five things that blood transports through the body.
a. _____
b. _____
c. _____
d. _____
e. _____

19. What is plasma? List 17 things that can be found circulating in plasma. _____
_____

1. _____   7. _____   13. _____
2. _____   8. _____   14. _____
3. _____   9. _____   15. _____
4. _____   10. _____   16. _____
5. _____   11. _____   17. _____
6. _____   12. _____

20. List the three types of blood cells, describing the basic function of each.
a. _____
b. _____
c. _____

21. Why is blood typed and crossmatched before being given to a patient? _____
_____
_____
_____

22. Why is the Rh factor especially important with a pregnancy or a transfusion? _____

_____

_____

_____

_____

23. Each line contains four different spellings of a word. Underline the correctly spelled word.

a. excelerator	axcelerater	accelerator	accelerater
b. aneurysm	aneruism	anurysm	anurism
c. bradicardia	bradycardea	bradecardia	bradycardia
d. endecardium	endocardium	endocardeum	endecardeum
e. erythrocyte	erithrocyte	erythrocite	erithrocite
f. hemaglobin	hemoglobin	hemogloben	hemagloben
g. eschemea	eschemia	ischemea	ischemia
h. murmer	murrmur	murmur	murmmur
i. myocardium	myocardeum	myacardium	myacardeum
j. phelebitis	phlebities	phlebitus	phlebitis
k. tachycardea	tachycardia	tachicardia	tachicardea
l. varecose	varicose	veracose	vericose
m. arrhythmea	arrhythmia	arrhthmia	arrhthmya
n. ischemic	eshcemic	ishemic	ishcemic

24. Match the cardiovascular tests (Column I) with the appropriate purpose for conducting (Column II).

COLUMN I

_____ a. Arteriograph
_____ b. Cardiac catheterization
_____ c. Doppler ultrasonography
_____ d. Echocardiograph
_____ e. Electrocardiograph
_____ f. Holter monitor
_____ g. Venogram
_____ h. Muga Scan

COLUMN II

1. To evaluate cardiac function and structure, and to detect defects by means of sound waves
2. To detect irregularly occurring symptoms or evaluate status of a recovering cardiac patient
3. Detects condition of deep veins of the legs, especially deep vein thrombosis
4. To inject dye to indicate the status of blood flow, malformed vessels, and aneurysm, or hemorrhage
5. To evaluate major blood vessels to determine deep vein thrombosis, peripheral aneurysms, and occluded carotid arteries
6. To identify heart rhythm, electrolyte imbalance, and conduction abnormalities
7. To visualize by fluoroscope the internal heart structure and activity and to visualize the coronary arteries
8. Determine condition of myocardium

25. Identify the major symptom in Column II with the disease or disorder in Column I.

COLUMN I

_____ a. Anemia
_____ b. Aneurysm
_____ c. Angina
_____ d. Arrest
_____ e. Arrhythmia
_____ f. Arteriosclerosis
_____ g. Atherosclerosis
_____ h. Athletic heart syndrome
_____ i. CVA
_____ j. CHF
_____ k. Coronary artery disease
_____ l. Embolus
_____ m. Endocarditis
_____ n. Hypertension
_____ o. Hypotension
_____ p. Leukemia
_____ q. Murmur
_____ r. MI
_____ s. Myocarditis
_____ t. Pericarditis
_____ u. Phlebitis
_____ v. Sickle cell anemia
_____ w. Stasis ulcer
_____ x. Thrombophlebitis
_____ y. Varicosities

COLUMN II

1. Sharp, sudden pain at sternum radiating to back of shoulders and arms; decreases when erect or leaning forward
2. A circulating foreign substance in a blood vessel
3. Irregular heart rhythm
4. Fatty deposits on the lining of blood vessels
5. Severe chest pain from a coronary artery spasm
6. Pounding heartbeats after exercise, enlarged heart, slow pulse
7. Blood pressure consistently above normal
8. Congestion of blood in the circulatory system, edema of extremities and lungs
9. Tightness of chest, substernal chest pain radiating down left arm, nausea and vomiting, perspiration, fainting
10. Lack of red blood cells or hemoglobin
11. Rigid arterial walls; causes hypertension
12. Confusion, weakness of one side, visual changes, paralysis, personality change
13. A bulging arterial wall which produces palpitations or tissue death
14. Complete sudden cessation of heart action
15. Mild chest soreness, fever, dyspnea, palpitations, feeling of pressure
16. Vegetative growths on inner heart structures
17. Abnormally shaped red blood cells, enlarged liver, pallor, painful crisis periods
18. Skin breakdown from inadequate circulation
19. Excessive WBC, bruising, fatigue, painful lymph nodes
20. Inflamed vein lining with thrombus formation, severe pain, fever, chills, and discoloration of involved extremity
21. Dilated, twisted veins, inefficient valves, leg cramps
22. A gurgling or swishing sound heard upon auscultation of the heart
23. Localized inflammation of a vein
24. Severe crushing pain radiating through chest to neck and jaw and down left arm; nausea, dyspnea
25. Consistently low blood pressure

26. Find the 32 words hidden in the puzzle:

adenitis
ambulate
anemia
angina
aorta
arterioles
artery
atrial
atrium
bicuspid
capillary

cardiac
coronary
diastole
exudate
heart
hemoglobin
infarct
ischemia
leukemia
lymph
mitral

murmur
nodes
plasma
spleen
systole
tachycardia
vagus
valve
ventricle
venule

```
A L E U K E M I A V E N U L E
V N H E M O G L O B I N I W V
A D E N I T I S C H E M I A E
G N A M B U L A T E C T G C N
U E R I I A T I N F A R C T T
S X T T C A T C N G D N E S R
S U O R A R O A T R I U M Y I
C D O A R T E R Y D A N X S C
O A T L E E R D T L S R A T L
R T P Q B R V I C A T X R O E
O E S I E I D A A H O P M L P
N L U P L O C C L L A U E A
A O D Y L L R U P V E Y R Y R
R E D A X E A R S C E P M E P
Y L U E D S E R T P O A U P A
P P L A S M A N Y H I R R Y H
R E L T A C H Y C A R D I A P
```

B. CRITICAL THINKING SITUATIONS: WHAT WOULD YOU SAY? WHAT WOULD YOU DO?

1. A female patient calls and is very concerned because she has just noticed a couple of lumps in her left axilla. They are not tender and seem to be shaped like a large bean. _____

_____

_____

2. A male patient who has angina calls to report that he has been experiencing severe chest pains off and on for the past two days. He is perspiring profusely and has had constant pain for the past twenty minutes. He has used four nitroglycerin tablets, but this time they are not working. _____

_____

_____

_____

_____

3. A female patient has been under treatment for two years for hypertension. She has lost 50 pounds and is getting regular exercise and watching her diet. Last time she was in the office, over 3 months ago, her blood pressure had been normal for about six months and she thought she was cured. Today, it is elevated again.

_____
_____
_____
_____
_____

4. You have gone to your spouse's company picnic. About one-half hour after eating several people began playing ball. A man made a hit and ran to first base, but then he grabbed his chest and fell to the ground. He complained of a crushing chest pain that went up to his jaw and down his left arm. He was also nauseated, perspiring, and short of breath. _____

_____
_____
_____
_____

After your instructor has returned your work to you, make all necessary corrections and place in a 3-ring notebook for future reference.

ASSIGNMENT SHEET

Chapter 11
Unit 9: THE IMMUNE SYSTEM

Note: This material is challenging. Concentrate on what you read and write and it will be easier. Keeping your immune system strong is vital to your health and well-being. The more you understand, the better your chances of avoiding severe illness.

A. MIXED QUIZ: FILL IN THE BLANKS IN THE FOLLOWING SENTENCES.

1. All blood cells originate in the _____ and initially develop from _____ .
   Erythrocytes develop from _____ and mature in the bone marrow. Granulated white blood cells develop from _____ stem cells. One type of agranulocyte, the _____ , develops from a _____ stem cell into two major classes, _____ , which mature in the _____ , and _____ , which mature in the _____ . Mononuclear phagocyte stem cells become the _____ which circulate in the blood and then enter the tissues to become _____ . Phagocytes are cells that _____ and _____ . Neutrophils carry _____ with _____ to destroy microorganisms. Eosinophils and basophils release _____ onto _____ or _____ in their environment.

2. Name the organs of the immune system.
   a. _____   f. _____
   b. _____   g. _____
   c. _____   h. _____
   d. _____   i. _____
   e. _____   j. _____

3. Answer each of the following questions:
   a. To what family do antibodies belong? _____
   b. How many classes of immunoglobins are there? _____
   c. What do B cells become after joining with an antigen? _____
   d. What do B cells produce after undergoing antigen-antibody complex? _____
   e. Into what do clone cells develop? _____

4. Answer using very brief responses.
   a. When antibodies change their shape, what may be exposed? _____
   b. What is complement? _____
   c. What does complement cascade create? _____
   d. What is the action caused by the combination of antibodies and complement system called? _____

   _____
   This type of immunity is the resistance to disease produced by _____ .

5. Fill in the blanks.
   The process of antibody-mediated response and other chemicals also cause an _____ .
   Basophils and mast cells release _____ which _____ and makes them more _____ . This _____ blood flow and allows _____ to seep into the surrounding tissues. This results in _____ , _____ , and _____ .

6. T cells act directly with their targets in action called _____ or _____ . T cells function in two ways; one type, the Helper T, also called by its marker _____ , activates _____ , ____ , _____ , and _____ . Suppressor cells are a subset of _____ . Killer T cells, also called _____ , act directly on _____ or _____ cells, and any other cell that has a _____ _____ and an _____ marker.

7. Natural killer cells (NK) are deadly _____ that contain _____ filled with _____ . They are called natural because they do not need to recognize a specific antigen like other T cells to kill the invading antigen. In AIDS, this cell activity is _____ . NK cells _____ to their targets and deliver a _____ of _____ to produce _____ in a cell's membrane which _____ the cell.

8. There are two branches of immune response, _____ , which results from B cell activity and _____ which results from _____ activity. Response can also be _____ , which means the _____ encounter or _____ with _____ encounters. A primary response requires _____ to ____ days to develop. Antibody-mediated responses act against _____ and _____ , _____ , and _____ . It cannot react to microorganisms already with a cell's _____ . Only those in _____ or _____ to a cell's _____ . Secondary response requires _____ or _____ days because of the _____ with memory. T cell primary response is _____ which attacks _____ , _____ , and _____ , _____ and _____

9. Why do killer cells cause rejection of an organ transplant? _____
_____

10. What stops an immune response? _____

11. List the four things that affect the status of the immune system.

   a. _____   c. _____
   b. _____   d. _____

12. List twelve elements and personal characteristics which influence the components of the immune system.

   a. _____   g. _____
   b. _____   h. _____
   c. _____   i. _____
   d. _____   j. _____
   e. _____   k. _____
   f. _____   l. _____

13. a. How do immunizations and vaccines provide protection against antigens? _____
_____

   b. Active immunity means _____
   c. Passive immunity means _____

14. Name the body fluids in which the AIDS virus survives the best.
   a. _____
   b. _____
   c. _____

15. How long after infection will it be before antibodies to the HIV proteins can be detected in the blood? _____
_____

16. Where does the virus go? _____

17. List the symptoms of HIV symptomatic infection.

   a. _____   f. _____
   b. _____   g. _____
   c. _____   h. _____
   d. _____   i. _____
   e. _____

18. Name the three opportunitistic diseases which AIDS patients may develop and other usual diseases and disorders which often occur.

1. _____   _____
2. _____   _____
3. _____   _____

   _____   _____
   _____   _____
   _____   _____
   _____

19. Beginning in 1993, the United States Department of Health and Human Services established new criteria for diagnosing AIDS. Name the 3 CD4 T lymphocyte categories and their respective cell counts.

1. _____
2. _____
3. _____

20. Name the clinical categories which describe symptoms. _____

21. Using the classification system in Table 11-6 in the textbook, identify the letter and number for the following combinations of symptoms.

   a. T cell count of 200-499 μL and Category C conditions _____
   b. T cell count of <200 μL and Category A conditions _____
   c. T cell count of ≥500 μL and Category B conditions _____

22. Name the diagnostic tests which verify the presence of HIV antibodies.

   a. _____
   b. _____
   c. _____

23. What are the two main ways to acquire AIDS?

   a. _____
   b. _____

24. List other ways to transmit the AIDS virus.

   a. _____   f. _____
   b. _____   g. _____
   c. _____   h. _____
   d. _____   i. _____
   e. _____   j. _____

25. Name four high-risk behaviors.

   a. _____   c. _____
   b. _____   d. _____

26. What can trigger allergic symptoms?

   a. _____   f. _____
   b. _____   g. _____
   c. _____   h. _____
   d. _____   i. _____
   e. _____   j. _____

27. What occurs when a person experiences anaphylactic shock? _____

_____

28. What kind of events might cause cancer cells to develop from mutation?

a. _____   d. _____

b. _____   e. _____

c. _____   f. _____

29. Differentiate between carcinogen and carcinogenesis. _____

_____

30. List some known carcinogens.

a. _____   e. _____

b. _____   f. _____

c. _____   g. _____

d. _____

31. Cancer cells are classified according to their origin. Tumors from epithelial tissues are known as _____ ; those from connective, muscle or bone tissue are called _____ . Cancer cells are also called _____ cells.

32. List the diagnostic procedures used to detect cancer.

a. _____   f. _____

b. _____   g. _____

c. _____   h. _____

d. _____   i. _____

e. _____

33. What are oncogenes? _____

34. What do oncogenes do? _____

35. Name the three major therapies used to treat cancer.

a. _____

b. _____

c. _____

36. Listed below are symptoms of (1) AIDS; (2) allergies; (3) cancer; (4) CFS; (5) Lupus; and (6) rheumatoid arthritis. Put the correct disease number on the line in front of the symptoms.

a. ___ sneezing, runny nose, congestion, difficult breathing

b. ___ nagging cough or hoarseness, change in wart or mole

c. ___ HIV virus antibodies are present

d. ___ persistent flush of cheeks, disc-like lesions on face, neck and scalp

e. ___ decrease in eosinophils, focal atelectasis, positive skin tests

f. ___ sore that will not heal, lump or thickened area, unusual bleeding, change in bowel or bladder habits

g. ___ loss of weight, chills and fever, night sweats, diarrhea, fatigue, persistent dry cough

h. ___ low grade fever, unexplained muscle weakness or pain, sleep disturbances

i. ___ stiff, painful joints, joint deformity, eventual joint destruction

j. ___ sore throat, swollen glands, headaches, depression, inability to concentrate

k. ___ red scaly rash, skin and joint involvement, period of remission

l. ___ tender, painful, hot, enlarged joints

37. Fill in the spaces from the Words to Know.

           _ _ _ **I** _ _ _ _   (belongs to immunoglobulin family)

_ _ _ _ _ _ **M** _ _ _   (starts a chain reaction)

    _ _ **M** _ _ _ _   (type of immunity)

      _ _ _ **U** _   (organism)

       _ **N** _ _ _ _ _   (foreign matter)

       _ **E** _ _ _ _   (harmless)

_ _ _ _ - _ _ _ _ _ _ _   (T-Cell activated)

    _ _ _ _ **S** _ _   (small sample)

      _ _ **Y** _ _ _   (an organ)

_ _ _ _ _ _ **S** _ _ _   (cancer cell)

     _ _ **T** _ _ _ _ _ _   (secondary growth)

     _ **E** _ _ _ _ _ _ _   (controlled)

   _ _ _ **M** _ _ _ _ _ _ _ _   (a drug treatment)

38. Match the words to know with the definitions.

COLUMN I

_____ a) allergens
_____ b) anaphylaxis
_____ c) antibody
_____ d) antigen
_____ e) autoimmune
_____ f) benign
_____ g) clone
_____ h) complement
_____ i) cytotoxic
_____ j) histamine
_____ k) hyperthermia
_____ m) interferon
_____ n) mutation
_____ o) oncogenes
_____ p) neoadjuvant chemotherapy
_____ q) permeable
_____ r) phagocytes
_____ s) Raynauds phenomenon
_____ t) retrovirus
_____ u) syndrome
_____ v) vaccine

COLUMN II

1. A substance released by basophils and mast cells
2. engulf and destroy antigens
3. A family of proteins that fight viruses and activate macrophages
4. The use of heat to raise body temperature
5. a group of symptoms or signs occurring at the same time in a particular disease or disorder
6. a cancer treatment given before surgery
7. protein substances belonging to the immunoglobulin family which neutralize antigens and destroy cells
8. a symptom of white or blue fingers when subjected to the cold
9. treated microorganisms given to induce immunity
10. particles in the air or foods we eat that cause reactions
11. more easily passed through, as is fluid leaving a blood vessel
12. a nonmalignant growth
13. an organism with RNA genetic material
14. a foreign material
15. a severe allergic reaction leading to circulatory collapse and death
16. a duplicate of the original
17. a group of 25 inactive enzyme proteins present in the blood
18. genes which transform normal into cancer cells
19. killer cells capable of destroying cells
20. antibodies which react against a person's own normal tissue
21. the changing of the genetic material within a cell

B. CRITICAL THINKING SITUATIONS: WHAT WOULD YOU DO? WHAT WOULD YOU SAY?

1. You notice one of your co-workers looks and acts very tired. Recently she has lost about 15 pounds and has had a cold. She has a little congestion in her chest which is making her short of breath and causing her to cough. When you talk to her about it she breaks down and cries telling you she is HIV positive and is having a hard time dealing with it. She doesn't want you to tell anyone, especially the doctor, because she has to work to take care of herself and her child. She's afraid she will lose her job. _____

   _____

   _____

   _____

   _____

   _____

2. A neighbor has just been diagnosed as having lung cancer. He says he is not going to go through chemotherapy or radiation because he will just end up dying anyhow. He believes these treatments just make you feel worse while you are waiting for the inevitable. Instead he is going to take the advice of a friend and send away for a cancer cure that's available in Mexico. _____

   _____

   _____

   _____

   _____

   _____

3. A patient in her late 20s has just been told she has systemic lupus erythematosus. She has heard the disease is life-threatening and she is frightened. _____

   _____

   _____

   _____

After your instructor has returned your work to you, make all necessary corrections and place in a 3-ring notebook for future reference.

ASSIGNMENT SHEET

Chapter 11
Unit 10: THE DIGESTIVE SYSTEM

A. MIXED QUIZ

1. Define digestion. _____

_____

2. List the raw materials the body requires to promote good health.
   a. _____   e. _____
   b. _____   f. _____
   c. _____   g. _____
   d. _____

3. List, in order, the organs of the alimentary tract through which food passes.
   a. _____   d. _____
   b. _____   e. _____
   c. _____   f. _____

4. Identify the organs of digestion on the following illustration.

Ascending colon

Cecum

Descending colon

Esophagus

Gallbladder

Liver

Pancreas

Pharynx

Rectum

Sigmoid colon

Small intestine

Stomach

Teeth

Tongue

Transverse colon

Vermiform appendix

Oral cavity — — —

Lips (cheil/o) — — —

_____

_____

Sublingual gland —

Diaphragm (phren/o) —

_____

Cystic duct — — —

_____

_____

_____

of large intestine

Ileum of

_____   _____

_____

_____

Parotid gland

_____

Submandibular gland

_____

_____

Hepatic duct

Pylorus of the stomach

_____

_____ of large intestine

Jejunum of small intestine (jejun/o)

_____ ___ of large intestine

_____ ___ of large intestine

5. List the accessory digestive organs of the mouth; explain their function in the digestive process.

a. _____

b. _____
   _____
   _____

c. _____
   _____
   _____
   _____

6. a. What are the initial teeth called? _____

   b. When do they appear? _____

   c. Initial teeth are lost beginning about age _____ and are replaced by _____

   d. Identify the four types of "secondary" teeth and their specific duties.

      a) _____

      b) _____

      c) _____

      d) _____

7. How is swallowing accomplished? _____

_____

_____

_____

8. Label the process of swallowing on the illustration.

Air Sinus
Epiglottis
Food
Hard Palate
Jawbone
Larynx
Pharynx
Soft Palate
Tongue
Trachae

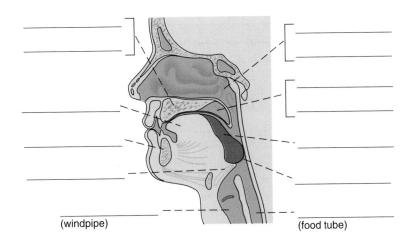

(windpipe)   (food tube)

9. How is food moved through the esophagus? _____
_____

10. Describe the structure of the stomach and explain its function. _____
_____
_____
_____
_____
_____
_____
_____

11. Describe the structure of the small intestine, naming its sections and explaining its function. ____
_____
_____
_____
_____

12. What functions does the liver perform, including the relationship with the portal circulation?
   a. _____
   b. _____
   c. _____
   d. _____
   e. _____
   f. _____
   g. _____
   h. _____
   i. _____
   _____

13. What role does the gallbladder play and how is it related to the liver? _____
_____
_____
_____

14. Label the following illustration.
    Common bile duct
    Cystic duct
    Duodenum
    Gallbladder
    Hepatic duct
    Liver
    Pancreas

15. Explain why the duodenum is vital to digestion. _____
    _____
    _____

16. Describe the location and function of the pancreas. _____
    _____
    _____
    _____

17. Where in the body are nutrients absorbed, and how is it accomplished? _____
    _____
    _____
    _____
    _____

18. Explain the function of the colon and name its five sections.
    The colon absorbs excess liquid from the chyme and eliminates the leftover waste products.
    a. _____   d. _____
    b. _____   e. _____
    c. _____

19. What function does the rectum perform? _____
    _____

20. Describe the structure and function of the anal canal. _____
    _____
    _____

21. Label the illustration below.

Anal Canal

Anus

Ascending Colon

Cecum

Descending Colon

External Anal Sphincter Muscle

Hepatic Flexor

Ileocecal Valve

Ileum

Internal Anal Sphincter Muscle

Rectum

Sigmoid Colon

Splenic Flexure

Tranverse colon

Vermiform Appendix

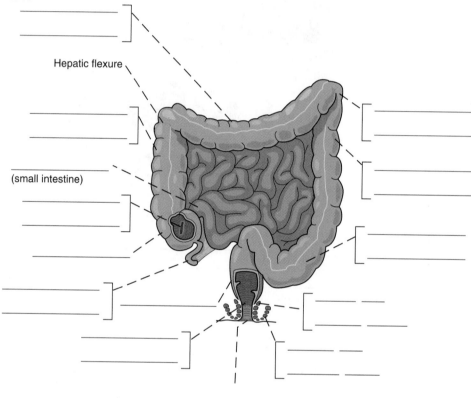

Hepatic flexure

(small intestine)

22. Multiple Choice: Each letter indicates a type of test that is performed. The numbers that follow show potential results of the test. Circle the correct number.

a. Cholecystography

1. properly functioning gallbladder

2. non-functioning gallbladder

3. cholelithiasis

4. bile duct obstruction

5. 2, 3, and 4

6. all of these

b. Barium swallow

1. condition and function of esophagus

2. esophageal varices

3. diverticulitis

4. esophageal stricture

5. duodenal ulcer

6. 1, 2, and 4

c. Upper GI series

1. gastric ulcer

2. tumor of stomach

3. diverticulitis

4. duodenal ulcer

5. polyp of the colon

6. ulcerative colitis

7. all but 5 and 6

8. all of these

d. Lower GI series

   1. tumors of colon
   2. polyps
   3. ulcerative areas
   4. diverticula
   5. duodenal ulcer
   6. gastric ulcer
   7. hemorrhoids
   8. 1, 2, 3, and 6
   9. 1, 2, 3 and 4
   10. 5, 6, and 7

e. Gastroscopy

   1. view growth for biopsy
   2. remove foreign objects
   3. obtain cells for study
   4. photograph sites
   5. chemical damage determination
   6. 1, 2, and 5
   7. 2, 3, and 4
   8. all of these

f. Nuclear and ultrasonography studies

   1. screen for disease processes
   2. locate infarcts
   3. locate cysts, tumors
   4. outlines organ shape
   5. detects functioning liver
   6. 2, 3, and 4
   7. all of these

g. Occult blood test

   1. detects mucus in feces
   2. detects blood in feces
   3. determines location bleeding
   4. determines enzymes in stool
   5. 1, 3, and 4
   6. 2
   7. 2, 3, and 4
   8. all of these

h. Proctoscopy

   1. hemorrhoids
   2. colitis
   3. polyps of the sigmoid
   4. fistulas
   5. rectal abscess
   6. 1, 2, and 4
   7. 1, 4, and 5
   8. 2, 3, and 5

i. Sigmoidoscopy

   1. inflammation and infection
   2. ulcerations
   3. tumors
   4. polyps
   5. duodenal ulcers
   6. condition of ileocecal valve
   7. 2, 4, and 5
   8. 3, 5, and 6
   9. 1, 2, 3, and 4

23. Match the following diseases or conditions, (Column I) with the appropriate symptoms or description (Column II).

COLUMN I

_____ a. Anorectal abscess or fistula
_____ b. Cirrhosis
_____ c. Colitis
_____ d. Colostomy
_____ e. Diarrhea
_____ f. Diverticulitis
_____ g. Esophageal varices
_____ h. Anal fissure
_____ i. Gastroenteritis
_____ j. Hemorrhoids
_____ k. Hepatitis
_____ l. Hiatal hernia
_____ m. Inguinal hernia
_____ n. Ileostomy
_____ o. Pancreatitis
_____ p. Paralytic ileus
_____ q. Peptic ulcer
_____ r. Polyp
_____ s. Pruritus ani
_____ t. Pyloric stenosis
_____ u. Spastic colon
_____ v. Ulcerative colitis

COLUMN II

1. Frequent liquid stools
2. Enlarged spleen, ascites, bloody emesis and stools, reduced platelets
3. Dilated anal veins, painful defecation, bleeding
4. Protruding mass at inguinal area or loop of intestine in scrotum
5. Tenderness and discomfort of the colon
6. Jaundice, hepatomegaly, loss of appetite, fatigue, clay-colored stools, weight loss
7. Absence of peristalsis, abdominal distention, distress, vomiting
8. Severe epigastric pain, not relieved by vomiting; a rigid abdomen, rales, tachycardia, fever, cold perspiring extremities
9. Asymptomatic growths protruding from the intestinal lining
10. Painful, throbbing lump near the anus, with or without drainage
11. Fever, nausea and vomiting, abdominal cramps, travelers' diarrhea
12. Forceful vomiting, dilation of stomach, emptying difficulty contents of stomach into duodenum
13. Recurrent bloody diarrhea with mucus and exudate, weight loss, weakness, anorexia, nausea, vomiting, abdominal pain
14. Itching of anal area, especially following bowel movement, reddened and skin, weeping and thickened skin, darkening of tissue
15. Lack of appetite, indigestion, nausea, vomiting, nosebleeds, bleeding gums, enlarged firm liver, jaundice, ascites
16. Alternating periods of constipation and diarrhea, lower abdominal pain, daytime diarrhea, mucus stools
17. A single or double opening on abdomen through which solid fecal material passes
18. Heartburn, epigastric pain relieved by food, a weight gain, bubbling hot water sensation
19. Opening of small intestine into the abdomen through which liquid stool is expelled
20. Bulging pouches in the intestine which cause abdominal pain, nausea, flatus, irregular bowel movements, high white blood cell count
21. Burning rectal pain with a few drops of blood with passing of stool, sentinal pile
22. Heartburn, regurgitation, vomiting, fullness, stomach spasms, difficult swallowing, gastric reflux

24. Unscramble the following Words to Know.

a. _ _ _ _ _ _ _ _   EDPAXINP
b. _ _ _ _ _ _ _ _ _   HSIORCISR
c. _ _ _ _ _ _ _   ICOTSIL
d. _ _ _ _ _ _ _ _   EHARIDRA
e. _ _ _ _ _ _ _ _ _   EIGISOTND
f. _ _ _ _ _ _ _ _   UNDMEUOD
g. _ _ _ _ _ _ _ _ _   HSUOGSAEP
h. _ _ _ _ _ _ _ _ _ _ _   DLBALRAGLDE
i. _ _ _ _ _ _ _ _ _   SETIHATIP
j. _ _ _ _ _ _ _ _ _   EILCOELAC
k. _ _ _ _ _ _ _   UISNNIL
l. _ _ _ _ _ _ _ _   UCJADNIE
m. _ _ _ _ _ _   UANSAE
n. _ _ _ _ _ _ _ _   ARNPAESC
o. _ _ _ _ _ _ _   IDSMGIO
p. _ _ _ _ _ _ _ _   ESOSNTSI
q. _ _ _ _ _ _ _   HCTASMO
r. _ _ _ _ _ _   UOEGTN
s. _ _ _ _ _ _ _   SVIERAC

B. CRITICAL THINKING SITUATIONS: WHAT WOULD YOU DO? WHAT WOULD YOU SAY?

1. Joe is a weight lifter. He has been trying to increase his dead lift amount before the national competition. He has developed a tender area in his right groin which seems to protrude at times. _____

_____

2. Nancy has not felt well the past two days. She had a generalized pain in her abdomen that got increasingly more uncomfortable and seemed to localize in the lower right quadrant. She was nauseated and didn't feel like eating. However, overnight the pain went away and she is feeling better. A friend suggested it was probably just PMS. _____

_____

3. A male patient called to schedule an appointment. He is complaining about what he thinks is an ulcer. Almost every time he eats he gets a feeling of fullness and chest pain. He usually has heartburn and sometimes brings food up into his throat which causes a burning sensation. You cannot schedule him for two weeks because the doctor is out of town. _____

_____

_____

_____

After your instructor has returned your work to you, make all necessary corrections and place in a 3-ring notebook for future reference.

ASSIGNMENT SHEET

Chapter 11
Unit 11: THE URINARY SYSTEM

A. MIXED QUIZ

1. List the three main functions performed by the urinary system, explaining the meaning of each function.
   a. _____
   b. _____
   c. _____

2. Identify the organs of the urinary system; describe their physical characteristics.
   a. _____
   _____
   b. _____
   _____
   _____
   c. _____
   _____
   d. _____
   _____
   _____

3. Label the following illustration.

   Aorta
   Inferior vena cava
   Hilum
   Left kidney
   Left ureter
   Right kidney
   Urethra
   Urinary bladder

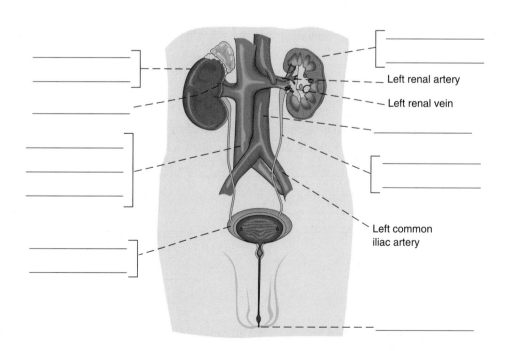

Left renal artery

Left renal vein

Left common iliac artery

4. How does the urinary system work with the other body systems to accomplish its job? _____

_____

_____

_____

_____

_____

5. How is the interior of the kidney constructed? _____

_____

_____

6. Label the following illustration.

Cortex

Hilum

Medulla

Renal artery

Renal papilla

Renal pelvis

Renal pyramid

Ureter

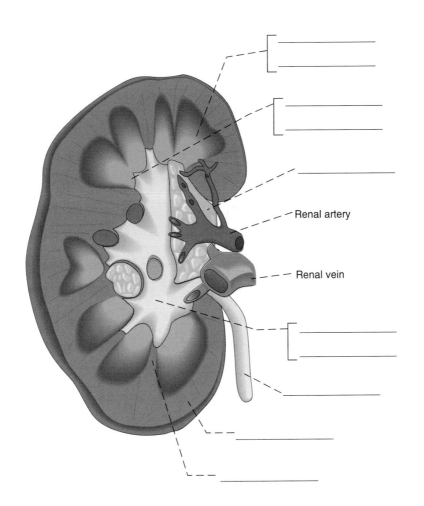

Renal artery

Renal vein

7. List the parts of the nephron and describe the function of each part.
   a. _____
   b. _____
      _____
   c. _____
      _____
   d. _____
      _____

8. Label the following illustration.
   Afferent arteriole
   Ascending limb-loop of Henle
   Bowman's capsule
   Collecting tubule
   Descending limb-loop of Henle
   Distal convoluted tubule
   Efferent arteriole
   Glomerulus
   Peritubular capillaries
   Proximal convoluted tubule

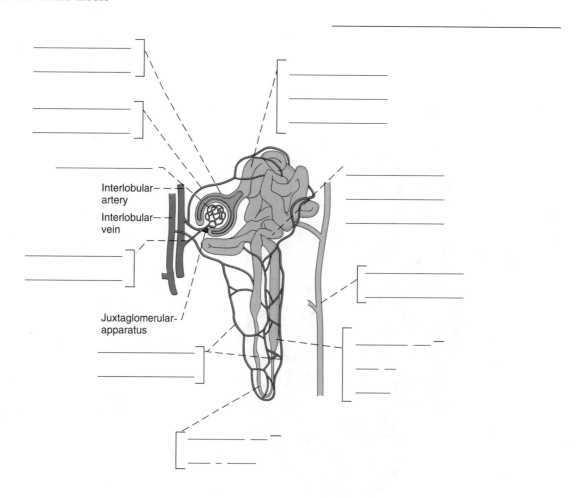

Interlobular artery

Interlobular vein

Juxtaglomerular apparatus

9. Describe kidney dialysis and identify two major types or methods. _____

_____

_____

_____

_____

_____

_____

_____

10. What are the two main categories of diagnostic examinations? Give one example of each type and explain how it is performed, and for what reason. _____

_____

_____

_____

11. List the symptoms of renal calculi.
   a. _____
   b. _____
   c. _____
   d. _____
   e. _____
   f. _____
   g. _____

12. Match the following diseases and disorders (Column I) to the appropriate symptom (Column II).

COLUMN I

___ a. Cystitis
___ b. Glomerulonephritis
___ c. Nephrotic syndrome
___ d. Polycystic kidney disease
___ e. Pyelonephritis
___ f. Renal failure
___ g. Stricture
___ h. Calculi
___ i Uremia

COLUMN II

1. Urgency, dysuria, nocturia, hematuria, ammoniac or fishy odor to urine, high fever, chills, flank pain, fatigue
2. Small stream of urine, prolonged urination time
3. Oliguria, azotemia, severe electrolyte imbalance, acidosis, uremia, other body system involvement
4. Frequency, dysuria, bladder spasms, sharp stabbing pain upon urination
5. Severe pain beginning in kidney, moving to groin area, nausea, vomiting, chills, and fever
6. Generalized dependent edema, pleural effusion, ascites, lethargy, fatigue, pallow, swollen external sexual organs
7. Urine products in the blood, coma, toxic waste levels in blood, eventual death
8. Moderate edema, proteinuria, hematuria, oliguria, fatigue, urinary casts, hypertension
9. Pointed nose, small chin, floppy low set ears, inner eyelid folds, eventually widened body, swollen tender abdomen, life-threatening bleeding, ureteral spasms

13. Unscramble the following words from the Words to Know.

a. _ _ _ _ _ _ _ _   ORATNICU

b. _ _ _ _ _ _ _   DELBRAD

c. _ _ _ _ _ _ _ _   LRAGOIUI

d. _ _ _ _ _ _ _   EYACSLC

e. _ _ _ _ _ _ _ _   YAUPILOR

f. _ _ _ _ _ _ _ _   ISYTICTS

g. _ _ _ _ _ _ _ _   AYISLSDI

h. _ _ _ _ _ _ _   RIYSADU

i. _ _ _ _ _ _ _ _ _   NERTNOITE

j. _ _ _ _ _ _ _ _ _   ENRETSOIC

k. _ _ _ _ _ _ _ _ _   RTEISRTUC

l. _ _ _ _ _ _ _   HUATRER

m. _ _ _ _ _ _ _   ONHEPNR

n. _ _ _ _ _ _ _   UILALCC

o. _ _ _ _ _ _ _ _ _ _ _   IOYPITLHRST

14. Complete the following puzzle.

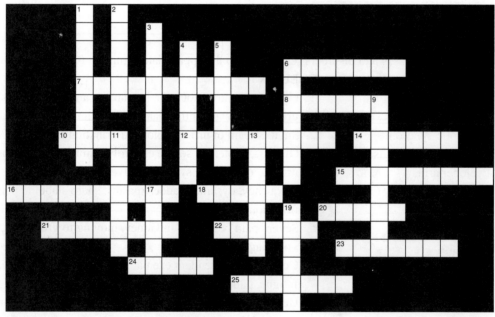

DOWN

1. To separate waste from the blood
2. Absence of urine
3. Urine left after voiding
4. Artificially clean the blood
5. System in this unit
6. Contains glomerulus
9. A narrowing
11. Painful urination
13. Calyx (pl)
17. Waste product of the kidneys
19. The organ that removes wastes from the blood

ACROSS

6. Kidney stones
7. The act of passing urine
8. To droop
10. To urinate
12. A narrowing
14. Tube from kidney
15. To produce from the blood
16. Renal capillary
18. Greek word for cup
20. Notched area of kidney
21. Bladder inflammation
22. Urine products in the blood

23. Drains urine from the bladder
24. Pertaining to the kidney
25. Sudden urge to void

15. Fill in the blanks from the list of Words to Know.

_ _ U _ _ _	(absence of urine)
_ _ _ R _ _ _ _ _	(separate and remove)
_ I _ _ _ _	(retroperitoneal organ)
_ _ _ _ _ N _ _ _ _ _	(expel from body)
_ _ _ A _ _ _ _ _	(presence of blood)
_ _ _ _ _ R _ _ _ _	(cluster of capillaries)
<u>S</u> Y <u>S</u> <u>T</u> <u>E</u> <u>M</u>	(group of organs)

16. Name the three types of incontinence

    a. _____

    b. _____

    c. _____

17. Nine treatments to improve the control of urine are mentioned in the textbook. List them.

    a. _____

    b. _____

    c. _____

    d. _____

    e. _____

    f. _____

    g. _____

    h. _____

    i. _____

B. CRITICAL THINKING SITUATIONS: WHAT WOULD YOU DO? WHAT WOULD YOU SAY?

1. A female patient who had a cystoscopic examination last week called saying that for the last couple of days, everytime she urinates it is very painful. She is having to pass urine very frequently and it looks like there is a little blood in it now. She wonders if this is normal. _____

_____

_____

_____

2. A male patient is complaining of periods of severe pain in his lower abdomen. He is nauseated and has vomited a couple of times. He also has a fever. He believes he has the flu and is requesting the doctor to phone in a prescription. When questioned he revealed he wasn't passing much urine, but he didn't think that was unusual since he is not taking in much fluid. _____

_____

_____

After your instructor has returned your work to you, make all necessary corrections and place in a 3-ring notebook for future reference.

ASSIGNMENT SHEET

Chapter 11
Unit 12: THE ENDOCRINE SYSTEM

A. MIXED QUIZ

1. Explain the difference between an exocrine and an endocrine gland, giving an example of each. _____

_____

_____

_____

2. What types of body functions are affected by hormones?

   a. _____   d. _____

   b. _____   e. _____

   c. _____   f. _____

3. List the nine glands discussed in the unit, identifying the location of each gland.

   a. _____

   b. _____

   c. _____

   d. _____

   e. _____

   f. _____

   g. _____

   h. _____

   i. _____

4. Identify the endocrine glands on the following illustration.

Posterior view

Cortex
Medulla

(Islets of Langerhans)

5. Complete the following chart.

GLAND	LOCATION	HORMONES SECRETED
Pituitary-anterior lobe		
-posterior lobe		
Thyroid		
Parathyroid		
Adrenal-medulla		
cortex		
Pancreas		
Thymus		
Pineal body		
Ovaries		
Testes		

6. Identify the hormones secreted by the gonads and the functions of each. _____
   _____
   _____
   _____

7. Explain what hormone secretion abnormality causes the following conditions.
   a. Giantism/Gigantism _____
   b. Dwarfism _____
   c. Acromegaly _____
   d. Goiter _____
   e. Tetany _____
   f. Diabetes _____
   g. Cretinism _____
   h. Cushing's syndrome _____
   i. Myxedema _____

8. How are hormones interrelated? _____
   _____
   _____
   _____

9. What diagnostic examinations are used to confirm the following conditions
   a. Diabetes _____
   b. Thyroid dysfunction _____
   c. Pregnancy _____
   d. Cushing's syndrome _____

10. List the symptoms, characteristics, and usual course of action taken in the following condition or diseases.
   a. Cretinism _____

   b. Cushing's Syndrome _____
   _____

   c. Diabetes mellitus _____

   d. Myxedema _____
   _____

11. What role does insulin play in the blood?
   a. _____
   b. _____

12. What factors contribute to the development of diabetes?
   a. _____
   b. _____
   c. _____
   d. _____
   e. _____

13. Define the following Words to Know using the glossary.
   a. adrenaline _____
   _____

   b. diabetes mellitus _____
   c. estrogen _____
   d. gonad _____
   e. hormone _____
   f. hypoglycemia _____
   g. ovary _____
   _____

   h. progesterone _____
   i. testes _____
   j. testosterone _____
   _____

14. Find the 21 words hidden in the puzzle.

acromegaly
adrenal
adrenaline
aldosterone
cretinism
dwarfism
endocrine

estrogen
exocrine
giantism
gland
goiter
gonad
hormone

ovary
pineal
pituitary
puberty
testes
tetany
thymus

```
R  I  O  G  O  N  A  D  A  W  T  D  C
A  C  R  O  M  E  G  A  L  Y  U  E  P
V  D  I  I  W  E  S  D  D  L  T  I  U
M  N  R  T  E  S  T  R  O  G  E  N  B
C  T  W  E  Q  Z  C  E  S  V  T  H  E
E  R  E  R  N  I  O  N  T  P  A  O  R
N  G  E  S  T  A  L  A  E  I  N  R  T
D  L  I  T  T  E  L  L  R  T  Y  M  Y
O  A  E  A  I  E  C  I  O  U  P  O  T
C  N  E  R  N  N  S  N  N  I  I  N  H
R  D  O  W  Q  T  I  E  E  T  N  E  Y
I  D  W  A  R  F  I  S  M  A  E  I  M
N  K  L  V  C  O  P  S  M  R  A  E  U
E  X  O  C  R  I  N  E  M  Y  L  W  S
```

B. CRITICAL THINKING SITUATIONS: WHAT WOULD YOU DO? WHAT WOULD YOU SAY?

1. A patient who is under care for diabetes calls to get something for the infection in her big toe. She had had an ingrown toenail that she cut out and it has gotten red and swollen. _____

   _____

   _____

   _____

2. An individual who is new in town calls to make an appointment. His chief complaints: he has no energy and he is always thirsty, which of course makes him drink more and have to urinate more frequently. He says he doesn't think it's anything serious, probably just an enlarged prostate gland, so he can wait a couple of weeks to get in. _____

   _____

   _____

After your instructor has returned your work to you, make all necessary corrections and place in a 3-ring notebook for future reference.

ASSIGNMENT SHEET

Chapter 11
Unit 13: THE REPRODUCTIVE SYSTEM

A. MIXED QUIZ

1. What is the difference between asexual and sexual reproduction? _____
_____

2. Explain the process of differentiation of the reproductive organs; compare the male to female organs.
_____
_____
_____
_____
_____
_____

3. Describe the fertilization of an ovum. _____
_____
_____
_____
_____

4. Fill in the blanks.
A male infant develops if the zygote contains a _____ chromosome. At about the 7th or 8th
week, the _____ begin to develop within the _____ . During the 8th or 9th month
the _____ move from the _____ through the _____ into the
_____

5. List the nine male sex organs or structures, describing their location and function.
a. _____
b. _____
c. _____
d. _____
_____
e. _____
f. _____
_____
g. _____
_____
h. _____
i. _____

6. Identify the structures on the following illustration.

Anal opening
Bulbourethral gland or Cowper's gland
Ejaculatory duct
Epididymis
Penis
Prepuce
Prostate gland
Rectum

Scrotum
Seminal vesicle
Spermatic cord
Symphysis pubis
Testis
Vas deferens (2 times)
Urethra
Urinary bladder

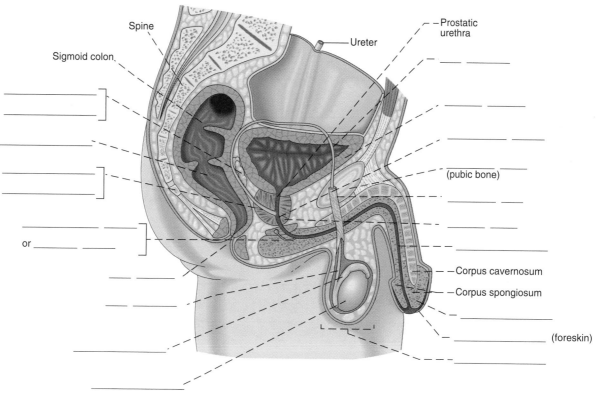

7. How do pituitary hormones affect the function of the testes? _____
_____
_____

8. List the secondary male sex characteristics.
   a. _____   e. _____
   b. _____   f. _____
   c. _____   g. _____
   d. _____

9. List, in order, the structures through which sperm pass.
   a. _____
   b. _____
   c. _____
   d. _____
   e. _____

10. What is the composition of semen?

    a. _____

    b. _____

    c. _____

    d. _____

11. List the four diseases and disorders of the male reproductive system; define the condition and identify the main symptoms and/or cause of the condition.

    a. _____

    _____

    b. _____

    _____

    c. _____

    _____

    _____

    d. _____

    _____

    _____

12. List the eight female sexual structures and describe their location and function, as identified.

    a. _____

    b. _____

    _____

    c. _____

    _____

    d. _____

    _____

    e. _____

    f. _____

    _____

    g. _____

    h. _____

13. Identify the internal structure on the following illustration.

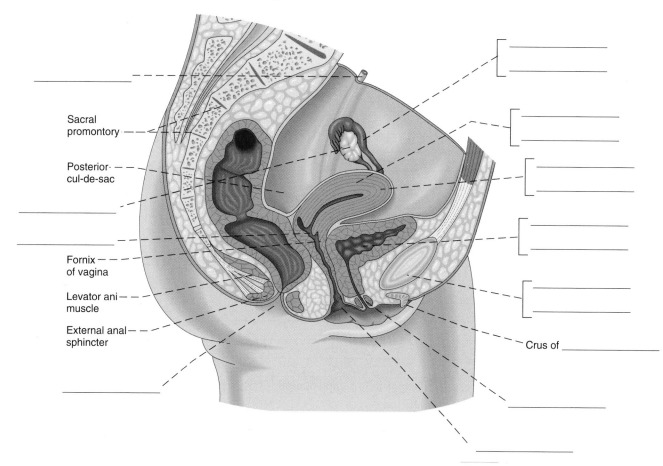

Sacral promontory

Posterior cul-de-sac

Fornix of vagina

Levator ani muscle

External anal sphincter

Crus of _____

14. Identify the external structures on the following illustration.

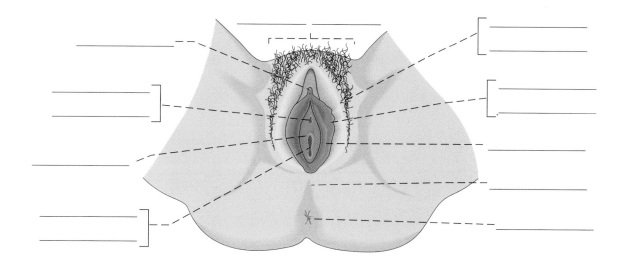

15. How do hormones from the pituitary gland affect the development of the female reproductive organs? _____

_____

_____

16. List the female secondary sex characteristics.

a. _____

b. _____

c. _____

d. _____

e. _____

f. _____

g. _____

h. _____

i. _____

17. Describe the process involved with ovum maturation and release and development of the corpus luteum.

_____

_____

_____

_____

_____

_____

18. Trace the pathway of an egg from expulsion to implantation if fertilized or to the exterior if not.

a. _____

_____

b. _____

19. List the four phases of the menstrual cycle, state the process which is occurring in each phase, and explain the purpose of menstruation.

a. _____

_____

b. _____

_____

c. _____

_____

_____

_____

d. _____

_____

_____

20. Identify the period of time during a pregnancy when the following occurs.

a. embryonic stage- _____

b. called a fetus- _____

c. systems complete, fingernails- _____

d. sex can be determined- _____

e. movement felt- _____

f. heartbeat detectable, half way- _____

g. weighs less than two pounds- _____

h. opens eyes- _____

i. hears sounds- _____

j. assumes head down position- _____

k. reaches five pounds- _____

l. weighs 7 1/2 lbs. and is 20 in. long- _____

21. Using Nagle's rule, calculate the expected delivery date for the following first days of last menstrual periods.

a. February 6, 1998- _____

b. January 15, 1998- _____

c. July 4, 1997- _____

d. September 29, 1997- _____

e. December 25, 1997- _____

22. List the usual signs and symptoms of early pregnancy.

a. _____   d. _____

b. _____   e. _____

c. _____   f. _____

23. List symptoms which occur later in pregnancy.

a. _____   e. _____

b. _____   f. _____

c. _____   g. _____

d. _____   h. _____

24. Describe the characteristics of the three stages of labor.

First a. _____

b. _____

Second a. _____

b. _____

c. _____

d. _____

Third a. _____

b. _____

25. List 8 reasons to use contraceptives.

a. _____

b. _____

c. _____

d. _____

e. _____

f. _____

g. _____

h. _____

26. Name 10 methods of contraception.

a. _____   h. _____

b. _____   i. _____

c. _____   j. _____

d. _____   k. _____

e. _____   l. _____

f. _____   m. _____

g. _____   n. _____

27. List the warning signals which may indicate a malignancy of the breast.

    a. _____

    b. _____

    c. _____

    d. _____

    e. _____

    f. _____

28. Name female organs other than the breast where cancer develops, identifying the major symptoms.

    a. _____

        1. _____

        2. _____

    b. _____

        1. _____

        2. _____

        3. _____

    c. _____

        1. _____

        2. _____

        3. _____

        4. _____

        5. _____

        6. _____

    d. _____

        1. _____

        2. _____

        3. _____

29. Match the following test (Column I) with its description (Column II).

    COLUMN I

    _____ a. Diaphanogram

    _____ b. Mammograph

    _____ c. Maturation index

    _____ d. Papanicolaou test

    _____ e. Pregnancy test

    _____ f. Ultrasonography

    _____ g. Colposcopy

    _____ h. Hysteroscopy

    COLUMN II

    1. Examination with an instrument connected to a monitor to view the endometrium

    2. Determines hormonal level from cells scraped from vaginal walls

    3. High frequency sound waves which detect and aid in the diagnosis of breast irregularities

    4. A urine specimen test to detect the presence of HCG

    5. Utilizes infrared light to detect and photograph various tissue structures of the breast

    6. Examination of cervical secretions for cancer cells

    7. An X ray of the breast

    8. An examination of the cervix following a questionable pap smear

30. Define the following diseases or disorders of the female reproductive system and briefly describe key symptoms.

a. abortion _____

_____

b. cervical erosion _____

_____

c. cervicitis _____

d. cystic breast disease _____

_____

e. cystocele _____

_____

f. dysmenorrhea _____

_____

g. endometriosis _____

_____

h. fibroids _____

_____

i. hysterectomy _____

j. malignancy of breast _____

_____

k. ovarian cyst _____

_____

l. PMS _____

_____

m. polyp _____

n. rectocele _____

_____

31. Identify the main characteristics of each of the following disease conditions.

a. chlamydia _____

_____

b. gonorrhea _____

_____

_____

c. herpes _____

_____

d. NGU _____

e. P.I.D. _____

_____

_____

f. syphilis (4 stages) 1) _____

2) _____

_____

_____

3) _____

4) _____

g. trichomoniasis _____

_____

h. vaginitis _____

32. Each line contains four different spellings of a word. Underline the correctly spelled word.

a. circumcision   circomcision   circumsision   circumcisun
b. dysmenorrhea   dismemorrea   dismenorehea   dysmenorrea
c. epididimus   epididimis   epididymis   epididymus
d. genetalea   genetalia   genitalea   genitalia
e. menapause   menopause   menaplaus   menoplaus
f. menorrhagia   menarrhagia   menorrhagea   menarrhagea
g. prostratectomy   prostatectemy   prostetectomy   prostatectomy
h. syfhillis   syphillis   syphilis   syphelis

33. Complete the puzzle with words from the list of Words to Know.

_ _ _ R _ _	(pelvic organ)
_ _ _ _ E _ _ _ _ _	(wall of uterus)
_ _ _ P _ _ _ _ _ _ _ _ _ _	(improper location of testes)
_ _ _ R _ _ _	(muscle growth)
_ _ _ _ _ _ O _ _ _ _ _	(pertains to menstruation)
_ _ _ D _ _ _ _ _ _	(coiled tube)
_ _ _ _ U _ _ _ _ _ _	(foreskin surgery)
_ _ _ _ _ C _ _	(the beginning)
S Y S T E M	(group of organs)
_ _ _ _ _ _ _ _ _ _ I _ _ _ _	(protozal)
_ _ _ V _ _	(entrance to uterus)
_ _ _ _ E _ _ _ _ _	(removal of mammary gland)

B. CRITICAL THINKING SITUATIONS: WHAT WOULD YOU DO? WHAT WOULD YOU SAY?

1. A sixty-five year old male patient wants the doctor to call in a prescription for him to get rid of his kidney infection. He has been having to urinate frequently, even getting up at night, and then he still dribbles sometimes in between. His brother had about the same problems and that's what he had. _____

_____

_____

2. You have a good relationship with your teenage daughter. She tells you some of the kids at school have been talking about birth control. One of the girls said she didn't need anything because she always douched right after she had sex. She buys those premixed disposable units at the supermarket. She also thinks that will prevent her from getting AIDS. _____

_____

_____

3. A 35-year-old female called to see if she should see the doctor. She had found a lumpy place on her left breast, but it didn't hurt or anything. Her friend told her that it was probably just cysts at her age and don't worry about it. _____

_____

_____

_____

After your instructor has returned your work to you, make all necessary corrections and place in a 3-ring notebook for future reference.

ASSIGNMENT SHEET

Section IV: THE CLINICAL MEDICAL ASSISTANT
Chapter 12: PREPARING FOR CLINICAL DUTIES

Unit 1: GUIDELINES FOR THE PERSONAL SAFETY AND WELL-BEING OF STAFF AND PATIENTS

Review the objectives and text for each unit before completing the assignment sheet for that unit in this chapter. When all sheets for the chapter have been completed, remove them from this workbook and give them to the instructor for evaluation.

A. BRIEF ANSWER

1. What should the medical assistant consider of patients when assisting with procedures? _____

_____

_____

2. Besides being apprehensive about procedures, what else may a patient be afraid of? _____

_____

3. List the types of patients who will need the undivided attention of the medical assistant? _____

_____

_____

4. Why should people leave assistance dogs (or other assistance animals) alone? _____

_____

5. How should you speak to patients, and why? _____

_____

6. What special instructions should you give to a patient who is blind? deaf? _____

_____

_____

B. TRUE OR FALSE: Place a "T" for True or "F" for False in the space provided.

_____ 1. There should be a scheduled time weekly for inspection of the entire medical facility.

_____ 2. Medical facilities are prime targets for pathogenic organisms to grow.

_____ 3. Asepsis is the state of being free from all pathogenic microorganisms.

_____ 4. Periodic remodeling of a medical facility should be done only after furniture and carpets become a safety hazard.

_____ 5. A disinfectant spray should be kept in a convenient place to disinfect small areas and to help eliminate unpleasant odors.

_____ 6. The ideal temperature setting is 78° F for a medical facility.

_____ 7. Small toys are not recommended in the pediatric area of the reception room because babies might swallow them.

_____ 8. Soap and water should be used each and every time you wash your hands.

_____ 9. If you wear gloves for assisting with invasive procedures, you will not need to wash your hands as often.

_____ 10. Emergency exits should be clearly posted with easy to follow paths for evacuation in each room of the medical facility.

C. BRIEF ANSWER

1. List the reasons for wearing latex gloves.

   a. _____
   _____

   b. _____
   _____

   c. _____
   _____

2. What information should be documented in case of an accident at a medical facility? _____
   _____

3. Explain what you should do after you have used a tissue to catch a sneeze. _____
   _____

4. What should you do (and what should you tell patients to do) if stricken with a case of the flu/bad cold? _____
   _____

5. What is a foamed alcohol preparation used for in the medical facility? _____
   _____

6. Why should hand lotion be available to the medical assistant in a medical facility? _____
   _____

D. FILL IN THE BLANKS

1. A _____ eliminates the possibility of dropping a bar of soap in the sink or on the floor when performing the handwashing procedure.
2. When performing the handwashing procedure a _____ should be used to dislodge microorganisms around cuticles and under the fingernails.
3. You should use a _____ to turn on and off faucets for handwashing.
4. Disposable gloves are available with or without _____
5. Scratches, paper cuts, and breaks in the skin should be covered with a _____ after handwashing and before gloving.
6. Spills should be cleaned up immediately to prevent _____.
7. Lab test results should be recorded _____ on charts and in logs to ensure accuracy.
8. Disposable sharp instruments, lancets, syringes and needles (intact) should be discarded in a _____ _____ after use.
9. Electrical appliances and wiring should be checked periodically for faulty operation and tagged for _____
10. _____ phone numbers should be posted near the phone.
11. Loose fitting clothing and jewelry can contribute to _____ while working with machines or equipment.
12. _____ chemicals should be kept away from flames and gas lines.

After your instructor has returned your work to you, make all necessary corrections and place in a 3-ring notebook for future reference.

ASSIGNMENT SHEET

Chapter 12: PREPARING FOR CLINICAL DUTIES
Unit 2: INFECTION CONTROL

A. WORD SCRAMBLE

1. _ _ _ _ _ _ _ _ _ _ _ _ _   HRDBUZISAOAO
2. _ _ _ _ _ _ _ _   TICAREAB
3. _ _ _ _ _ _ _   SELAMIA
4. _ _ _ _ _ _ _ _ _ _   YORMPGOOHL
5. _ _ _ _ _ _ _ _ _ _   UCTESPBSELI
6. _ _ _ _ _ _   ORPSSE
7. _ _ _ _ _ _ _ _ _ _   TNESISAERC
8. _ _ _ _ _ _ _   PSSASIE
9. _ _ _ _ _ _ _ _   EOPHAGTN
10. _ _ _ _ _ _ _ _ _ _ _   EFNCONINTME
11. _ _ _ _ _ _ _   RLEDTPO

B. MATCHING: Read the definition in Column II and then find the matching answer in Column I. Place the letter of the correct answer in the space provided.

COLUMN I   COLUMN II

_____   1. Cholera   a. Fungus condition
_____   2. Autotrophs   b. Can live independently
_____   3. Obligate parasite   c. Feed on organic matter
_____   4. Tinea pedis   d. External parasites
_____   5. Viruses   e. From contaminated food/water
_____   6. Escherichia coli   f. Disease producing microorganisms
_____   7. Dysentery   g. Feed on inorganic matter
_____   8. Facultative parasites   h. Grow best in the absence of oxygen
_____   9. Ticks and fleas   i. Non-pathogen
_____   10. Heterotrophs   j. Smallest of microorganisms
_____   11. Pathogens   k. Completely dependent on host
_____   12. Anaerobes   l. Common cause urinary tract infections
                                 m. Protozoa

C. BRIEF ANSWER

1. Name the common pathogens known to man. _____

2. What are the growth requirements for microorganisms? _____
_____

3. What precautions must be taken to prevent disease transmission? _____
_____

4. Explain the infection cycle. _____
_____

5. What is droplet infection? _____
_____

6. List good health habits which are helpful in resisting disease, and explain why they are beneficial. _____

_____

7. Name a disinfectant and an antiseptic that is commonly used in the medical office. _____

_____

8. What is most commonly used in preparing a patient's skin for injection or surgery procedures? _____

_____

9. What is sterilization? _____

10. Describe the proper method of cleaning instruments. _____

_____

_____

11. Why is it advisable to soak instruments? _____

_____

12. What purpose does a brush serve in cleaning instruments? _____

_____

13. Why should precautions be taken in the storage of instruments? _____

14. Why is autoclaving the most desirable form of sterilization? _____

15. Explain the precautions to be taken when you are exposed to all blood and body fluids. (These precautions are known as the "blood and body fluid standard/universal precautions.") Why is it vitally important to follow these precautions carefully? _____

_____

_____

_____

_____

16. How are used needles, scalpels, and other sharp instruments to be handled? Why? _____

_____

_____

17. How should waste be treated before it is disposed of from a medical office or clinic? _____

_____

18. Name the two most feared communicable diseases that health care facilities must strive to prevent transmitting to the public. _____

19. What must the health care worker perform both before and after gloving? _____

D. MATCHING: Read the disease in Column I and then match with the common name in Column II. Place the letter of the correct answer in the space provided.

COLUMN I   COLUMN II

_____ 1. Varicella   a. Pinworms

_____ 2. URI   b. Scabies

_____ 3. Conjunctivitis   c. Chicken pox

_____ 4. Pediculosis   d. Scarlet fever

_____ 5. Herpes simplex   e. Hepatitis B

_____ 6. Enterobius vermicularis   f. Common cold

_____ 7. Scarlatina   g. Fever blister

                                            h. Head lice

                                            i. Pinkeye

E. FILL IN THE BLANK

1. Antibacterial agents, antibiotics, corticosteroids depending on the causative agent, is the treatment for _____ .

2. Cleansing of areas with antibacterial soap and water and topical and/or oral antibiotics is the treatment for _____ .

3. Topical application of drying medications and antibiotics for secondary infections is the treatment for _____ .

4. 2-3 weeks, usually 13-17 days, is the incubation period for _____ .

5. In one week nits (eggs) hatch; in two weeks they mature. This describes the incubation period for _____ .

6. Bed rest, antipyretics, topical antipruritics, is the treatment for _____ .

7. 14-50 days is the incubation period for both _____ and _____ .

8. Blister-like lesions which later become crusted and itchy are symptoms of _____ .

9. Antibiotics, analgesics, antipyretics, increase in fluid intake, plus bed rest is the treatment for _____ .

10. Strawberry tongue, rash of skin and inside of mouth, high fever, nausea and vomiting are symptoms of _____ .

F. BRIEF ANSWER (refer to Table 12-1 in your textbook):

1. List the symptoms of conjunctivitis. _____

_____

2. How is impetigo transmitted? _____

3. What is the treatment for hepatitis A and hepatitis B? _____

_____

4. How long is the incubation period for aseptic meningitis? For bacterial meningitis? _____

_____

5. Describe the symptoms of varicella. _____

_____

6. Explain the treatment for pediculosis and *why* it is important to follow it carefully. _____

_____

_____

_____

_____

_____

_____

_____

7. List the symptoms of herpes simplex, and tell how it is transmitted. _____

_____

8. What is the incubation period of pinworms and how are they transmitted? _____

_____

9. What are the symptoms of enterobius vermicularis and how is it treated? _____

_____

_____

10. List the symptoms of aseptic meningitis and of bacterial meningitis. _____

_____

_____

11. How is aseptic meningitis transmitted? Bacterial meningitis? _____

_____

12. What is the treatment of aseptic meningitis? Bacterial meningitis? _____

_____

_____

13. What are the symptoms and treatment of influenza? _____

_____

14. List the symptoms and treatment of the common cold. _____

_____

15. What is the means of transmission and the incubation period of the common cold? _____

_____

16. How is conjunctivitis transmitted? _____

17. What are the symptoms of hepatitis A? Of hepatitis B? _____

_____

18. How is hepatitis A transmitted? Hepatitis B? _____

_____

19. What are symptoms of pediculosis and how is it transmitted? _____

_____

20. List the symptoms and treatment of scabies. _____

_____

21. How is scabies transmitted and what is the incubation period? _____

_____

22. How are strep throat and scarlet fever transmitted and how long are the incubation periods? _____
_____
_____

23. List the symptoms of strep throat and scarlet fever and the treatment for each. _____
_____
_____
_____
_____

24. List the communicable diseases that should be reported to the local health department (besides STDs).
_____
_____

25. List the symptoms of AIDS. _____
_____
_____

26. What is the incubation period for AIDS? _____

27. What are the symptoms of Haemophilus influenzae type B? _____
_____

28. How is Haemophilus influenzae type B transmitted? _____
_____

G. CROSSWORD

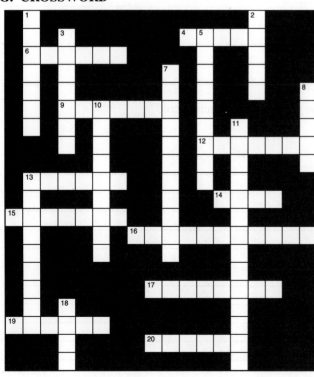

ACROSS

4. Every day
6. Latex barrier for hands
9. Regular habit
12. Free from septic matter
13. Destroyed only by autoclaving
14. Rinse used instruments in _____ water
15. Protection
16. Helps reduce the spread of diseases
17. Do over and over
19. Prior to
20. To do again

DOWN

1. Clean and sanitary
2. Circle
3. Management
5. Destroys microorganism using steam under pressure
7. Safety measures
8. Used in washing hands/instruments
10. Global
11. Duty
13. Free of all living organisms
18. Infected person/animal

H. CRITICAL THINKING SITUATIONS: WHAT WOULD YOU SAY? WHAT WOULD YOU DO?

1. One of your co-workers is most negligent about handwashing. It bothers you because you realize how easily diseases can be transmitted from person to person. _____

   _____

2. You notice that there are several patients in the reception area waiting to be seen by the physician. One of them is sneezing and coughing, and appears to be very ill. _____

3. As you remove a suture pack from the autoclave, you notice that the sterilization indicator tape has not changed color. _____

4. You are checking instruments in preparation for autoclaving. You notice that two of the hemostats have loose hinges and a towel clamp is rusty. _____

   _____

ACHIEVING SKILL COMPETENCY

Reread the TPO for each procedure and then practice the skills listed below, following the procedure in your textbook.

   Hand Washing - Procedure 12-1
   Wrap Items for Autoclave - Procedure 12-2

When you feel you have mastered the performance of the skill, sign your name on the appropriate evaluation sheet and give it to your instructor to indicate you are prepared to perform the procedure for evaluation.

After your instructor has returned your work to you, make all necessary corrections and place in a 3-ring notebook for future reference.

ASSIGNMENT SHEET

CHAPTER 13: BEGINNING THE DATA BASE
Unit 1: MEDICAL HISTORY

A. WORD SCRAMBLE

1. _ _ _ _ _ _ _ _ _   TCRUBEMNE
2. _ _ _ _ _ _ _ _ _ _ _ _   LIEBANMRATOIS
3. _ _ _ _ _ _   EGARIT
4. _ _ _ _ _ _ _   MPYSTMO
5. _ _ _ _ _ _   RVEXET
6. _ _ _ _ _   YDRMEE
7. _ _ _ _ _ _   CILETI
8. _ _ _ _ _ _ _   TUSTRAE
9. _ _ _ _ _ _ _ _   HSIDCTAP

B. BRIEF ANSWER

1. Why must assistance be given to patients in completing the medical history form? _____

_____

2. Where should the medical assistant interview patients to obtain medical history information? _____

_____

3. Describe how additional questions on the medical history form regarding AIDS and hepatitis should be worded. _____

_____

4. What additional questions should be asked of patients regarding AIDS and hepatitis to determine if further investigation should be made as to the health status of that patient? _____

_____

_____

5. Define the following terms.
   a. CC (chief complaint) _____
   b. PI (present illness) _____

   _____

   c. ROS (review of systems) _____

   _____

   d. PH (past history) _____

   _____

   e. FH (family history) _____

   _____

   f. PSH (personal-sociocultural history) _____

   _____

6. Explain why medical history forms vary in detail and length. _____

_____

7. What is a genogram and why is it helpful to physicians? _____

_____

_____

8. Why must the patient's height and weight be recorded at the initial visit? _____

_____

9. Why is it important to keep an accurate record of the patient's weight? _____

_____

10. Why must the medical assistant note which method is used when recording a child's length? _____

11. List three purposes that the growth chart serves. _____

_____

12. Why must head circumference be measured and recorded until a child is 36 months of age? _____

13. What type of measuring tape is used to measure head circumference? _____

14. What is usually requested for adults when taking the chest measurement? _____

_____

C. SPELLING: Each line contains four different spellings of a word. Underline the spelled word and use it in a sentence.

1. measurement	measurement	measuremit	measeurment
2. traiage	treaige	triage	trauge
3. abnormalities	abnormalidies	abnarmalities	abnormalitaes
4. stadure	statere	stateure	stature
5. recumbent	recumbant	recombent	racumbent
6. infermation	informashion	information	infarmation
7. simptom	symptom	symptome	symptim
8. haight	heite	height	hieght
9. interview	intraview	innerview	inerveiw
10. circumference	circomfrence	circumferance	circumferince

1. _____
2. _____
3. _____
4. _____
5. _____
6. _____
7. _____
8. _____
9. _____
10. _____

D. SITUATIONS: What would you say? What would you do?

1. A new co-worker is interviewing a new patient at the reception window asking medical history questions and completing the form in earshot and view of everyone in the office. What would you do? _____

_____

2. This same new worker is found erasing several items on the completed medical history form. What advice do you offer and why? _____

_____

3. A two-year-old patient is being very uncooperative with routine height and weight measurements. _____

_____

_____

_____

_____

ACHIEVING SKILL COMPETENCY

Reread the TPO for these procedures and then practice the skills listed below, following the procedures in your textbook.

Procedure 13-1   Interview Patient to Medical History Form Completion
Procedure 13-2   Measuring Height
Procedure 13-3   Measure Recumbent Length of Infant
Procedure 13-4   Weighing Patient on Upright Scale
Procedure 13-5   Weighing Infant
Procedure 13-6   Measure Head Circumference
Procedure 13-7   Measure Chest Circumference

When you feel you have mastered performance of a skill, sign your name on the appropriate evaluation sheet and give it to your instructor to indicate you are prepared to perform the procedure for evaluation.

After your instructor has returned your work to you, make all necessary corrections and place in a 3-ring notebook for future reference.

ASSIGNMENT SHEET

Chapter 13: BEGINNING THE DATABASE
Unit 2: TRIAGE

A. ESSAY ANSWER
1. Discuss the origin of triage. _____
2. Where in the medical office should triage be performed? _____

   _____
3. Explain phone triage. _____

   _____

   _____
4. State the purpose of progress notes in the patient chart. _____

   _____
5. What type of questioning should be used during patient interviews to obtain information regarding their medical condition? _____

   _____
6. Discuss what you should cover with patients at each office visit? _____

   _____
7. List the categories for determining the urgency of a patient's condition. _____

   _____

   _____
8. What is the best way for compliance of physician's instructions to patients? _____

   _____

B. COMPLETE THESE STATEMENTS
1. The French word triage means to _____.
2. In many medical facilities, small _____ provide privacy to patients during triage.
3. In the medical office there should be a _____ of action developed regarding telephone and face-to-face triage.
4. All office personnel must be familiar with standard first aid procedures and _____.
5. You should _____ patients to write down their questions to discuss with the doctor so they will not forget.

C. MATCHING

COLUMN I	COLUMN II
____ 1. prioritize	a. careful; dedicated and thorough
____ 2. trivial	b. permission to make decision using your own judgment
____ 3. dispatch	c. sort in order of importance
____ 4. discretion	d. to combine together in a united whole
____ 5. conscientious	e. of little importance
	f. send; convey

ASSIGNMENT SHEET

Chapter 13
Unit 3: VITAL SIGNS

This unit contains many important concepts and skills to be mastered; therefore, this workbook unit will be divided into four sections.

SECTION 1–TEMPERATURE CONTROL AND MEASUREMENT
A. FILL IN THE BLANKS

1. Identify the four vital signs indicating what body function is being measured.

   a. (e.g.) blood pressure   measures   the force of the heart

   b. _____   measures   _____

   c. _____   measures   _____

   d. _____   measures   _____

2. Vital sign findings should be recorded _____

   _____

3. The body loses heat through _____ and _____ .

4. The balance between heat production and heat loss determines the _____ .

5. Temperature is usually the _____ in the morning and the _____

   in the afternoon and evening.

6. Complete the following paragraph which explains how temperature is controlled in the body.

   Temperature in the body is controlled by the _____ in the _____

   of the brain. When receptors sense the presence of excess heat, the _____ produce

   _____ which _____ from the surface of the skin, causing the

   body to _____ . The surface blood vessels _____ which allows

   more blood to be in contact with the surface of the skin. The blood _____ heat,

   thereby _____ the blood in the vessels. When receptors sense a lack of heat, the surface

   blood vessels _____ to _____ heat loss. Small papillary muscles

   _____ producing _____ to help _____ the

   body. Shivering and chills will cause body heat to _____ .

7. Explain briefly how a fever develops (use 5 steps).

   a. _____

   b. _____

   c. _____

   d. _____

   e. _____

8. Fill in the blanks for the correct Fahrenheit temperature when referring to classifications of fevers.

   a. Slight = _____ °F

   b. Moderate = _____ °F

   c. Severe = _____ °F

   d. Dangerous = _____ °F

   e. Fatal = _____ °F

9. The column of mercury shown on the thermometer reads a "normal" 98.6~° on the Fahrenheit scale. At each arrow, read the temperature and enter the finding at the corresponding space.

| a. _____ | c. _____ | e. _____ | g. _____ | i. _____ |
| b. _____ | d. _____ | f. _____ | h. _____ | j. _____ |

10. The column of mercury on the thermometer reads a "normal" 37~° on the Celsius scale. At each arrow, read the temperature and enter the finding at the corresponding space.

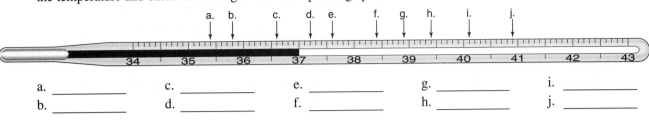

a. _____   c. _____   e. _____   g. _____   i. _____

b. _____   d. _____   f. _____   h. _____   j. _____

11. List the five thermometer types.

1. _____

2. _____

3. _____

4. _____

5. _____

12. Name situations when oral temperature measurement is contraindicated.

a. _____

b. _____

c. _____

d. _____

e. _____

13. Match the following terms (Column I) with their meanings (Column II).

COLUMN I

_____ a. Afebrile
_____ b. Axillary
_____ c. Febrile
_____ d. Oral
_____ e. Sublingual
_____ f. Fever
_____ g. Celsius
_____ h. Rectal
_____ i. Calibration
_____ j. Stem
_____ k. Disinfectant
_____ l. Contraindicated

COLUMN II

1. A metric measurement
2. By mouth
3. Numbered markings
4. Not appropriate
5. Thermometer section
6. Fever
7. Underarm
8. Germicide
9. Without fever
10. Beneath tongue
11. Elevated body heat
12. Anal
13. Fahrenheit
14. Anesthetic
15. Security

14. Convert the following Celsius temperatures to Fahrenheit.

a. 36.5°C = _____ °F   d. 35.7°C = _____ °F

b. 39.5°C = _____ °F   e. 36.8°C = _____ °F

c. 38.8°C = _____ °F   f. 37.4°C = _____ °F

15. Convert the following Fahrenheit temperatures to Celsius.

a. 96.8°F = _____ °C   d. 99.2°F = _____ °C

b. 97.4°F = _____ °C   e. 100.2°F = _____ °C

c. 98.6°F = _____ °C   f. 102.4°F = _____ °C

16. WORD SEARCH: There are 50 words hidden in the puzzle. Can you find them?

accuracy	collapse	febrile	lubricant	severe
afebrile	cooling	fever	mercury	shake
aseptically	contraindicated	findings	metric	slight
axillary	dangerous	fragile	moderate	stem
bulb	degrees	glass	mouth	stubby
buttocks	disinfectant	heat	normal	sublingual
calibration	electronic	holder	oral	subnormal
centigrade	elevation	infection	record	temperature
chills	fahrenheit	insert	rectal	tenths
chipped	fatal	inspect	security	thermometer

```
A G L A S S I E T V E E O F A T A L M M W Q I S T N D
C H I L L S O T B C L O B T P W I E L E V A T I O N V
O I Y T W C B N Y I C F I H E M K V Z T O P W I M G X
L G F J M I T O G P H C N E C M M I W R W S T U B B Y
L V A C C U R A C Y I U S R C V P S Y I E A S H A K E
A E A J K U R L R Y P T P M P O E E C C R V Y T Z X P
P N F A H F P U I X P B E O Q H C S R B K N L R W V C
S W E R T I C D L P E Y C M R T O W I A J L V C X I N
E N B P R R B V A G D D T E I Y Q L P U T M V X W O F
W I R C E B V X U N J H V T L W A L D I W U L W I O E
M V I M C O W G T E G H I E M C A L O E W P R T Z C V
B C L I T E N I P I U E S R C M V X U Y R W C E N L E
C F E S A I J L L Y T Q R X R S Z Y I N S E R T D E R
K H J R L N B S A W Q Z R O P U T V W L F U C B L S W
B G D O M U R B C I W R N P U F X C V N L I Y I V C S
U K O M L U B R I C A N T G H S W Q I K N A R X C V T
T C C O N T R A I N D I C A T E D E P O T B R C X I E
T D F A S C V B B N I O Y U I O R W R C E I O Y E C M
O S U B N O R M A L M T Q W E E O T C F K L H H T Y U
C E N T I G R A D E I O S D V C C S U B L I N G U A L
K E R E Y U I O O R S D D E L E I O L S D E M N V C S
S E R N K L M O U T H I S E L K L U S D R E C O R D I
U T Y T F G H C R T Y U I E R I B I O H E A T Y U I O
W E R H A S E P T I C A L L Y A K L A W E R T Y O I R
A S D S L S Z X C V B N M S D F T F I N D I N G S I A
D I S I N F E C T A N T E D E G R E E S G J K L Z X L
```

ACHIEVING SKILL COMPETENCY

Reread the TPO for each procedure and then practice the skills listed below, following the procedures in your textbook.

Procedure 13-8	Clean and Store a Mercury Thermometer
Procedure 13-9	Measure Oral Temperature with a Mercury Thermometer
Procedure 13-10	Measure Rectal Temperature with a Mercury Thermometer
Procedure 13-11	Measure Axillary Temperature with a Mercury Thermometer
Procedure 13-12	Measure Oral Temperature with Disposable Plastic Thermometer
Procedure 13-13	Measure Temperature Electronically

If Available—Measure Core Body Temperature with Infrared Tympanic Thermometer

When you feel you have mastered performance of a skill, sign your name on the appropriate evaluation sheet and give it to your instructor to indicate you are prepared to perform the procedure for evaluation.

SECTION 2—THE PULSE AND ITS MEASUREMENT

1. Define pulse and explain how it occurs. _____

   _____

2. Name and locate the five pulse points.

   a. _____
   b. _____
   c. _____
   d. _____
   e. _____

3. How is pulse rate determined; what is the normal adult rate? _____

   _____

4. List five factors which influence heart rate.

   a. _____
   b. _____
   c. _____
   d. _____
   e. _____

5. Stimulation of the sympathetic nervous system _____ heart rate. The parasympathetic nervous system _____ the heart rate.

6. List eight situations which cause the heart rate to increase.

   a. _____ e. _____
   b. _____ f. _____
   c. _____ g. _____
   d. _____ h. _____

7. List four situations which cause the heart rate to decrease.

   a. _____ c. _____
   b. _____ d. _____

8. Name the two qualities of the heartbeat which must be observed, defining the terms and listing the words used to describe the characteristics.

   a. _____
   b. _____

   _____

9. List eight times when apical pulse measurement would be indicated.

   a. _____ e. _____
   b. _____ f. _____
   c. _____ g. _____
   d. _____ h. _____

10. True or False: Place a "T" for true or an "F" for false in front of each of the following statements.

    _____ a. A patient would be sitting or lying down when the pulse is measured.
    _____ b. The radial pulse can be found at the inner wrist area on the little finger side.
    _____ c. The radial pulse is best felt by placing your thumb over the artery.
    _____ d. The pulse which can be felt in the radial artery is caused by the contraction of the aorta.
    _____ e. Apical pulse is located at the right fifth intercostal space.
    _____ f. A quick way to estimate the location of the apex is to position the right hand over the patient's chest and listen at the point under the thumb.

11. Fill in the blanks.

Pulse deficit can be determined by measuring _____ pulse and _____

pulse at the _____ . If a patient has a pulse deficit, the auscultated apical pulse rate is

_____ than the _____ pulse rate. This occurs because some of the

contractions are _____ .

12. Match the terms (Column I) with the correct meanings (Column II).

COLUMN I   COLUMN II

_____   a. Antecubital   1. Excessively slow heart rate

_____   b. Apex   2. Feel by touching

_____   c. Arrhythmia   3. Inner elbow area

_____   d. Auscultate   4. A pulse point on the instep of the foot

_____   e. Brachial   5. Excessively rapid heart rate

_____   f. Bradycardia   6. A pulse point at the inner wrist

_____   g. Carotid   7. A pulse point near the trachea

_____   h. Femoral   8. Lower edge of the heart

_____   i. Palpate   9. To listen

_____   j. Pulse deficit   10. A pulse point at the inner elbow

_____   k. Radial   11. Without a regular pattern of beats

_____   l. Tachycardia   12. A pulse point at the groin

                              13. The difference between apical and radial pulse

                              14. Weak heart volume

13. WORD SCRAMBLE: Unscramble the following terms.

a. _ _ _ _ _   RTEHA

b. _ _ _ _   EBTA

c. _ _ _ _ _ _ _ _   TCNTAROC

d. _ _ _ _ _ _ _ _   LYOISTSC

e. _ _ _ _ _ _   LIACAP

f. _ _ _ _ _   SLUEP

g. _ _ _ _ _ _ _ _ _ _   HRAMTIRHYA

h. _ _ _ _ _ _ _   ATCRDIO

i. _ _ _ _ _ _   ALRIDA

j. _ _ _ _ _ _ _ _   HLRAIBAC

k. _ _ _ _ _ _ _   MROAFLE

l. _ _ _ _ _ _   EYTARR

m. _ _ _ _   TREA

n. _ _ _ _ _ _   YHTRMH

o. _ _ _ _ _ _   LVEMOU

ACHIEVING SKILL COMPETENCY

Reread the TPO for these procedures and then practice the skills listed below, following the procedures in your textbook.

Procedure 13-15   Measure Radial Pulse

Procedure 13-16   Measure Apical Pulse

When you feel you have mastered performance of a skill, sign your name on the appropriate evaluation sheet and give it to your instructor to indicate you are prepared to perform the procedure for evaluation.

SECTION 3: RESPIRATIONS: OBSERVATION AND MEASUREMENT

C. BRIEF ANSWER

1. One respiration is the combination of one total _____ and one total _____.
   Two other terms which are frequently used and have the same meaning are _____ and
   _____.

2. When are respirations usually measured? _____
   _____

3. Why are respirations measured as if the pulse is being measured? _____
   _____

4. The quality of respirations must be observed. Normal respirations are _____, and
   _____.

5. Excessively rapid and deep respirations are known as _____.

6. Patients with difficult or labored breathing are said to have _____.

7. Noisy respirations are called rales, and are often present with diseases such as _____,
   _____, and _____.

8. Quality characteristics which are evaluated when respirations are measured are:
   a. Depth of inhalation which is described as _____, _____ or
   _____.
   b. Rhythm of respiration which is described as _____ or _____.

9. Absence of breathing is known as _____.

10. Describe the breathing pattern known as Cheyne-Stokes. _____
    _____
    _____

11. Normal respiration rate for an adult is _____ per minute.

12. Respiration rate is affected by:
    a. a _____
    b. e _____
    c. e _____
    d. i _____
    e. t _____

13. Fill in the temperature-pulse-respiration ratio below.

Temperature	Pulse	Respiration
99°F		
100°F		
102°F		
104°F		

14. Work the crossword puzzle using terminology concerning pulse and respiration.

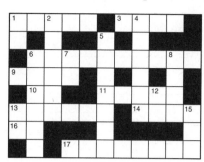

ACROSS

1. Organ which pumps blood
3. Contraction phase
6. Without rhythm
9. Lower heart edge
10. Part of the verb "to be"
11. One of the vital signs
13. Heart
14. A period of time
16. Father
17. A pulse point

DOWN

1. Mercury (abbr)
2. Sudden heart failure
4. Breathe out
5. Difficult breathing
6. Auscultated heart beat
7. Prescription (abbr)
7. A plan or thought
12. Senior (abbr)
13. Anterior-posterior (abbr)
14. Solution (abbr)

15. Each line contains four different spellings of a word. Underline the correctly spelled term.

a.	Cheyne-Stokes	Chain-Stokes	Cheyne-Stoakes	Chenye-Stokes
b.	dispnea	dispena	dyspnea	dyspnae
c.	eshale	exhale	exhail	exhaile
d.	expirashun	experation	expieration	expiration
e.	enhale	enhail	inhale	inhail
f.	inspiration	enspiration	ensperation	insperation
g.	resperation	respiration	rexpiration	rexperation

ACHIEVING SKILL COMPETENCY

Reread the TPO for the procedure and then practice the skill listed below, following the procedure in your textbook.

Procedure 13-17   Measure Respirations

When you feel you have mastered performance of a skill, sign your name on the appropriate evaluation sheet and give it to your instructor to indicate you are prepared to perform the procedure for evaluation.

After your instructor has returned your work to you, make all necessary corrections and place in a 3-ring notebook for future reference.

SECTION 4: BLOOD PRESSURE

D. BRIEF ANSWER

1. Name the four vital signs.

   a. _____

   b. _____

   c. _____

   d. _____

2. Define blood pressure. _____

   _____

3. What does blood pressure measurement evaluate?

   a. _____

   b. _____

   c. _____

   d. _____

4. Where is blood pressure measured? (be specific) _____

5. Name the two organs which maintain blood pressure in the body.

   a. _____

   b. _____

6. Explain briefly how blood pressure is maintained. _____

   _____

   _____

   _____

7. Name the two phases of the blood pressure, describing the corresponding action which occurs and the relative amount of pressure with each phase. _____

   _____

E. FILL IN THE BLANKS

8. Blood pressure is measured in _____ .

9. Blood pressure is measured by a _____ which has either an _____ dial or a column of _____ .

10. Normal adult systolic pressure is between _____ to _____ ; normal diastolic pressure is from _____ to _____ .

11. Blood pressure which is consistently high is called _____ .

12. Blood pressure which is consistently low is called _____ .

13. An elevated pressure without apparent cause is said to be _____ or _____ hypertension.

14. List six possible causes of hypertension.

   a. _____   d. _____

   b. _____   e. _____

   c. _____   f. _____

15. Define pulse pressure. _____

16. Using the "general rule of thumb" is the pulse pressure of the following examples too low, normal, or too high? (Note: a normal pulse pressure does not mean the blood pressure is within a normal range)

   a. 130/86 _____

   b. 160/90 _____

   c. 110/74 _____

   d. 200/110 _____

   e. 186/98 _____

   f. 120/100 _____

   g. 174/116 _____

17. Several equipment factors influence accurate measurement. Explain what each item indicates or would cause to occur.
    a. Leaking mercury or bubbles would cause _____ .
    b. Too small a cuff would cause _____ .
    c. Too large a cuff would cause _____ .
    d. Mercury meniscus below "O" indicates _____ .

18. True or False: Place a "T" for true or an "F" for false in front of each of the following statements.
    _____ a. Completely deflate the cuff before applying.
    _____ b. Blood pressure may be measured over a silky sleeve.
    _____ c. The cuff is placed around the arm with the arrow at the brachial artery.
    _____ d. Inflate cuff slowly until you no longer hear beats.
    _____ e. When you miss the systolic reading, immediately reinflate the cuff before all air pressure escapes.
    _____ f. The patient's arm should be extended straight down at the side when in sitting position.
    _____ g. Palpatory readings are done only when the pressure cannot be auscultated.

19. What does it mean to take a baseline reading? _____
_____

20. Define auscultatory gap. _____

21. What would cause you to think a patient might have an auscultatory gap: _____
_____

22. Work the crossword puzzle using terms learned in the unit.

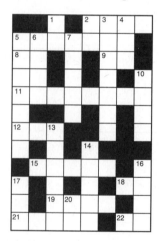

DOWN
  1. Bone
  2. Article; used in language
  3. Silver-colored liquid
  4. To take nourishment
  5. Fell
  6. 365 days
  7. Felt in arteries
 10. Contraction phase
 13. Pulse point at wrist
 14. Noisy respirations
 16. The number of times
 17. Three dimensional X-ray (abbr)
 20. Pelvic exam (abbr)

ACROSS
  2. End of prayer
  5. Difficult breathing
  8. Second word in music scale
  9. Right (abbr)
 11. Blood
 12. External organ of hearing
 15. Most desirable option
 18. Mother
 19. Bottom edge of heart
 21. Stories
 22. Barium enema (abbr)

B. MATCHING: Put the letter of the correct position from Column II in the proper blank in Column I.

COLUMN I

_____ 1. Back and posterior
_____ 2. Exercise post-partum
_____ 3. Proctoscopic
_____ 4. Eye, Ear, Nose, Throat
_____ 5. Anterior
_____ 6. Pelvic
_____ 7. Shock
_____ 8. Abdominal exam
_____ 9. Gynecologist
_____ 10. G.P./Internal Medicine
_____ 11. Ophthalmologist, Thoracic Surgeon, ENT Specialist
_____ 12. Proctologist
_____ 13. No specialty
_____ 14. G.P./Orthopedist/Internist
_____ 15. G.P./Internal Medicine/Gynecologist

COLUMN II

a. Genupectoral
b. Sims'/Knee-Chest
c. Semi-Fowler's/Fowler's
d. Horizontal/Recumbent/Supine
e. Prone
f. Trendelenburg
g. Dorsal Recumbent
h. Lithotomy

C. MATCHING: Put the letter of the correct position from Column I in the proper blank in Column II.

COLUMN I

_____ 1. Horizontal Recumbent
_____ 2. Dorsal Recumbent
_____ 3. Prone
_____ 4. Sims'
_____ 5. Knee-chest
_____ 6. Semi-Fowler's
_____ 7. Lithotomy
_____ 8. Trendelenburg

COLUMN II

a. Lying flat on table with buttocks at lower end of table and feet supported in stirrups
b. One left side with leg flexed slightly and right leg flexed sharply to chest
c. On back with feet elevated
d. On knees and chest with head to one side, knees separated
e. Flat on back, legs together
f. Sitting with head of table elevated to 45~° angle
g. Flat on stomach, head to one side
h. Flat on back, feet flat on table, knees flexed

D. IDENTIFICATION

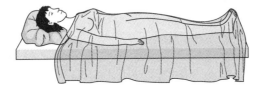

1. _____

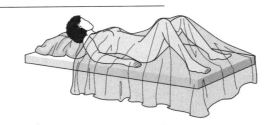

1. _____

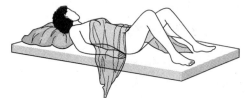

1. _____

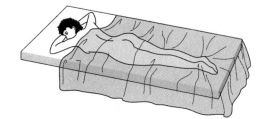

2. _____

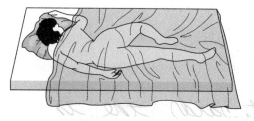

3. _____

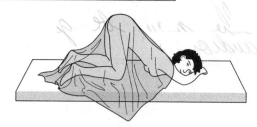

4. _____

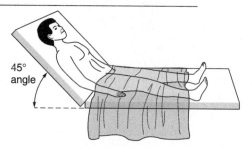

45°
angle

5. _____

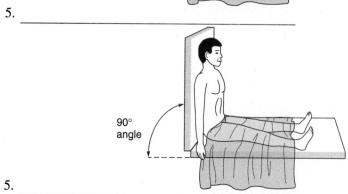

90°
angle

5. _____

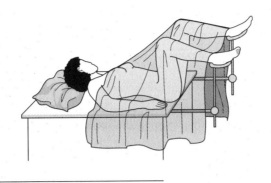

6. _____

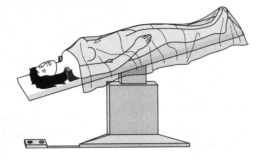

7. _____

E. CROSSWORD PUZZLE

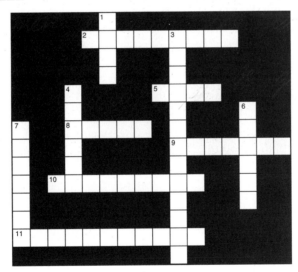

ACROSS

2. pelvic
5. chest, proctoscopic exam
8. back, posterior
9. same as Sims'
10. same as Supine
11. eye, ear, nose, throat

DOWN

1. proctoscopic exam
3. shock
4. anterior
6. relax abdomen
7. eye, ear, nose, throat

F. CRITICAL THINKING SITUATIONS: What would you say? What would you do?

1. A female patient in her 80s seems to be very confused as you explain to her that you want her to undress and wear a gown and drape in preparation for a complete physical examination. _____

_____

ACHIEVING SKILL COMPETENCY

Reread the TPO for each procedure and then practice the skills listed below, following the procedures in your textbook.

Procedure 14-8	Assist Patient to Horizontal Recumbent Position
Procedure 14-9	Assist Patient to Prone Position
Procedure 14-10	Assist Patient to Sims' Position
Procedure 14-11	Assist Patient to Knee-Chest Position
Procedure 14-12	Assist Patient to Semi-Fowler's Position
Procedure 14-13	Assist Patient to Lithotomy Position

When you feel you have mastered performance of a skill, sign your name on the appropriate evaluation sheet and give it to your instructor to indicate you are prepared to perform the procedure for evaluation.

After your instructor has returned your work to you, make all necessary corrections and place in a 3-ring notebook for future reference.

ASSIGNMENT SHEET

Chapter 14: PREPARING PATIENTS FOR EXAMINATIONS
Unit 3: PREPARING PATIENTS FOR EXAMINATIONS

A. BRIEF ANSWER

1. Define subjective and objective symptoms and give three examples of each.

   _____

   _____

   _____

2. List each section of a physical examination and describe how the physician conducts the exam.
   See text pages 524 to 529 for description of the physical examination.

3. Describe the role of the MA in the patient examination process.

   _____

   _____

   _____

4. List various patient education tips for various sections of the patient examination.

   _____

   _____

5. What are the nine sections of the abdominal cavity?

   _____

   _____

6. List the internal organs located in each of the nine sections of the abdomen.

   _____

   _____

   _____

7. Define the Problem Oriented Medical Record (POMR) system.

   _____

   _____

8. Explain how data is recorded with the POMR system.

   _____

   _____

9. What are progress notes?

   _____

   _____

10. List the warning signs for adults and children.

   _____

11. What are the standard physical examination schedules for adults and children?

   _____

B. MATCHING: Match the definitions

Column I

____ 1. Sphygmomanometer
____ 2. Speculum
____ 3. Tonometer
____ 4. Tape measure
____ 5. Stethoscope
____ 6. Guaiac test paper
____ 7. Tuning fork
____ 8. Percussion hammer
____ 9. Ophthalmoscope
____ 10. Otoscope
____ 11. Goose neck lamp
____ 12. Tongue depressor

Column II

a. Used to elicit an involuntary response
b. Provides light necessary for inspection
c. Used to view tiny capillaries behind retina
d. Used to check sense of smell
e. Instrument used to examine inner ear
f. Used for indirect auscultation
g. Instrument used to inspect a body cavity
h. Permits visual inspections of mouth/throat
i. Measures intraocular pressure to determine glaucoma
j. Physician uses this instrument to assess patient's hearing
k. Test for occult blood in stool
l. For measuring chest and extremities
m. Used to obtain blood pressure readings in both arms

C. IDENTIFICATION: Identify these instruments used in examinations.

1. _____
2. _____
3. _____
4. _____
5. _____
6. _____

7. _____
8. _____
9. _____
10. _____
11. _____

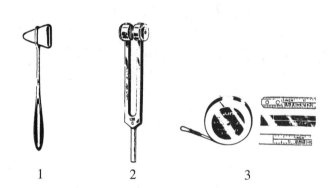
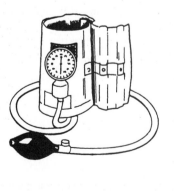
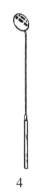
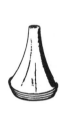
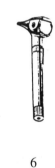

1   2   3   4   5   6

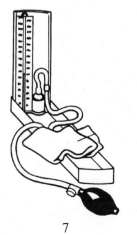
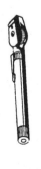
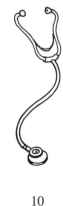
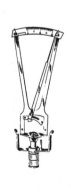

7   8   9   10   11

D. COMPLETION

1. Direct percussion is termed _____ and is done by striking the finger against the patient's body.
2. Pitch, quality, duration, and resonance are terms that refer to _____.
3. Direct _____ is done by placing your ear directly over a body area to hear sounds within.
4. _____ of problems in the SOAP method of recording patient information means documenting measurement of the patient's symptoms.
5. Referrals, medications, surgery, therapy, exercise, or other orders to return a patient to better health are all part of the _____ in the SOAP method.

E. MORE MATCHING

Column I

_____ 1. Percussion
_____ 2. Progress notes/report
_____ 3. Palpation
_____ 4. Objective symptoms
_____ 5. Manipulation
_____ 6. First part of physical exam
_____ 7. Romberg test
_____ 8. General appearance
_____ 9. Set of procedures
_____ 10. Auscultation
_____ 11. Red ink
_____ 12. Inspection
_____ 13. Writer
_____ 14. Mensuration
_____ 15. Subjective findings

Column II

a. Includes measurement, vital signs, and vision screening
b. Takes dictation during patient's exam
c. Plan of treatment
d. Visual exam of body's various parts
e. You can't see; patient feels
f. Listening to body sounds
g. Heel-to-shin test
h. Measurement of chest and extremities
i. The tapping of the fingers over a body area to produce sounds
j. The forceful passive movement of a joint to determine range of motion
k. Applying fingers/hands against the skin to feel underlying tissues/abnormalities
l. Record patient's subsequent visits on these
m. Check balance to detect muscle abnormality
n. Describes patient's overall state of health
o. Alerts of allergy or other vital information
p. Complete physical exam
q. Can be seen by all

After your instructor has returned your work to you, make all necessary corrections and place in a 3-ring notebook for future reference.

ASSIGNMENT SHEET

Chapter 14
Unit 4: ASSISTING WITH SPECIAL EXAMINATIONS

A. WORD PUZZLE: SOLVE THIS PUZZLE USING THE WORDS TO KNOW IN THIS UNIT.

```
        _ _ S _ _ _ _ _
        _ _ _ _ I _ _ _
        _ _ _ _ G _ _ _ _ _
        _ _ _ M _ _ _ _
        _ _ _ O _
      _ _ _ _ I _ _ _ _ _ _
        _ _ D _ _ _ _ _ _ _ _ _ _
        _ O _ _ _ _
    _ _ _ _ _ _ _ _ S
        _ _ C _ _ _
      _ _ _ _ _ O _ _ _ _
    _ _ _ _ _ _ P _ _ _ _ _
        _ Y _ _ _ _ _ _
```

B. BRIEF ANSWER

1. What instructions must be given to patients in preparation for a sigmoidoscopy? _____

   _____

2. What might result if patients are not completely informed about preparations for a diagnostic examination such as a sigmoidoscopy? _____

   _____

3. Why is air sometimes introduced into the colon during a sigmoidoscopy?_____

4. What advice can you give to patients in regard to flatulence they may experience following a sigmoidoscopy? _____

C. MATCHING

COLUMN I

_____ 1. Triage
_____ 2. Pap test
_____ 3. Women age 35 +
_____ 4. Proper preparation
_____ 5. Douching
_____ 6. LMP
_____ 7. Maturation index
_____ 8. Plain enema
_____ 9. Slow deep breaths
_____ 10. Flatulence
_____ 11. Constipation
_____ 12. BSE

COLUMN II

a. Necessary for successful examination
b. Relax abdominal muscles
c. Record first day of last menstrual period
d. Normally relieved with lots of fluids
e. Ascertain reason for patient's visit
f. Part of preparation for sigmoidoscopy
g. Cytological test to detect cervical cancer
h. Advise female patients to do routinely following her period
i. Used to obtain a smear of interior cervix
j. Should schedule routine mammographies
k. Washes away natural vaginal secretions
l. Hormonal evaluation
m. For relief, lie in prone position with pillow across mid abdomen

D. COMPLETION

1. _____ is a diagnostic examination of the interior of the sigmoid colon.
2. During the sigmoidoscopy it may be necessary to use a _____ pump to remove mucus or fecal material that is obstructing the view of the colon.
3. Patients who cannot tolerate the knee-chest position for a sigmoidoscopy may be asked to move into the _____ position for the exam.
4. A plain cleansing _____ is required before the sigmoidoscopy procedure is performed.
5. A cytologic screening test to detect cancer of the cervix is the _____ test.
6. Patient scheduled for a Pap test should not _____ 24-48 hours prior to their appointment or the smear may be reported as negative only because _____ cells have been washed away.

E. IDENTIFY THESE INSTRUMENTS:

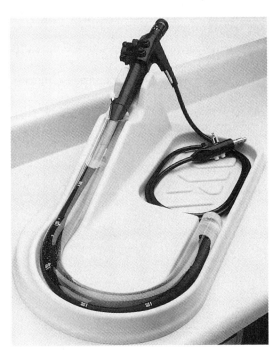

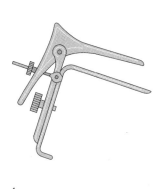

1._____

2._____

3. List all necessary supplies/equipment for:

   a. Pap test/Pelvic examination

     _____
     _____
     _____
     _____
     _____

   b. Sigmoidoscopy

     _____
     _____
     _____
     _____

F. CRITICAL THINKING SITUATION: What would you say? What would you do?

   1. A female patient in her mid-30s is scheduled for a complete physical examination including a Pap test. As you are getting the gown and drape sheet out, she tells you that she is so glad she had time this morning to douche before taking her shower because she wanted to be fresh and clean for the exam. _____

     _____
     _____
     _____

ACHIEVING SKILL COMPETENCY

   Reread the TPO for each procedure and then practice the skills listed below, following the procedure in your textbook.

   Procedure 14-14   Assist with a Gynecological Examination and Pap Test

   Procedure 14-15   Assist with Sigmoidoscopy

   When you feel you have mastered performance of a skill, sign your name on the appropriate evaluation sheet and give it to your instructor to indicate you are prepared to perform the procedure for evaluation.

   After your instructor has returned your work to you, make all necessary corrections and place in a 3-ring notebook for future reference.

ASSIGNMENT SHEET

Chapter 15: SPECIMEN COLLECTION AND LABORATORY PROCEDURES
Unit 1: THE MICROSCOPE

Review the objectives and text for each unit before completing the assignment sheet for that unit in this chapter. When all the sheets for the chapter have been completed, remove them from this workbook and give them to the instructor for evaluation.

1. _ _ _ _ _ _   TENUMI
2. _ _ _ _ _ _ _ _ _ _   ECOJTBVEI
3. _ _ _ _ _ _ _ _   DECONNSE
4. _ _ _ _ _ _ _ _ _   NRBILOUCA
5. _ _ _ _ _ _ _ _ _ _   HECNTIACIN
6. _ _ _ _ _ _ _ _ _ _ _ _   IDTEIRNEMAET
7. _ _ _ _ _ _ _ _   NEIMPSCE
8. _ _ _ _ _ _ _   YMGNFAI
9. _ _ _ _ _ _ _ _ _ _   NCMOTPEESA
10. _ _ _ _ _ _ _ _ _   LMOAOCNUR
11. _ _ _ _ _ _ _ _ _ _   CPIETOIRFN

B. COMPLETION

1. The _____ is used to examine objects which cannot be seen with the naked eye.
2. Eyeglasses are not necessary when performing microscopic work because the microscope may be focused to _____ for all visual defects except _____ .
3. A monocular microscope has _____ eyepiece and a binocular microscope has _____ .
4. The microscope should be transported carefully by holding it by the _____ and supporting it with your other hand under the _____ .
5. The shortest objective lens of the microscope magnifies objects _____ larger than can be seen with the naked eye.
6. The _____ power lens of the microscope magnifies objects 40X larger than can be seen with the naked eye.
7. The _____ regulates the amount of light directed on the magnified specimen.
8. The _____ may be raised or lowered in focusing the specimen.
9. The ocular lenses of the microscope should be cleaned with _____ .
10. The _____ dial helps focus the specimen in detail.

Name _____

C. IDENTIFICATION: Label the parts of the microscope:

1. _____
2. _____
3. _____
4. _____
5. _____
6. _____
7. _____
8. _____
9. _____
10. _____

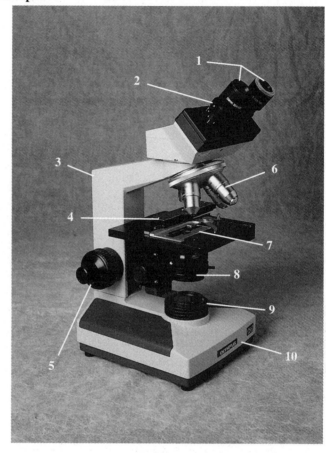

D. COMPLETION

1. Gloving is always a must when handling _____ blood or body fluid specimens.
2. When splashing of any blood/body fluids could be possible while you are working, you should wear
   _____ , _____ , _____ (or _____),
   _____ .
3. Basic proper handwashing _____ and _____ any/all procedures must
   become a habit for all health workers for self-protection from disease _____ .
4. Any break in the skin should be covered with a bandage after handwashing and before _____
   for self-protection against possible _____ .
5. It is important to recap or close bottles, jars, tubes, etc., immediately after use to avoid _____ ,
   _____ , and _____ .
6. Spills should be cleaned up _____ to avoid accidents.
7. Immediate recording of lab results helps to ensure _____ .
8. For better _____ you should work in a well-lighted, properly ventilated, uncluttered, quiet
   area.
9. All sharp items that are disposable should be discarded in a _____ container.
10. _____ should never be broken off or handled after use, but placed intact in a puncture-proof
    biohazardous container.
11. All _____ waste should be discarded in proper containers. .
12. The health care worker should make _____ of all electrical appliances and equipment
    for frayed wires or faulty operation and _____ for repair if needed.
13. Accidents should be reported to your _____ immediately.
14. Emergency telephone numbers should be posted near the _____ in the lab.

15. Before using any electrical appliance or equipment, you should make sure that your hands are _____.

16. First aid items should be available in the lab for _____ use.

17. Loose-fitting or bulk clothing and jewelry should not be worn when working in the lab because it could contribute to _____.

18. Every lab should have an emergency _____, which is functional in preventing further damage to the eyes from chemical splashes.

19. Use gas or air valves and bunsen burners/flames with caution, away from _____ chemicals.

20. Broken glass or any sharp, unusable item should be placed in a sturdy cardboard box or puncture-proof container marked " _____ " and placed in the proper waste receptacle.

21. Marking broken glass or unusable sharp items will protect unsuspecting custodial personnel from _____.

22. The health care worker must _____ lean into the work area in working with flame or chemicals to avoid self-injury or accidents.

23. Chemicals should be poured at _____ to avoid injury and accidents.

24. _____ eat, drink, chew gum, smoke, or place hands or fingers to mouth or place any item in your mouth while working.

25. It is a good practice to designate a " _____ " and a " _____ " area in your lab and enforce this policy to avoid confusion about items.

E. ESSAY ANSWER

1. List the basic recommended standard precautions for health care providers.

_____

a. _____

_____

b. _____

c. _____

d. _____

e. _____

f. _____

2. How can health care providers set a good example for patients regarding health habits? _____

_____

_____

3. When and how and why should you clean up spills in the lab or facility? _____

_____

_____

_____

4. How do you clean up spilled blood (or other body fluids)? _____

_____

_____

_____

_____

5. Why should patients be given both verbal and written instructions for procedures/tests? _____

_____

_____

_____

_____

ACHIEVING SKILL COMPETENCY

Reread the TPO for this procedure and then practice the skill listed below, following the procedure in your textbook.

Procedure 15-1   Using the Microscope

When you feel you have mastered performance of a skill, sign your name on the appropriate evaluation sheet and give it to your instructor to indicate you are prepared to perform the procedure for evaluation.

After your instructor has returned your work to you, make all necessary corrections and place in a 3-ring notebook for future reference.

ASSIGNMENT SHEET

Chapter 15
Unit 2: CAPILLARY BLOOD TESTS

A. FILL IN THE BLANKS: Use the Words to Know in this unit.

1. _ _ _ _ _ _ _ _ E _ _ _ _ _ _ _ _ _ _ _
2. _ _ _ _ _ _ _ R _ _
   P H E N Y L K E T O N U R I A
3. _ T _ _
4. _ H _ _ _ _ _ _ _ _ _ _ _
5. _ _ R _ _ _ _ _ _ _
6. _ _ _ _ _ O _ _ _ _ _ _ _
7. P _ _ _ _ _
8. _ _ _ O _ _ _ _ _ _
9. _ I _ _ _ _ _ _ _ _ _ _ _
10. _ _ E _ _ _ _
11. _ _ _ _ _ S _ _
12. _ I _ _ _ _ _
13. _ _ _ _ _ _ _ S _

B. COMPLETE THE FOLLOWING STATEMENTS

1. Laboratory instructions must be followed exactly in _____ , _____ , _____ , and sending all specimens for analysis.
2. The medical assistant should alert the physician of abnormal laboratory findings by circling or underlining them in _____ .
3. Skin puncture is performed to obtain a _____ blood specimen.
4. Capillary blood tests are performed when _____ of blood is required.
5. _____ is a congenital disease due to a defect in the _____ of the amino acid, phenylalanine.
6. PKU tests are required by law in _____ and in _____ .
7. H and H is an abbreviation for _____ and _____ .
8. A skin puncture site should be approximately _____ deep to allow sufficient blood flow for capillary tests.
9. The microhematocrit fills quickly by _____ .
10. The three layers which blood is separated into after centrifugation in a microhematocrit tube are _____ , _____ , and _____ .
11. The hematocrit is expressed as the _____ of the total blood volume in cubic centimeters of erythrocytes packed by _____ .
12. When performing skin puncture procedures, the first drop of blood is blotted away because it may contain _____ or _____ .
13. The normal hematocrit range for adult males is _____ and for adult females _____ .
14. The function of the red blood cell is to transport _____ and carry _____ from the cells.
15. Patients who complain of lack of energy or fatigue may possibly be suffering from _____ .

16. _____ should be worn when working with blood or any body fluids.

17. The purpose of a GGT (standard glucose tolerance test) is to determine a patient's ability to metabolize
_____ .

18. Many physicians order a _____ GTT.

19. Patients scheduled for a GTT must _____ from midnight or 8 to 12 hours before the test.

20. It is a possibility that patients feel weakness and may faint during a _____ .

21. During a GTT, the blood glucose level falls as _____ is secreted into the blood in reaction to the glucose that has been ingested.

22. The normal blood glucose range is _____ .

23. The _____ is made preferably with fresh whole blood.

24. Name the five types of white blood cells in a differential count.

a. _____   d. _____

b. _____   e. _____

c. _____

25. Draw, color, and label each of the blood cells of the differential WBC count.

26. Draw, color, and label RBCs and platelets (refer to Fig. 15-23).

C. IDENTIFICATION: Label this centrifuged microhematocrit tube.

D. TRUE OR FALSE: Place a "T" for True or an "F" for False in front of each of the following statements.

_____ 1. A blood smear should have an even distribution of cells and end in a feathered tip.

_____ 2. A blood smear can be made with either venous or capillary blood.

_____ 3. The best blood smears are those that are made with old blood from the refrigerator.

_____ 4. Both fasting blood and urine samples are taken in a GTT.

_____ 5. Patients may come and go during a GTT as long as they are on time every hour to have the test performed.

E. MATCHING: Match the definitions

Column I

_____ 1. Capillaries
_____ 2. 12 to 16 grams/100 ml blood
_____ 3. Hematology
_____ 4. PKU test
_____ 5. Skin puncture sites
_____ 6. Hematocrit
_____ 7. Centrifugal action
_____ 8. Fasting
_____ 9. 14 to 18 grams/100 ml of blood
_____ 10. Phenylalanine
_____ 11. Fasting blood glucose range
_____ 12. Hemoglobin
_____ 13. 5,000 to 10,000
_____ 14. Anemia
_____ 15. Differential

Column II

a. Limited to neonates
b. Packed red blood cells
c. Separates blood components
d. Arteries
e. Convey blood from arteries to other venules
f. An amino acid
g. Normal hemoglobin range for females
h. Study of blood and its components
i. Ring/great finger, ear lobe, infant's heel or great toe
j. Erythrocytes
k. Decrease in the number of RBCs
l. Normal hemoglobin range for males
m. Nothing to eat or drink for specified time
n. 80 to 120 mg/100 ml of blood
o. Normal WBC count range
p. Carbon dioxide
q. Iron carrying protein components in blood
r. Test to determine the number of each type of WBCs

F. IDENTIFICATION: Identify these blood cells:

1. _____

2. _____

3. _____

4. _____

5. _____

6. _____

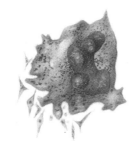

7. _____

G. CROSSWORD PUZZLE

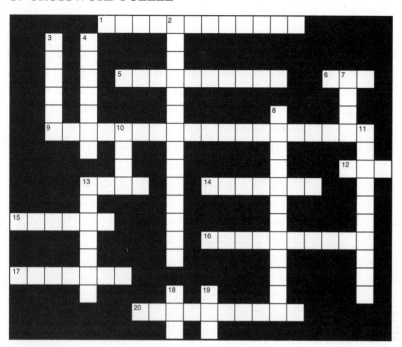

ACROSS

1. Test to determine the number and percentage of WBCs
5. Must never open while spinning
6. Physicians' office laboratory
9. The body's system that removes worn out RBCs
12. Leukocyte
13. Immediately!
14. Sugar
15. Used for skin puncture
16. Volume of packed RBCs
17. Secreted by the Islets of Langerhans
20. Sum of all physical and chemical changes in the body

DOWN

2. Formation of RBCs
3. Relinquish; exemption
4. New born infant
7. Occupational Health and Safety Administration
8. Process of WBCs eating foreign cells
10. Clinical Laboratory Improvement Amendment
11. Place where diagnostic tests are performed
13. Needles used for skin puncture should be this
18. Glucose tolerance test
19. Erythrocyte

H. BRIEF ANSWER

1. What is the purpose of wearing latex gloves in performing laboratory procedures? _____

_____

2. List the regulatory bodies that govern the POL and explain why this is necessary. _____

_____

_____

3. List lab practices that yield quality assurance in the POL. _____

_____

4. What are waivered tests? _____

_____

5. List three laboratory tests from each of the sections in Table 15-1 of your textbook. Use reference books to explain the purpose of each test and patient preparation as indicated for each. _____

_____

6. What are the practices health care providers should follow to ensure reliable and accurate data and quality health care to patients? _____

    a. _____

    b. _____

    c. _____

    d. _____

    e. _____

7. For tests performed in the POL, what should the log book include?

    a. _____

    b. _____

    c. _____

    d. _____

    e. _____

ACHIEVING SKILL COMPETENCY

Reread the TPO for these procedures and then practice the skills listed below, following the procedure in your textbook.

Procedure 15-2	Puncture Skin with Sterile Lancet
Procedure 15-3	Obtain Blood for PKU Test
Procedure 15-4	Determine Hematocrit (Hct) Using Microhematocrit Centrifuge
Procedure 15-5	Hemoglobin (Hb) Determination Using the Hemoglobinometer
Procedure 15-6	Screen Blood Sugar (Glucose) Level
Procedure 15-7	Count Erythrocytes (RBCs) Manually
Procedure 15-8	Count Leukocytes (WBCs) Manually
Procedure 15-9	Making a Blood Smear

When you feel you have mastered performance of a skill, sign your name on the appropriate evaluation sheet and give it to your instructor to indicate you are prepared to perform the procedure for evaluation.

After your instructor has returned your work to you, make all necessary corrections and place in a 3-ring notebook for future reference.

ASSIGNMENT SHEET

Chapter 15
Unit 3: VENOUS BLOOD TESTS

A. SPELLING: Each line contains four different spellings of a word. Underline the correctly spelled word.

1. Coageulate	Coagulate	Coagulade	Cogulate
2. Consiousness	Conseousness	Consciousness	Consciouseness
3. Elasticity	Elasticiety	Elastisity	Elosticity
4. Angorge	Engarge	Ingorge	Engorge
5. Hemolysis	Himolysis	Hemolisis	Hemolyesis
6. Hemotoma	Hematoma	Himotoma	Hemitoma
7. Legable	Ledgible	Legoble	Legible
8. Prothrombin	Prothromben	Prothrombon	Prothrambin
9. Tournequet	Tourniquiet	Tourniquet	Tournaquat
10. Venipuncture	Veniapuncture	Venapuncture	Venipunkture

B. BRIEF ANSWER

1. The surgical puncture of a vein is termed _____.

2. A means of promoting better palpation and sometimes visual position of the vein is a _____.

3. A _____ is a collection of blood just under the skin.

4. Applying _____ immediately following venipuncture will reduce the possibility of a hematoma.

5. The two methods for obtaining venous blood specimens are

   a. _____

   b. _____

6. The breakdown of blood cells is termed _____.

7. Blood drawn in blue stoppered tubes should be done within _____ hours.

8. Tubes used to collect whole blood for various tests contain a(n) _____.

9. _____ is a clear, light yellow liquid which is obtained from whole blood which has been allowed to clot and then _____.

10. Information necessary to perform various blood tests for patients should contain

   a. _____

   b. _____

   c. _____

   d. _____

   e. _____

   f. _____

   g. _____

   h. _____

   i. _____

11. _____ should be written on the lab request form if results are needed immediately.

12. Cell deterioration may be prevented by _____ the blood specimen if it must be kept for over _____ hours.

13. The rate at which red blood cells settle in a particular calibrated tube within a given amount of time is called a(n) _____.

14. _____ is required to perform an ESR and should be done within two hours after it is obtained.

15. The SED rate is useful in the diagnosis and evaluation of diseases of the _____ and in _____ , _____ and collagen's patients.

16. List the four most commonly used colors to code blood specimen tubes and tell what they stand for.

    a. _____

    b. _____

    c. _____

    d. _____

17. During the venipuncture procedure the tourniquet must never be left on the patient's arm longer than _____ .

C. MATCHING: Match these commonly performed lab tests with their normal values:

Column I

Column II

_____ 1. Hemoglobin a. 4 to 5 mEq/L

_____ 2. BUN b. 5,000 to 10,000/cu mm

_____ 3. LDL cholesterol c. 130 to 200 mg/dl

_____ 4. Sed Rate d. 35.5 to 49%

_____ 5. CO e. 11 to 13 sec

_____ 6. Triglyceride f. 80 to 120 mg/dl

_____ 7. RBC count g. 132 to 142 mEq/L

_____ 8. Creatinine h. 3.5 to 7.5 mg/dl

_____ 9. Potassium i. 0 to 10 mm/hr

_____ 10. Total cholesterol j. 90 to 130 mg/dl

_____ 11. Hematocrit k. 8 to 20 mg/dl

_____ 12. Uric acid l. 12 to 16 g/dl

_____ 13. WBC count m. 98 to 106 mEq/L

_____ 14. Glucose n. 0 to 15 mm/hr

_____ 15. Pro time o. 40 to 150 mg/dl

_____ 16. HDL cholesterol p. 3.5 to 5.5 × 10/cu mm

_____ 17. ESR Wintrobe method q. 150,000 to 350,000/cu mm

_____ 18. Sodium r. 0.7 to 1.4 mg/dl

_____ 19. Platelet count s. 25 to 32 mEq/L

_____ 20. Chloride t. 0 to 20 mm/hr

u. 45 to 65 mg/dl

D. BRIEF ANSWER

1. In compliance with quality control and quality assurance regulations, what information must be kept in the POL log book?

    a. _____

    b. _____

    c. _____

    d. _____

    e. _____

    f. _____

2. Explain how to package blood specimens for analysis to out-of-town/state laboratories. _____

_____

_____

3. What is the purpose of a Saf-T-click shielded blood needle adapter? _____

_____

4. How does the Saf-T-click shielded blood needle adapter work? _____

_____

E. TRUE OR FALSE: Place a "T" for True or an "F" for False in front of each of the following statements.

_____ 1. Veins carry blood to the heart.

_____ 2. Some patients feel anxious about blood tests and may experience nausea.

_____ 3. A patient should have the arm supported for the venipuncture procedure.

_____ 4. Laws regarding venipuncture are the same everywhere.

_____ 5. Veins have some elasticity and will give somewhat when depressed.

_____ 6. Gentle mixing of blood with an anticoagulant in a figure-eight motion helps prevent hemolysis.

_____ 7. The needle guard should be kept over the needle to protect it from contamination and to prevent injuries.

_____ 8. The bevel of the needle should be down when inserting it for the venipuncture procedure.

_____ 9. Following the syringe method of venipuncture, the entire syringe and needle must be placed (intact) in a puncture-proof receptacle.

_____ 10. The same pair of gloves may be worn all day as long as one performs proper handwashing technique before and after each procedure.

_____ 11. All breaks in the skin must be covered with a bandage to protect the health care worker from transmitting or contracting disease.

_____ 12. Health care workers should make it a habit to practice standard universal precaution recommendations.

ACHIEVING SKILL COMPETENCY

Reread the TPO for this procedure and then practice the skills listed below, following the procedure in your textbook.

Procedure 15-10   Obtain Venous Blood with Butterfly Needle Method
Procedure 15-11   Obtain Venous Blood with Sterile Needle and Syringe
Procedure 15-12   Obtain Venous Blood with Vacuum Tube
Procedure 15-13   Complete an ESR Using the Wintrobe Method

When you feel you have mastered performance of a skill, sign your name on the appropriate evaluation sheet and give it to your instructor to indicate you are prepared to perform the procedure for evaluation.

After your instructor has returned your work to you, make all necessary corrections and place in a 3-ring notebook for future reference.

ASSIGNMENT SHEET

Chapter 15
Unit 4: BODY FLUID SPECIMENS

A. MATCHING: Match the Words to Know in Column I with their meanings in Column II.

Column I	Column II
_____ 1. Amber	a. Quantity not sufficient
_____ 2. Caustic	b. Urination
_____ 3. Occult	c. Clear urine after centrifugation
_____ 4. Crenated	d. Cloudiness
_____ 5. Feces	e. Examination of urine
_____ 6. Micturition	f. Last menstrual period
_____ 7. Dextrose	g. Rusty color of urine
_____ 8. Random	h. Diagnostic
_____ 9. Supernatant	i. Shrunken (RBC)
_____ 10. Turbidity	j. Hidden
_____ 11. Urinalysis	k. Glucose/sugar
_____ 12. UTI	l. Can burn
_____ 13. LMP	m. Stool
_____ 14. QNS	n. Unplanned
	o. Calibrated
	p. Urinary tract infection

B. BRIEF ANSWER

1. Explain
   a. Clean-catch midstream urine specimen. _____

   _____

   b. Catheterization. _____

   _____

   c. Infant urine collection. _____

   _____

2. The three parts of a complete urinalysis are:
   a. _____
   b. _____
   c. _____

3. Distilled water has a specific gravity of _____

4. _____ are chemically treated paper which react with urine to determine the presence of waste substances in the body.

5. Urine specimens should be kept _____ until analysis can be performed to avoid the growth of _____ or _____ .

6. Each specimen sent for laboratory analysis must have a _____ completed and attached to it for proper processing.

7. When performing urinary catheterization, the health care worker must always wear _____ .

8. Standard (Universal) precautions state that all health care workers should wear gloves when working with any _____ and _____ .

C. MULTIPLE CHOICE

_____ 1. To avoid bacteria growth and decomposition of cells, urinalysis should be performed within

    a. 1 hour   b. 45 minutes   c. 2 hours   d. 4 hours

_____ 2. Catheterization is performed

    a. to obtain a sterile urine specimen for analysis   c. to instill medication into the bladder
    b. for relief of urinary retention   d. all of these

_____ 3. The normal range of specific gravity of urine is

    a. 1.000-1.500   b. 1.010-1.025   c. 1.020-1.025   d. 1.030-1.035

_____ 4. Urine with a strong ammonia-like odor may be alkaline from a high concentration of

    a. bacteria   b. fungus   c. sugar   d. blood

_____ 5. The pH range for normal urine is from

    a. 1-3   b. 3-5   c. 5-7   d. 7-9

_____ 6. Ketone (acetone) bodies present in urine are the result of metabolized

    a. fat   b. sugar   c. starches   d. bulk

_____ 7. Before performing any urine test the specimen should first be

    a. centrifuged   b. heated   c. stirred   d. refrigerated

_____ 8. Cancer is detected from sputum specimens by the

    a. Gram stain   b. gentian violet   c. Wright stain   d. Papanicolaou
                               stain   stain

_____ 9. Examination of fecal material (stool specimens) may determine the presence of

    a. microbial organisms   b. ova   c. occult blood   d. All of these

D. BRIEF ANSWER

1. What patient education would you give to patients regarding:
    a. the respiratory system _____

    _____

    b. the digestive system _____

    _____

2. How do you collect a specimen for drug/alcohol analysis? _____

_____

3. What should you make patients aware of in completing the form for substance analysis? _____

_____

4. List all who should receive a copy of the substance analysis form.
    a. _____   d. _____
    b. _____   e. _____
    c. _____

5. What information should be included regarding samples for substance analysis?

   a. _____

   b. _____

   c. _____

   d. _____

   e. _____

6. What does the substance analysis screen for? _____

_____

E. CRITICAL THINKING SITUATIONS: What would you say? What would you do?

1. A 10-year-old patient needs to have his hemoglobin checked. He wants you to use his little finger to obtain the blood sample. _____

_____

2. A patient calls to ask if she can run errands in between the times that you take blood and urine samples for her GTT scheduled for tomorrow morning. _____

_____

3. A patient calls to inform you that the scheduled first morning urine sample will have to be dropped off after work tomorrow. _____

_____

ACHIEVING SKILL COMPETENCY

Reread the TPO for these procedures and then practice the skills listed below, following the procedure in your textbook.

Procedure 15-14	Catheterize Urinary Bladder
Procedure 15-15	Test Urine with Multistix>> 10 SG
Procedure 15-16	Determine Glucose Content of Urine with Clinitest Tablet
Procedure 15-17	Obtain Urine Sediment for Microscopic Examination
Procedure 15-18	Instruct Patient to Collect Sputum Specimen
Procedure 15-19	Instruct Patient to Collect Stool Specimen

   When you feel you have mastered performance of a skill, sign your name on the appropriate evaluation sheet and give it to your instructor to indicate you are prepared to perform the procedure for evaluation.

   After your instructor has returned your work to you, make all necessary corrections and place in a 3-ring notebook for future reference.

ASSIGNMENT SHEET

Chapter 15
Unit 5: BACTERIAL SMEARS AND CULTURES

A. COMPLETION

1. _____ is a gelatinlike substance, mixed with sheep's blood that encourages the growth of microorganisms in a petri dish.
2. Gram-positive bacteria take a _____ color from the Gram-stain procedure.
3. _____ bacteria take a red or pink color from the counter stain in the Gram-stain procedure.
4. The purpose of Gram-staining is to make heat-fixed bacteria visible for _____ examination.

B. BRIEF ANSWER

1. Explain how to obtain a bacteriological smear. _____
   _____
   _____
2. Explain how to heat-fix a bacteriological smear for staining. _____
   _____
3. Why is heat-fixing necessary? _____
   _____
   _____
4. What is the purpose of culturing? _____
   _____
5. Why are culture plates placed upside down in the incubator? _____
   _____
   _____
6. Name the diseases caused by Gram-positive bacteria. _____
   _____
7. Name the diseases caused by Gram-negative bacteria. _____
   _____
   _____
8. Why is it necessary to stain bacteria? _____
   _____
9. How are bacteria identified? _____
   _____
10. Why must all solutions be recapped immediately after each use? _____
    _____
    _____
11. Why must gloves be worn when working with bacterial smears and cultures? _____
    _____
    _____
    _____
    _____
12. What patient education could you offer a patient while preparing or obtaining a throat culture? _____
    _____
    _____
    _____
    _____

C. MATCHING: Place the correct letter from Column II on the line to the left of Column I.

Column I

_____ 1. Breaks infection cycle
_____ 2. Staphylococci
_____ 3. Nasopharyngeal culture
_____ 4. Diplococci
_____ 5. Streptococci
_____ 6. Incubation period for cultures
_____ 7. Blue flame
_____ 8. Alcohol/acetone
_____ 9. Destroys specimen
_____ 10. Spore forming bacteria

Column II

a. Bacteria that form pairs
b. 23-48 hours
c. Hottest
d. Proper handwashing and sterile technique
e. Excessive heating
f. Form grape-like clusters
g. NPC
h. Bacteria appearing in chains
i. Crystal violet
j. Helpful in removing dye
k. Immersion oil
l. Have capsule-like coverings

D. CROSSWORD PUZZLE CLUES

ACROSS

5. Means passed through a flame
7. Nutrient for microorganisms
8. Gram-positive bacteria stain
10. Gram-negative bacteria stain
12. Cultures streaked with a fine wire _____
14. Means of isolating disease-causing organisms
15. Must be sterile to obtain sample
16. Clear plastic dish with lid
20. Wear latex gloves to obtain a bacteriological _____
21. Have certain characteristic formations and shapes
23. Blue part is the hottest
24. Abbreviation for identification
25. Fill with dye for gram stain

DOWN

1. What a bacteriological smear is made on
2. Bacteria are classified by
3. Purpose of the bacteriological smear is to identify _____
4. Take care in handling
6. Crystal violet
9. Gelatin-like substance
11. Provides proper growth temperature for cultures
13. Roll specimen on to slide to _____ microorganisms
17. Use in gram stain procedure
18. Bacteria in clusters
19. Purpose of procedure is for identification of bacteria
22. Allow specimens to _____ dry

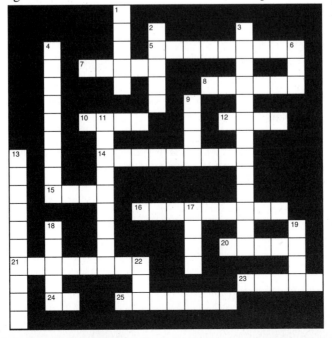

E. IDENTIFY THESE BACTERIAL SHAPES

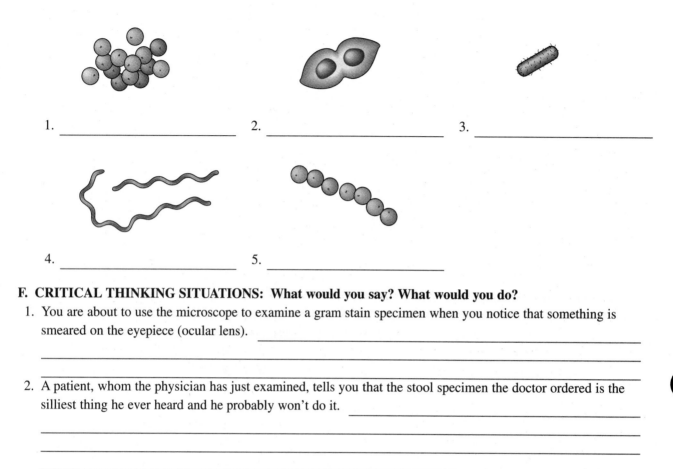

1. _____   2. _____   3. _____

4. _____   5. _____

F. CRITICAL THINKING SITUATIONS: What would you say? What would you do?

1. You are about to use the microscope to examine a gram stain specimen when you notice that something is smeared on the eyepiece (ocular lens). _____
   _____
   _____

2. A patient, whom the physician has just examined, tells you that the stool specimen the doctor ordered is the silliest thing he ever heard and he probably won't do it. _____
   _____
   _____
   _____

ACHIEVING SKILL COMPETENCY

Reread the TPO for these procedures and then practice the skills listed below, following the procedure in your textbook.

Procedure 15-21	Prepare Bacteriological Smear
Procedure 15-22	Obtain a Throat Culture
Procedure 15-23	Prepare a Gram Stain

When you feel you have mastered performance of a skill, sign your name on the appropriate evaluation sheet and give it to your instructor to indicate you are prepared to perform the procedure for evaluation.

After your instructor has returned your work to you, make all necessary corrections and place in a 3-ring notebook for future reference.

ASSIGNMENT SHEET

Chapter 16: DIAGNOSTIC TESTS, X-RAYS, AND PROCEDURES
Unit 1: DIAGNOSTIC TESTS

A. WORD SEARCH: Find the words listed below:

ALLERGY	HISTAMINE
INJECTION	SERUM
DILUTE	ADRENALINE
INTERPRET	ITCH
ANTIBODY	SYMPTOM
HYPERSENSITIVE	WHEAL
EXTRACT	SYSTEMATIC
CONTACT DERMATITIS	VENOM
NOTE	GAUGE
EOSINOPHIL	TIME
KIT	SHOCK

```
G  E  D  C  A  R  T  J  P  F  J  K  T  G  K  L  B  T
A  O  I  N  J  E  C  T  I  O  N  M  U  N  G  J  L  H
L  R  L  K  R  A  O  A  J  L  S  V  D  H  L  K  B  W
L  K  U  C  J  S  N  B  I  N  T  E  R  P  R  E  T  C
E  X  T  R  A  C  T  E  J  P  Z  N  P  F  L  O  B  P
R  Z  E  C  R  H  A  N  T  I  B  O  D  Y  D  S  R  W
G  L  V  A  M  B  C  R  D  O  A  M  K  A  B  I  F  D
Y  B  Q  D  P  T  T  N  S  E  R  U  M  W  G  N  C  C
N  S  T  R  B  C  D  A  J  T  J  T  W  H  C  O  U  K
H  Y  P  E  R  S  E  N  S  I  T  I  V  E  K  P  I  Z
I  N  S  N  A  P  R  S  Y  Z  L  T  I  A  D  H  U  O
S  R  E  A  G  K  M  K  M  K  Y  C  O  L  P  I  H  K
T  I  M  L  L  R  A  B  P  M  E  H  T  K  F  L  N  T
A  L  O  I  O  H  T  C  T  O  G  A  G  O  W  O  R  I
M  S  Y  N  T  D  I  F  O  E  A  B  C  S  E  S  U  M
I  B  K  E  Z  N  T  N  M  Z  U  H  I  H  O  H  H  E
N  O  T  E  D  E  I  G  R  E  G  K  Z  O  A  O  E  K
E  V  E  S  B  O  S  Y  S  T  E  M  A  T  I  C  E  C
K  I  Q  T  Z  L  P  C  R  E  O  D  U  P  N  K  I  T
```

Name _____

B. TRUE OR FALSE: Answer the following statements with "T" for True or "F" for False.

_____ 1. A positive allergic reaction to a skin test is shown by a raised area on the skin called a wheal.

_____ 2. Wheals are measured in inches.

_____ 3. Reactions to scratch tests usually occur within the first 20 minutes.

_____ 4. Intradermal tests are sometimes used by physicians to determine medicine sensitivity or immunization needs.

_____ 5. The patch test is read after a 12 hour and a 20 hour time period.

C. SENTENCE COMPLETION

1. _____ are utilized to determine allergic reactions in patients.

2. Desirable sites for the _____ test are the arms and back.

3. The _____ test is done to determine the cause of contact dermatitis.

4. In performing the intradermal test, the antigen is introduced into the dermal layer of skin in dosages of _____ to _____ by sterile technique.

5. For accurate test results the expiration date of the _____ should be checked each time before use.

6. It may be necessary to _____ small children to successfully perform skin tests.

7. A life-threatening allergic reaction must be counteracted with an injection of _____ to prevent anaphylactic shock.

8. Symptoms of _____ initially include intense anxiety, weakness, sweating, and shortness of breath.

9. Patients refer to desensitizing injections of allergy serum as _____ .

10. It is a good practice to alternate arms of patients who have frequent allergy serum injections to prevent _____ .

11. The medical assistant's role in diagnostic tests and procedures is to _____ and _____ patients.

D. MATCHING

_____ 1. antibody   A. released in allergic/inflammatory reactions
_____ 2. immune   B. of or pertaining to the whole body
_____ 3. venom   C. immunizing agent that produces antibodies
_____ 4. histamine   D. protected or exempt from a disease
_____ 5. systemic   E. a protein substance carried by cells to counteract effects of an antigen
_____ 6. antigen   F. pertaining to tissue
_____ 7. extract   G. a poisonous secretion
                       H. a substance distilled or drawn out of another substance

E. ESSAY ANSWER

1. List patient education regarding allergy injections.

_____
_____
_____
_____

2. Explain how you would advise a new allergy patient about scheduling desensitizing injections and other instructions.

_____
_____
_____
_____

ACHIEVING SKILL COMPETENCY

Reread the TPO for these procedures and then practice the skills listed below, following the procedure in your textbook.

Procedure 16-1	Perform a Scratch Test
Procedure 16-2	Apply a Patch Test

When you feel you have mastered the performance of the skill, sign your name on the appropriate evaluation sheet and give it to your instructor to indicate you are prepared to perform the procedure for evaluation.

After your instructor has returned your work to you, make all necessary corrections and place in a 3-ring notebook for future reference.

ASSIGNMENT SHEET

Chapter 16: DIAGNOSTIC TESTS, X-RAYS, AND PROCEDURES
Unit 2: CARDIOLOGY PROCEDURES

A. MATCHING: Match the definitions from Column II with the correct terms in Column I.

Column I

_____ 1. Artifacts
_____ 2. Somatic
_____ 3. Segment
_____ 4. Repolarization
_____ 5. Purkinje
_____ 6. Augmented
_____ 7. Sedentary
_____ 8. Galvanometer
_____ 9. Precordial
_____ 10. Voltage
_____ 11. Interval
_____ 12. Electrode
_____ 13. Standardization
_____ 14. Impulse
_____ 15. Stylus

Column II

a. Enlarged
b. Electrocardiogram
c. Little activity
d. Additional electrical activity
e. Changes impulses into mechanical motion
f. Chest leads
g. Difference in electrical potential
h. Fibers which cause muscles of the ventricle to contract
i. Momentary surge of current
j. Provides a reliable reading
k. Muscle voltage artifacts
l. Provides printed representations of EKG paper
m. Period when heart momentarily relaxes
n. Bectrolyte
o. Metal sensors which pick up electrical impulses
p. Portion of EKG between two waves
q. Length of a wave

B. MULTIPLE CHOICE: Select the correct letter for the following statements and place it on the line to the left of the number.

_____ 1. The EKG is interpreted by the _____ .

   a. lab technician   b. medical assistant   c. physician   d. nurse practitioner

_____ 2. The first impulse recorded on the graph paper in the EKG cycle is the _____ wave.

   a. T   b. P   c. R   d. Q

_____ 3. The routine EKG consists of _____ leads.

   a. 6   b. 10   c. 8   d. 12

_____ 4. The patient must be _____ for a good tracing to be obtained.

   a. sleeping   b. standing   c. relaxed   d. unconscious

_____ 5. Metal electrodes should be cleaned with _____ .

   a. mild detergent/   b. alcohol/ether   c. baking soda/water   d. mild detergent/silver
      scouring powder   polish

_____ 6. A proper amount of _____ must be used with each metal electrode to provide maximum

    a. alcohol   b. electrolyte   c. oil   d. powder

_____ 7. The _____ of the EKG is necessary to enable a physician to judge deviations from the

    a. length   b. quality   c. standardization   d. augmentation

_____ 8. The usual standardization mark is _____ in size.

    a. 1 mm wide   b. 2 mm wide   c. 1 mm wide   d. 2 mm wide
      and 10 mm high   and 5 mm high   and 5 mm high   and 10 mm high

_____ 9. If the tracing is too large, the _____ button should be turned down to one half.

    a. sensitivity   b. stylus   c. selector   d. on/off

_____ 10. The tracing paper is normally run at a speed _____ mm/second.

    a. 15   b. 25   c. 50   d. 75

C. IDENTIFICATION: Label these diagrams of the ECG cycle:

1. Place the correct letter for each wave of the ECG tracing on the line next to the number in the following:

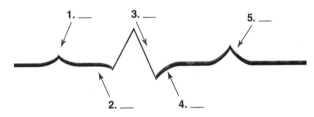

2. Label the numbered lines below with the correct name of each area of the electrical conduction through the heart:

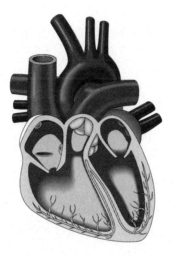

D. COMPLETION

1. All muscle movement produces _____.
2. The current enters the electrocardiograph through the wires to reach the _____.
3. The amplifier _____ the electrical impulses.
4. Electrical impulses are transformed into mechanical motion by the _____.
5. A _____ produces printed representations on EKG paper.
6. An electrical impulse originates in the modified myocardial tissue in the _____.
7. The first impulse recorded on the EKG paper from the atrial contraction is known as the _____.
8. When the muscles of the ventricles contract, the _____ of waves are produced on the EKG paper.
9. During the recovery of the ventricles the _____ is produced.
10. A routine EKG consists of _____ leads.
11. _____ means to make larger.
12. Chest leads are also called _____ leads.
13. AC or _____ current interference is caused by additional electrical activity.
14. The standardization mark is included in an EKG to provide a _____ reading.
15. The tracing paper is normally run at a speed of _____ per second.

E. CROSSWORD PUZZLE

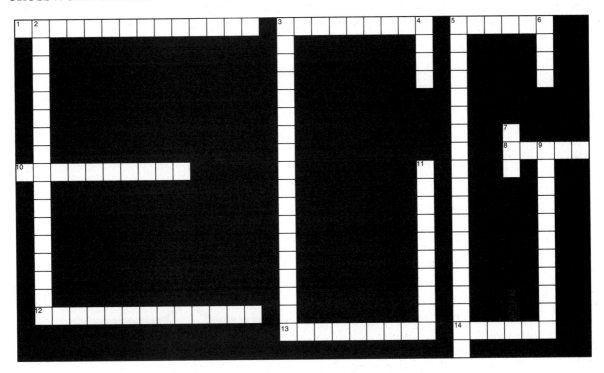

ACROSS
1. Time of recovery before heart contracts again
3. Pick up electrical current from patient
5. Produces a printed representation on ECG paper
8. Precordial is another name for _____ leads
10. Irregular heartbeat
12. Ambulatory EKG
13. Inactivity
14. Slight/distant

DOWN
2. Instrument used to record electrical impulses of the heart
3. Permanent record of heart's electrical activity
4. An EKG tech does lots of these
5. These provide a basis for physicians to judge deviations from the standard
6. Immediately!
7. Abbr. for electrocardiogram
9. Used to provide maximum electrical conduction
11. Study of the heart

F. TRUE OR FALSE: Answer the following statements with "T" for True or "F" for False.

_____ 1. In the electrical conduction system, the first area of the heart to receive the electrical impulse is the purkinje fibers.

_____ 2. Shivering from being nervous or cold can cause somatic tremor.

_____ 3. A rhythm strip indicates to the physician the size of a patient's heart.

_____ 4. For better electrode contact the skin sites should be rubbed vigorously to increase circulation.

_____ 5. For single and multi-channel computerized electrocardiographs, you simply press "auto" to run a 12 lead ECG.

_____ 6. It is necessary to shave dense chest hair for placement of electrodes.

_____ 7. Stress test ECGs are performed routinely on all patients.

_____ 8. A fetal monitor is a walking or 24-hour ECG.

_____ 9. Patients should keep a diary of their activities and symptoms during a 24-hour electrocardiogram.

_____ 10. It is important to check the batteries and proper working order of the Holter monitor before applying the device to a patient.

G. Fill in the missing information from this diagrammatic representation of cardiac impulses on EKG tracing: (A) Course of electrical impulses (B) Cardiac muscle reaction to impulses (C) EKG tracing of impulse waves (D) Phases of cardiac cycle

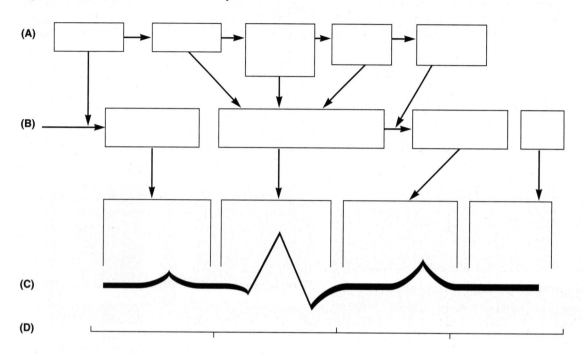

H. CRITICAL THINKING SITUATION: What would you say? What would you do?

1. A patient is being prepped for an EKG and appears to be very apprehensive. She is apparently intimidated by the machine and the wires and expresses a great fear of electric shock.

_____

_____

ACHIEVING SKILL COMPETENCY

   Reread the TPO for this procedure and then practice the skill listed below, following the procedure in your textbook.

   Obtain Standard 12-Lead EKG/ECG

   When you feel you have mastered the performance of the skill, sign your name to the evaluation sheet and give it to your instructor to indicate you are prepared to perform the procedure for evaluation.

   After your instructor has returned your work to you, make all necessary corrections and place in a 3-ring notebook for future reference.

I. LABEL THE ECG TRACINGS: are they abnormalities or interference artifacts?

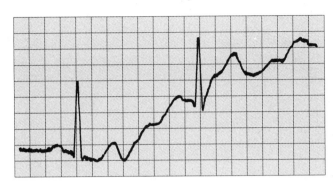

1. _____

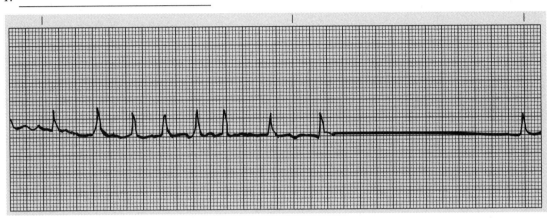

2 _____

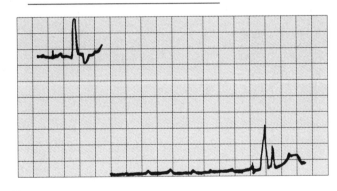

3. _____

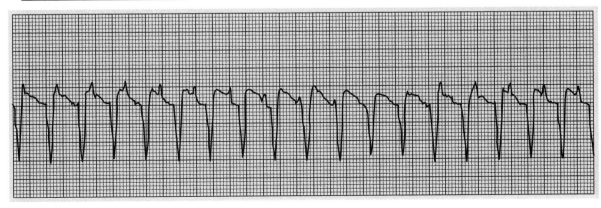

4. _____

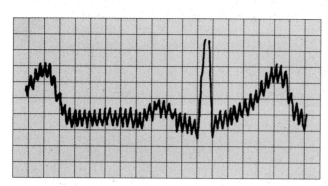

5. _____

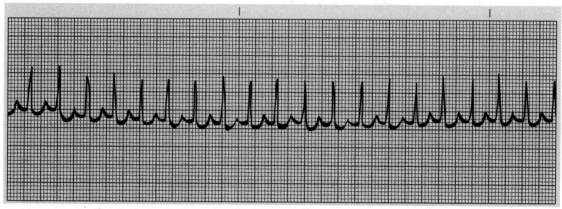

6. _____

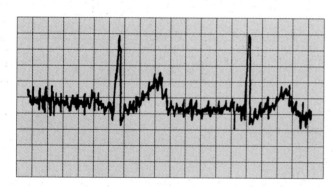

7. _____

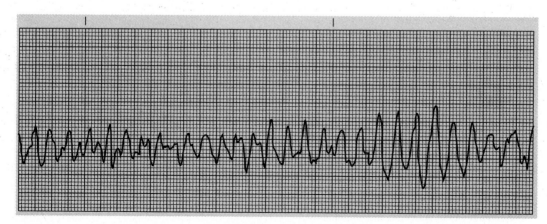

8. _____

ASSIGNMENT SHEET

Chapter 16: DIAGNOSTIC TESTS, X-RAYS, AND PROCEDURES
Unit 3: DIAGNOSTIC PROCEDURES

A. COMPLETION

1. The purpose of the _____ test is to determine the presence of _____ blood in the stool.
2. Vital capacity should equal _____ capacity plus _____ reserve.
3. _____ mouthpieces are used with vital capacity tests to prevent disease transmission.
4. Advising patients to list their concerns and bring them to their next appointment will _____ the number of phone consultations.

B. MATCHING: Match the definitions

Column I

_____ 1. dyspnea
_____ 2. maturity
_____ 3. ultrasound
_____ 4. intermittent
_____ 5. spirometry
_____ 6. resonance
_____ 7. expirations
_____ 8. Hemoccult Sensa
_____ 9. patient education
_____ 10. claustrophobia

Column II

a. coming and going
b. to sound again
c. breathing out; exhaling air
d. fear of being enclosed
e. guaiac reagent strip
f. yields more accurate test results
g. full development
h. difficulty breathing
i. measures hearing
j. measurement of air capacity of lungs
k. vibrations of sound waves

C. WORD SEARCH PUZZLE: Find the words listed below. After you complete the puzzle, use the words numbered 5, 7, 8,10,11,13,14, 16 in a sentence.

1. TEST
2. CONTRAST
3. EARLY
4. POLYPS
5. INVASIVE
6. PATIENT
7. ECHOES
8. GUAIAC
9. REAGENT

10. CLAUSTROPHOBIA
11. OCCULT
12. SPIROMETER
13. IMPLANTS
14. DIAPHANOGRAPHY
15. MAGNETIC
16. IMAGE
17. SONOGRAM

```
C M H M M M R E S A D A S D O S A C P F
J S S A R B R M S P I R O M E T E R B S
I M A G E H R B G L A L D J T N D H L K
L J A N I T K A L C P T I N V A S I V E
Y A C E X N L M P D H J T F R L F C L R
C P A T I E N T O Q A H C F B P Y C M B
M H M I F G S B M S N Y C P L M E G M C
R E C C L A U S T R O P H O B I A P D W
T K L A B E T V A U G C Q Z N P F E R K
S O N O G R A M H U R B C A T T A W B C
W M K B P C T A A G A S D U S R R A J T
P L B T L S G I R S P M H D L C B A P E
Z T F L O K A S H O H M I Y Q T C F S S
R S E O H C E Z S P Y L O P K L H B K T
```

5. Invasive _____
7. Echoes _____
8. Guaiac _____
10. Claustrophobia _____
11. Occult _____
13. Implant _____
14. Diaphanography _____
16. Image _____

D. TRUE OR FALSE: Answer the following statements with "T" for True or "F" for False.

_____ 1. In the spirometry procedure a clip is placed on some patients' noses to encourage them to breathe in deeply through the mouth.

_____ 2. One of your important duties in performing spirometry is to coach patients to completely expel all the air from their lungs quickly.

_____ 3. An oscilloscope is an instrument that shows a picture of converted electrical impulses from the patient during echocardiography.

_____ 4. High frequency sound waves are conducted through the use of a transducer in ultrasonic scanning.

_____ 5. Thermography is a measurement of heat patterns given off by the skin.

_____ 6. Diaphanography is performed by transillumination.

_____ 7. Hemoccult tests are only given to patients who have abdominal distress.

_____ 8. Patients are advised to avoid eating red meats 48 hours prior to and until all three specimens have been obtained for the Hemoccult Sensa test.

E. CRITICAL THINKING SITUATION: What would you say? What would you do?

1. One of your patients who was in for a CPE last month comes in to make an appointment for a family member. There is also a hemoccult test delivered. This completed test has been in the car for 3 weeks and is in a torn and tattered envelope.

_____

_____

_____

ACHIEVING SKILL COMPETENCY

Reread the TPO for this procedure and then practice the skill listed below, following the procedure in your textbook.

Perform a Hemoccult Test

When you feel you have mastered the performance of the skill, sign your name on the appropriate evaluation sheet and give it to your instructor to indicate you are prepared to perform the procedure for evaluation.

After your instructor has returned your work to you, make all necessary corrections and place in a 3-ring notebook for future reference.

ASSIGNMENT SHEET

Chapter 16: DIAGNOSTIC TESTS, X-RAYS, AND PROCEDURES
Unit 4: DIAGNOSTIC RADIOLOGICAL PROCEDURES

A. FILL IN BLANK: Use the Words to Know from Unit 4 in your text

```
_ _ _ _ _ _ _ M _ _ _ _ _ _ _
        _ _ _ _ A _ _ _ _
      _ _ M _ _ _ _ _ _ _ _ _
        _ _ _ M _ _ _ _ _
        _ _ _ O _ _ _ _ _ _ _
        _ _ _ _ G _ _ _
          _ _ R _ _ _
        _ _ _ _ _ A _ _ _ _ _
      _ _ _ _ _ _ P _ _ _ _ _
          _ _ H _ _ _ _ _
            _ _ _ Y
```

B. BRIEF ANSWER

1. What are roentgen rays?

   _____

   _____

2. What are therapeutic X rays used for?

   _____

3. What type of symptoms do patients experience if the gallbladder malfunctions?

   _____

4. What food should patients avoid if they have gallbladder trouble?

   _____

5. Why must the digestive tract be free of foods during an upper GI series?

   _____

   _____

6. Why is air-contrast sometimes ordered with a barium enema examination?

   _____

   _____

7. What is an IVP?

   _____

   _____

   _____

8. What is another term for KUB?

   _____

9. How are patients X-rayed for mammography?

   _____

   _____

10. Describe the method of radiology called a CAT (Computerized Axial Tomography) scan.

   _____

   _____

11. Describe echocardiography.

_____

_____

12. List the steps to prepare patients for a Barium Enema.

_____

_____

_____

13. Describe a barium swallow or upper Gl Series.

_____

_____

14. Explain why pregnant women should not have X rays.

_____

15. List X-ray procedures that do not require patient preparation.

_____

C. MATCHING

_____ 1. Therapeutic X-rays   a. Defines structures of urinary system

_____ 2. Mammography   b. Do not require patient preparation

_____ 3. Evacuants   c. Barium and water mixture

_____ 4. UGI series   d. Flat plate of abdomen

_____ 5. CAT scan   e. Breast self-examination

_____ 6. Bone studies   f. Performed with sterile catheter in conjunction with cystoscopy

_____ 7. IVP   g. Laxatives and enemas

_____ 8. KUB   h. X-ray of different angles of breast tissue

_____ 9. Contrast media   i. Used to treat cancer

_____ 10. Retrograde pyelogram   j. Generates images of tissue in slices about 1 cm thick

   k. Barium swallow

D. MULTIPLE CHOICE

_____ 1. A diagnostic aid frequently requested by physicians that needs no patient preparation is the:

   a. IVP   b. chest X-ray   c. UGI   d. cholecystogram

_____ 2. Diagnostic X rays are _____ in pregnant female patients, especially during the first trimester.

   a. contraindicated   b. indicated   c. important   d. common

_____ 3. Carbonated and alcoholic beverages should be avoided prior to X rays of the visceral organs because they produce:

   a. rashes   b. stones   c. delays   d. flatus

_____ 4. A voiding cystogram may be ordered along with a(n):

   a. UGI   b. KUB   c. IVP   d. BaE

_____ 5. Nuclear medicine is the branch of medicine that uses _____ in the diagnosis and treatment of patients.

   a. xeroradiography   b. radionuclides   c. radioactive materials   d. both B & C

_____ 6. Which X ray is helpful in determining the position of an IUD?

   a. IVP   b. UGI   c. MRI   d.KUB

_____ 7. Breast self-examination is recommended for women of all ages:

   a. daily   b. weekly   c. monthly   d. yearly

_____ 8. All women should have a baseline mammography between the ages of:

     a. 25-39   b. 35-39   c. 45-49   d. 55-59

_____ 9. To reduce the possible effects of swelling and soreness often caused from compression of the breasts during mammography you should instruct patient to omit _____ from their diets 7-10 days prior to the examination.

     a. salt   b. caffeine   c. fats   d. cholesterol

_____ 10. Compression of the breasts during mammography allows a much clearer picture of breast tissue and also requires the use of less:

     a. analgesics   b. time   c. radiation   d. flatus

E. CRITICAL THINKING SITUATION: What would you say? What would you do?

1. A male patient in his late 50s phones to tell you of his discomfort following his barium enema this morning. He says he feels bloated and constipated.

_____

_____

_____

After your instructor has returned your work to you, make all necessary corrections and place in a 3-ring notebook for future reference.

ASSIGNMENT SHEET

Chapter 17: MINOR SURGICAL PROCEDURES
Unit 1: MINOR SURGICAL PROCEDURES

A. WORD PUZZLE: Use the list of Words to Know from this unit.

1. _ _ _ _ _ _ _ _ I _ _ _ _ _ _
                    N

2.   _ C _ _ _ _ _ _ _
                  I

3.   _ _ _ _ S _ _ _ _ _ _
                  I

4.   _ _ _ _ O _ _ _ _
                  N

5. _ _ _ _ _ _ _ _ A _ _ _ _
                  N
                  D
                  D
                  R

6.   A _ _ _ _ _ _ _ _ _ _

7. _ _ _ _ _ _ _ _ I _ _ _
                  N

8 _ _ _ _ _ _ _ _ A _ _ _ _
                  G

9.   _ _ E _ _ _ _ _ _ _

B. BRIEF ANSWER

1. List what you must tell a patient in preparation for minor office surgery

   a. _____

   b. _____

   c. _____

   d. _____

2. What two things should the medical assistant do the day before the scheduled surgery?

   a. _____

   b. _____

3. What is the purpose of the skin preparation before a surgical procedure? _____

   _____

   a. _____

   b. _____

4. Why must the medical assistant be extremely careful to avoid nicking the patient's skin when performing a skin preparation? _____

   _____

5. What must the medical assistant do if asked to assist directly with a surgical procedure?

   _____

6. Other than directly assisting with a surgery procedure, when else should the medical assistant wear surgical gloves, and why? _____
_____

7. List the items included in the basic setup for most minor surgical procedures. _____
_____
_____
_____

8. What types of surgical procedures may the medical assistant be asked to assist with in the medical office/clinic? _____
_____
_____

9. What symptoms should patients look for and report following a surgical procedure?
_____
_____

10. What is the usual recommended post-op diet? _____

11. Why are follow-up visits necessary in patient care? _____

12. Other than the scheduled post-op visit, what can the medical assistant do to follow up with patients?
_____

13. What, in general, can the medical assistant advise patients to do following minor surgery?
_____
_____

14. How should the medical assistant instruct patients to care for the site of surgery. _____
_____

15. What is the purpose of an electrocautery device in minor office surgical procedures? _____
_____

16. Define cryosurgery and state its use. _____
_____

17. Give pre-op instructions to a patient scheduled for a minor surgical procedure. _____
_____

    a. _____
    b. _____
    c. _____
    d. _____
    e. _____

When patient arrives for the appointment:

    a. _____
    b. _____
    c. _____
    d. _____

18. Give post-op instructions to a patient following a minor office surgery.

    a. _____
    b. _____
    c. _____
    d. _____
    e. _____
    f. _____
    g. _____

19. List universal precaution barriers that must be worn by health care providers for invasive procedures.

_____

_____

20. Explain how to care for surgical instruments before use and following use. _____

_____

21. List the important information that must be recorded on the patient's chart regarding a surgical procedure.

_____

_____

22. List the items needed for a skin prep tray. _____

_____

_____

23. What is hemophilia? _____

24. Explain how to properly remove sutures and why. _____

_____

_____

_____

_____

_____

25. Describe how to remove skin staples. _____

_____

_____

26. Describe skin closures and how they are applied. _____

_____

_____

C. MATCHING: Place the correct letter answer from Column II on the line to the left of Column I.

Column I

_____ 1. Local anesthetic
_____ 2. Medical history
_____ 3. I & D
_____ 4. Before surgery
_____ 5. Formalin solution
_____ 6. Necessary
_____ 7. 30° angle
_____ 8. Application of antiseptic
_____ 9. Sterile transfer forceps
_____ 10. After surgery
_____ 11. 6 minutes
_____ 12. IUD
_____ 13. Antiseptic
_____ 14. D & C
_____ 15. Contaminated

Column II

a. Pre-operative
b. Used to place specimen into formalin solution
c. Surgical consent form
d. Dilatation and curettage
e. Post-operative
f. Incision and drainage
g. Skin preparation
h. Administered by physician
i. May help in determining possible allergic reactions
j. Reduces microbial growth
k. Used to preserve tissue specimen
l. Expiration date
m. Angle of shaving surgery site
n. Intrauterine device
o. Circular motions
p. Unsterile
q. Thorough surgical scrub

D. IDENTIFY:

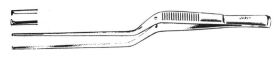

1. _____

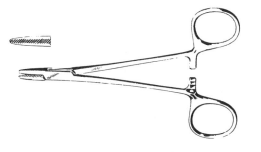

8. _____

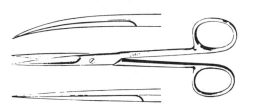

2. _____

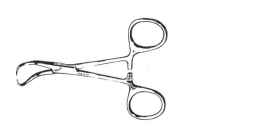

9. _____

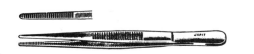

3. _____

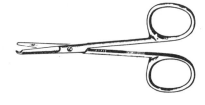

10. _____

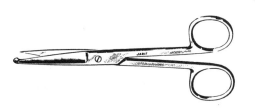

4. _____

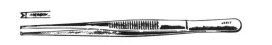

11. _____

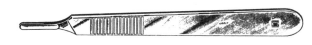

5. _____

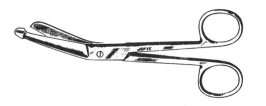

12. _____

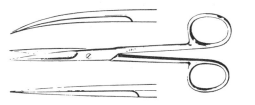

6. _____

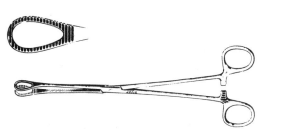

7. _____

E. MULTIPLE CHOICE

_____ 1. This process uses subfreezing temperature to destroy/remove tissue.
   a. electrocautery   c. diathermy
   b. cryosurgery   d. chemotherapy

_____ 2. Electrocoagulation is performed with a(n):
   a. cryo unit   c. hyfrecator
   b. autoclave   d. scalpel

_____ 3. A fenestrated sheet is one that has a(n):
   a. fold   c. stain
   b. pleat   d. opening

_____ 4. Autoclaved items remain sterile if they have been properly processed and protected from moisture for:
   a. 3 days   c. 3 weeks
   b. 30 days   d. 3 months

_____ 5. To reduce the possibility of infection for a surgical procedure skin preparation includes:
   a. cleaning the site with a soapy solution c. applying antiseptic solution
   b. shaving the skin   d. all of these

_____ 6. A serious blood clotting disease that occurs mostly in males is called:
   a. hemophilia   c. hematuria
   b. hemophobia   d. hemiplegia

_____ 7. A thorough initial surgical scrub must be performed for _____ minutes:
   a. 2   c. 6
   b. 4   d. 8

_____ 8. Assisting with surgical procedures not only requires knowledge and skill, but
   a. self-discipline   c. empathy
   b. personal integrity   d. all of these

_____ 9. In removing sutures you must be careful to pull the clipped suture _____ the incision to avoid stress on the incision site.
   a. away from   c. into
   b. toward   d. within

_____ 10. Tell patients who are to have skin staples removed that it is normal to feel a _____ sensation during the procedure.
   a. burning   c. nauseated
   b. tugging   d. stinging

_____ 11. Patients are normally requested to fast before surgical procedures because it lessens the possibility of the patient:
   a. bleeding a lot   c. being late
   b. talking too much   d. becoming nauseated

_____ 12. Included in the list of symptoms following a surgical procedure that should be reported to the physician are:
   a. unusual pain, burning or uncomfortable sensation   c. fever, nausea and vomiting
   b. bleeding or discharge   d. all of these

_____ 13. Following suture removal the patient should be instructed to report any sign of infection to the physician immediately and:
   a. keep the site clean and dry with a supportive bandage   c. soak the area four times a day
   b. wear sterile gloves   d. none of these

_____ 14. You should always check the patient's emergency room report for the following information regarding suture removal:

    a. the date and the number of sutures put in

    b. date of patient's tetanus booster

    c. the length of time the sutures were to be left in

    d. all of the above

_____ 15. An ace wrap is a supportive bandage that:

    a. gives an attractive appearance to the injury

    b. increases circulation of the injured area

    c. gives support to the injured limb

    d. B & C

F. WORD SEARCH PUZZLE: Find the words listed below in the word search puzzle.

patient	hemophilia	wart
gloves	polyp	fenestrated
biopsy	anesthesia	antiseptic
authorize	electrocautery	cryosurgery
pre-op	suture	taut
cauterize	histology	post-op

```
G L E X A T R E P A T I E N T R E A
L Q M L Q K B I O P S Y N L R E A S
O Z A B S M Z T L B S R A T K M F D
V K Z N U P A R Y T Z E D G F R B H
E R P K T H O T P M A G M K E B J I
S E W O U I B T G I E R P W N L A S
L Z F Q R H S S S F G U L B E R T T
K I H C E T G E T O L S B F S K C O
P R E O P W H M P X P O D P T S E L
Z O T S A T A U T T K Y N L R F C O
P H W B S G L R O Z I R Z S A X B G
Q T X E E L E C T R O C A U T E R Y
S U N O P Y A I L I H P O M E H E P
C A U T E R I Z E T X C M J D O F D
```

G. COMPLETION: Fill in what's missing in this list of sterile items used in a basic setup for most minor surgical procedures:

1. scalpel handle and _____
2. hemostats
3. _____
4. needles and _____
5. suture scissors
6. _____
7. probe
8. gauze squares
9. vial of _____ medication
10. _____
11. _____
12. towels
13. _____
14. tray

H. CRITICAL THINKING SITUATIONS: What would you say? What would you do?

1. As you are performing a skin prep on a patient for removing a sebaceous cyst from his scalp, he tells you that he is rather nervous about this procedure because he is a hemophiliac. _____

_____

2. A young lady returns to have sutures removed. As you take the bandage off you notice that the sutured laceration site is quite infected. _____

_____

3. You have not been able to clean and sterilize the instruments on the counter because you have been so busy with patient care. A co-worker picked up these instruments and says the doctor needs them for a surgical procedure stat! _____

_____

4. You have set up the suture tray for the physician to suture a 7-yearold's laceration of the right forearm. This child is most curious about everything he sees and asks many questions. The child's mother is with him. You must leave the room to answer a phone call. When you return, the child's mother is in the rest room and the child is touching some of the instruments on the suture tray. _____

_____

_____

_____

ACHIEVING SKILL COMPETENCY

Reread the TPO for these procedures and then practice the skills listed below, following the procedure in your textbook.

Procedure 17-1	Prepare Skin for Minor Surgery
Procedure 17-2	Put on Sterile Gloves
Procedure 17-3	Assist with Minor Surgery
Procedure 17-4	Assisting with Suturing a Laceration
Procedure 17-5	Remove Sutures

When you feel you have mastered performance of a skill, sign your name on the appropriate evaluation sheet and give it to your instructor to indicate you are prepared to perform the procedure for evaluation.

ASSIGNMENT SHEET

Chapter 18: ASSISTING WITH MEDICATIONS
Unit 1: PRESCRIPTION AND NONPRESCRIPTION MEDICATIONS

Review the objectives and text for each unit before completing the assignment sheet for that unit in this chapter. When all sheets for the chapter have been completed, remove them from this workbook and give them to the instructor for evaluation.

B. WORD PUZZLE: Use the following clues to solve this word puzzle.

1.   _ D _
2.   _ _ _ _ R _ _ _ _
3.   _ _ _ _ _ U _ _
4.   _ _ G _ _ _ _ _ _ _
5.   _ _ _ _ E _ _ _
6.   _ _ _ _ N _
7.   _ _ _ _ _ _ F _ _ _ _ _ _ _
8.   _ _ _ _ _ O _ _ _ _
9.   _ _ _ _ R _ _ _
10.   _ _ _ _ _ _ C _ _ _ _ _
11.   _ _ _ _ E _ _ _ _ _ _ _ _
12.   _ _ _ _ M _ _ _ _ _
13.   _ _ E _ _ _ _ _ _ _ _ _
14.   _ _ _ _ N _ _
15.   _ _ T _
16.   _ _ _ _ _ A _ _ _ _
17.   _ _ D _ _ _
18.   _ _ _ _ M _ _ _ _ _ _ _ _
19.   _ _ _ _ _ I _ _
20.   _ _ _ _ _ _ N _ _
21.   _ _ _ I _ _ _ _
22.   _ _ _ S _ _ _ _
23.   _ _ _ _ T _ _ _ _ _
24.   _ _ _ _ _ R _ _
25.   _ _ _ A _ _
26.   _ T _
27.   _ _ _ _ _ I _ _ _ _
28.   _ _ O _ _
29.   _ _ _ N _ _ _

CLUES

1. Medication reference
2. Mastery
3. To plan
4. Rule
5. Distribute
6. Quantity
7. Categorize
8. Monitored
9. Correct
10. Study of medicines/drugs
11. To shorten
12. One show fills prescriptions
13. Written order for medicine
14. A permit
15. Numerical calculations
16. Medicines
17. Command
18. Big word for drugs/medicines
19. Highly controlled substances
20. Consultation
21. Enrollment
22. To write an order for medicine
23. Chemical
24. Means
25. Amount of medicine to take
26. Needs no prescription
27. To give
28. Call
29. Caution

B. MATCHING: **Read the definition in Column II and then find the matching answer in Column I. Place the letter of the correct answer in the space provided.**

COLUMN I

_____ 1. Schedule I
_____ 2. Schedule II
_____ 3. Schedule III
_____ 4. Schedule IV
_____ 5. Schedule V
_____ 6. Hypnotic
_____ 7. Warning labels
_____ 8. Antipyretic
_____ 9. Diuretic
_____ 10. Anesthetic

COLUMN II

a. Low potential for addiction
b. Subject to state/local regulations
c. Special instructions on prescription
d. Produces lack of feeling
e. High potential for addiction
f. Increases excretion of urine
g. High psychological dependency
h. Not refilled without prescription
i. Produces sleep
j. Relaxes skeletal muscles
k. Reduces fever

C. SENTENCE COMPLETION

1. The _____ is a valuable resource which the medical assistant should keep handy in the medical office.

2. The medical assistant should keep abreast of the newest _____ which should have been approved by the FDA.

3. The _____ is a legal document.

4. When phoning in a prescription, to assure accuracy, you should ask the pharmacist to _____ the information to avoid dangerous misunderstandings.

5. All physicians who prescribe, dispense, or administer medication in the United States must register annually with the United States Department of Justice, _____ , under the Controlled Substance Act of 1970.

6. Commonly used medications must be rotated according to their _____ .

7. One of the most sensitive and important duties the medical assistant performs is _____ .

8. You must check with your employer regarding the _____ in your state before administering medications.

9. The OTC-PDR is a valuable reference to help you identify medicines that patients use for _____ .

10. When the physician moves the medical practice it must be reported to the nearest _____ .

11. DEA registration must be renewed every _____ years.

12. Physicians must be in compliance with the DEA requirements of the _____ to administer, dispense, or prescribe any controlled substance.

13. _____ prescriptions are primarily prohibited since there is very limited medical use for them.

14. For convenience in writing several medications orders at once, many physicians use the _____ medication prescription pads.

D. MATH REVIEW: Solve the following problems. Show all work and place the answer on the provided line.

Addition
1. $0.2 + 0.35 + 0.0037 =$ _____
2. $0.4 + 0.003 + 0.421 =$ _____
3. $0.222 + 0.0003 + 0.216 =$ _____
4. $3.15 + 0.237 =$ _____
5. $3.007 + 0.2 =$ _____

Subtraction
6. $0.2 - 0.03 =$ _____
7. $0.37 - 0.205 =$ _____
8. $2.5 - 1.8 =$ _____
9. $4.5 - 0.127 =$ _____
10. $5.5 - 5.017 =$ _____

Multiplication
11. $5 \times 0.4 =$ _____
12. $7 \times .137 =$ _____
13. $5 \times 3.5 =$ _____
14. $10 \times 0.07 =$ _____
15. $100 \times 0.0238 =$ _____

Division
16. $0.2 \div 100 =$ _____
17. $0.35 \div 25 =$ _____

18. $2.5 \div 3 =$ _____
19. $1.45 \div 15 =$ _____
20. $3.15 \div 10 =$ _____

Fractions

21. $^2/_5 + ^1/_8 =$ _____
22. $2^1/_2 - 1^3/_4 =$ _____
23. $^2/_3 \times ^1/_4 \times ^3/_5 =$ _____
24. $^1/_8 \div ^3/_5 =$ _____
25. (change to decimal) $^3/_4 =$ _____

Percentages

26. 25% of 4.8 = _____
27. 30% of 17 = _____
28. 15% of 36 = _____
29. 75% of 74 = _____
30. 63% of 97 = _____

Ratio/Proportion: Find x in the following

31. 5:200 :: x:40 _____
32. $^1/_2$:2 :: $^1/_4$:x _____
33. x:30 :: 4:10 _____
34. 0.05:x :: 0.15:30 _____
35. 20:60 :: x:50 _____

E. TRANSLATE INTO SENTENCE FORM THE FOLLOWING ABBREVIATIONS.

1. Rx$\bar{s}$ aq po pc qd PRN _____
2. Rx ss tab po tid $\bar{c}$ aq com ac _____
3. alt noc rep ad lib _____
4. pt DC Fe caps STAT _____
5. Give 2 T emul qid alt dieb _____
6. qns sol _____
7. G 1 tsp. H2O2 hs. _____
8. dil pulv /c aq ferv et f sat sol _____
9. Div dos et adde aq bull, 1 m elix, m et sig. _____

10. pt NPO/am Ba po/GI studies. _____

F. MULTIPLE CHOICE: Place the correct letter on the blank line for each of the following questions.

_____ 1. A medication which slows the blood clotting process is called a(n)
    a. anorexic   c. anticoagulant
    b. sedative   d. hormone

_____ 2. Bronchodilators are medications used to
    a. treat anemia   c. neutralize stomach acid
    b. stop diarrhea   d. promote easier breathing

_____ 3. Physicians prescribe antipyretics to
    a. prevent convulsions   c. elevate mood
    b. reduce fever   d. relieve tension

_____ 4. Medications which promote sleep/sedation are called
      a. antiemetics   b. antacids
      c. sedatives   d. vitamins

_____ 5. Antihistamines are prescribed to
      a. relieve cold/allergy symptoms   c. reduce heart beat rate
      b. suppress coughing   d. increase urinary output

_____ 6. Antitussives are medications which are used to
      a. treat hormonal disorders   c. fight infection
      b. suppress coughing   d. supplement vitamin deficiencies

_____ 7. To fight infection a physician may prescribe a(n)
      a. tranquilizer   c. bronchodilators
      b. cathartic   d. antibiotic

_____ 8. A heart depressant will
      a. reduce heart rate   c. prevent convulsions
      b. suppress appetite   d. stop vomiting/nausea

_____ 9. To promote evacuation of the bowel tract, a physician may prescribe a(n)
      a. sedative   c. cathartic
      b. antidiarrheal   d. tranquilizer

_____ 10. Respiratory stimulants are used to treat
      a. convulsions   c. vitamin deficiencies
      b. shock and drug poisoning   d. muscle/bone conditions

_____ 11. Iron compounds are prescribed to treat
      a. anemia   c. appetite disorders
      b. muscle/bone conditions   d. tension/anxiety

_____ 12. Analgesics are medications prescribed to
      a. promote sleep/sedation   c. relieve pain
      b. reduce fever   d. relieve tension/anxiety

_____ 13. An anticonvulsant is a medication that is used to
      a. suppress appetite   c. suppress coughing
      b. prevent convulsions   d. relieve anxiety

_____ 14. Muscle/bone conditions are often treated with
      a. tranquilizers   c. vitamins
      b. antibiotics   d. musculoskeletal relaxants

_____ 15. Antacids are prescribed to
      a. neutralize stomach acid   c. stop vomiting/nausea
      b. suppress appetite   d. supplement vitamin deficiencies

G. MATCHING: Match the color in Column I with the corresponding section of the *Physicians' Desk Reference* in Column II.

COLUMN I   COLUMN II

_____ 1. Yellow   a. Products in alphabetical order according to their classification
_____ 2. Pink   b. Current information about diagnostic products
_____ 3. White   c. Lists brand or (if desired) generic names of products
_____ 4. Blue   d. Generic or chemical names of products
_____ 5. Green   e. Picture identification
                      f. Complete product information

H. MATH REVIEW: Solve the following word problems.

1. Jessica, a medical assistant, earns $7.50 per hour for the first 40 hours per week. When she exceeds 40 hours in any work week, she is paid time and a half. One week during the winter flu season she worked 53 hours. When she received her paycheck, the gross amount was $397.53
   a. When Jessica works overtime, what is the hourly rate of pay?

   _____

   b. Based on the 53 hours, 13 of which were overtime, what should the gross amount be on her paycheck?

   _____

   c. Is the gross amount on the paycheck she received correct?

   _____

2. The Medical Supply Company is offering a 15% discount on sterile gloves purchased during their anniversary month. The regular cost of the sterile gloves is $37.50 per 100 gloves.
   a. What is the cost of 300 gloves without the discount?

   _____

   b. What is the cost of 300 gloves with the discount?

   _____

   _____

   c. How much is saved with the discount?

   _____

3. A medical assistant can type 250 words in 3 minutes. At the same rate, how long would it take this medical assistant to type 5000 words?

   _____

   _____

   _____

   _____

4. Two of Mrs. Smith's children have been diagnosed with conjunctivitis. The physician wrote a prescription for an antibiotic ophthalmic solution. It reads: 2 gtts TID in each affected eye for 5 days.
   a. If each child needs drops instilled in each eye, how many drops would be needed?

   _____

   _____

   _____

   _____

   b. How many household teaspoons would this be?

5. A medical assistant was asked by her physician-employer to check over a small order from the medical supply house that had arrived while the staff was out to lunch. To expedite the task, the physician handed the medical assistant a copy of the original order (see illustration following):

THE ORIGINAL ORDER

ITEMS	PER UNIT	TOTAL
2 boxes disposable gloves; 100 ct.	$3.75	$7.50
3 boxes syringes; 50 ct.	25.00	75.00
10 thermometers	1.50	10.50
12 boxes tissues	0.25	3.00
5 cartons tongue dep.; 100 ct.	1.38	6.90
6 bottles hand soap	1.77	17.70
		$130.60

THE FINAL BILL

ITEMS	PER UNIT	TOTAL
2 ctns., surg. gloves	$5.75	$11.50
3 ctns., disp. syr.	25.00	75.00
100 thermometers	1.50	150.00
12 boxes tissues	0.25	3.00
5 cartons tongue dep.	1.38	6.90
19 bottles, hand soap	1.77	17.70
		$264.15

The first obvious problem is that the totals do not match on the order and on the bill. An item count further reveals some discrepancies between the quantities shown on the bill and the items actually received. Specifically, only 10 boxes of tissues and 4 cartons of tongue depressors were delivered.

a. Double check each item on the original order; if any mathematical errors are found, correct them.

THE ORIGINAL ORDER

ITEMS	PER UNIT	TOTAL

b. Double check the final bill as shown: if any mathematical errors are found, correct them.

_____

c. Still working with the bill as shown, are there any further discrepancies beyond mathematical errors?

_____
_____
_____
_____

d. Now reconcile the count discrepancies with the corrected amounts shown on the bill.

_____
_____
_____
_____
_____

e. What procedure should be followed in paying the supplier for items actually ordered and received? What should be done with overages? With shortages? With incorrect items?

_____

_____

_____

6. Mrs. Brown, a patient of Dr. Johnston, has been diagnosed as suffering from refractory rickets. Dr. Johnston has prescribed the following treatment:

Ergocalciferol USP, Vitamin D_2 Tab, 100,000 USP units q6h for 14 days.

Ergocalciferol USP, Vitamin D_2 is available in either 50,000 USP units tablets or 8,000 USP units/ml drops. Dr. Johnston has decided to start Mrs. Brown on tablets. After 14 days of treatment, Dr. Johnston will test to determine if Mrs. Brown's serum calcium levels have returned to within normal limits. If so, therapy may be continued at a lower dosage.

a. How many tablets should be given q6h?

_____

b. How many tablets should be given Qid? _____

c. How many tablets should be ordered for the 14-day treatment? _____

7. After the 14-day treatment that Mrs. Brown took in problem 6, Dr. Johnston finds that her serum calcium levels are returning to normal limits. He decides to continue her on a treatment of Ergocalciferol USP, Vitamin D_2 at a reduced level for a period of one month. However, instead of tablets, the medication will be administered in liquid form. His new prescription is as follows:

Ergocalciferol USP, Vitamin D_2 gtt, 48,000 USP units, Bid for 30 days.

As stated in problem 6, Ergocalciferol USP, Vitamin D_2, is available in 8,000 USP units/ml drops; 60 ml bottle with dropper.

a. How many drops will be required for each dosage?

_____

b. How many drops are required for Mrs. Brown's daily dosage? _____

c. How many bottles of Ergocalciferol USP, Vitamin D_2 , will be needed to fill the entire prescription?

_____

_____

8. Bill Jones, a young boy weighing 73 $1/4$ pounds, has a mild ulcerative colitis condition which has been bothering him for several weeks. The physician recommended a treatment of Azulfidine and wrote the following prescription:

Azulfidine 30mg/Kg, q6h for 7 days.

Azulfidine is available in 500 mg 100s tablets.

a. How many ml of Azulfidine will Bill receive per day?

_____

b. How many tablets will be needed per dosage? For the whole prescription?

_____

_____

_____

9. Brad has a case history of chronic asthma. As a treatment of first choice, Brad's doctor has prescribed theophylline anhydrous. Since this is a rather strong medication, the dosage is individualized for Brad based on his body weight and age. Brad is 15 years old and weighs 121 pounds. The recommended dosage for ages 12-16 years is 18mg/Kg/day. The prescription is as follows:

$$18\text{mg/Kg/day p.o., not to exceed } 900 \text{ mg/day.}$$

Theophylline is available in 125 mg capsule form.

a. How many mg of theophylline would Brad receive based on 18mg/Kg/day p.o.?

_____
_____
_____
_____

b. Would this amount be the proper dosage? Yes or No.

_____

c. If not, what would be the amount of theophylline in mg Brad would receive per day based on the prescription?

_____

10. Bobby, a 10-year-old boy, was diagnosed as having strep throat. The physician ordered penicillin G potassium U 5,000,000 IM, stat. The recommended pediatric dosage is U 3,000,000-1,200,000 per day. Penicillin G potassium is available in U 5,000,000/ml. How many ml has the doctor prescribed for Bobby?

_____

CRITICAL THINKING SITUATIONS: What would you say? What would you do?

1. A patient stops in your office to pick up a prescription for his allergy. He mentions that if it's the same thing he got the last time, he might as well not take it. _____

2. One of your elderly patients calls to tell you that all of the prescriptions that she had filled at the pharmacy look different from what she usually takes. She mentions that they didn't cost as much and she's not going to take any of them because she thinks the doctor made a mistake. _____

_____
_____
_____

After your instructor has returned your work to you, make all necessary corrections and place in a 3-ring notebook for future reference.

ASSIGNMENT SHEET

Chapter 18: ASSISTING WITH MEDICATIONS
Unit 2: METHODS OF ADMINISTERING MEDICATIONS

A. FILL IN THE BLANK

1. Most oral medications are intended for absorption in the _____ .
2. The _____ method of administering medication involves placing the medication under the tongue.
3. Sublingual and buccal methods of administration introduce medication immediately into the

   _____ through membranes.
4. _____ medications are supplied as creams, suppositories, tablets, douches, foams, ointments, tampons, sprays, and salves.
5. Medications which are applies in various forms to the skin are termed _____ .
6. _____ medications are breathed into the respiratory tract.
7. _____ medications are given by means of injection.
8. The _____ is the most convenient method of medication.
9. The dosage of _____ drugs is determined by the body surface area of the patient.
10. Allergies and other vital information are noted on a patient's chart in _____ ink.

B. MATCHING: Read the definition in Column I and then find the matching answer in Column II. Place the letter of the correct answer in the space provided.

COLUMN I	COLUMN II
_____ 1. Buccal	a. Placed on a fleshy body part
_____ 2. Oxygen	b. Most common medication method
_____ 3. Package insert	c. Applied to the skin
_____ 4. Transdermal patch	d. Require categorized storage
_____ 5. Patient education	e. Placed in mouth between cheek/gums
_____ 6. Oral medication	f. Contains medication information
_____ 7. Topical	g. Inhalation treatment in emergencies
_____ 8. Prescription	h. Gains compliance with treatment plan
_____ 9. Sublingual	i. Requires physician's signature
_____ 10. Sample medications	j. Big part of medical assistant's job
	k. Placed under tongue

C. BRIEF ANSWER

1. List the points of the standard format checklist for administering medications. _____

   _____

2. How many times should you check a medication before you administer it and why? _____

   _____

3. Why is it a good idea to always check the medication container after administering medication? _____

   _____

4. What does technique mean regarding medications? _____
_____
_____

5. Explain what time has to do in regard to medications. _____
_____

6. Why is it important to check the expiration date on medications? _____
_____

7. Do the same guidelines apply to sample packets of medicines the same as to prescriptions? Explain your
   answer. _____
_____

After your instructor has returned your work to you, make all necessary corrections and place in a 3-ring notebook
for future reference.

ASSIGNMENT SHEET

Chapter 18: ASSISTING WITH MEDICATIONS
Unit 3: INJECTIONS AND IMMUNIZATIONS

A. FILL IN THE BLANK: Complete the following statements about preparing and injecting a dose of insulin.

1. In order to mix the insulin within the vial (bottle) you should gently _____ it between your fingers (hands).
2. The amount of air injected into the vial should be _____ to the insulin dose.
3. Too large an air bubble in the syringe will _____ the insulin dose.
4. Insulin injections should be administered at a(n) _____ angle.
5. It should take one less than _____ seconds to inject the insulin dose.
6. There is always a possibility of _____ shock when administering any medication.
7. Medication should only be administered to patients when a physician is available nearby should the patient exhibit any _____ .
8. The term _____ simply means under the skin.
9. _____ injections are used in allergy and tuberculin testing.
10. A small _____ will develop at the site of the intradermal injection giving evidence that the medication is in the dermal layer of the skin.
11. Following the intradermal injection, the patient must be observed for at least _____ minutes.
12. Subcutaneous injections are administered at a _____ angle of insertion.
13. Medications injected into the muscle tissue are termed _____ .
14. The purpose of the _____ method of injection is to inject irritating substances deep into the muscle layer of tissue and prevent leakage from following the path of the needle.
15. In the Z-track and subcutaneous methods of injection, the injection site should not be _____ after medication is administered.
16. The medical assistant is not qualified to administer the _____ method of injection.

B. IDENTIFICATION: Label the parts of this syringe.

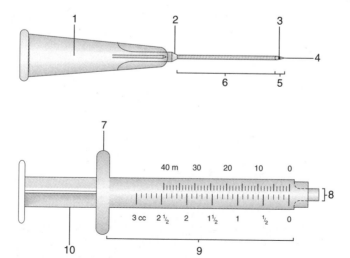

1. 1. _____
    2. _____
    3. _____
    4. _____
    5. _____
    6. _____
    7. _____
    8. _____
    9. _____
   10. _____

2. Label the <u>ANGLES</u> of injection in these pictures.

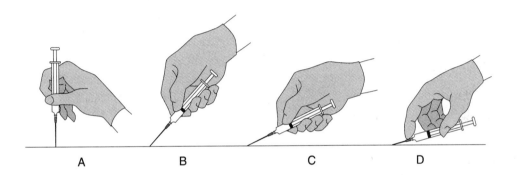

a. _____
b. _____
c. _____
d. _____

3. Identify the <u>TYPES</u> of injections that these pictures indicate.

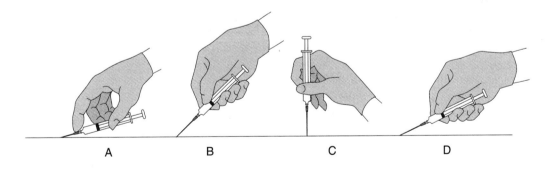

a. _____
b. _____
c. _____
d. _____

C. BRIEF ANSWER

1. Name the tissue layers and sites of injection for intradermal, intramuscular, and subcutaneous. _____

_____
_____
_____
_____

2. Explain how to reassure a patient in preparing for an injection. _____

_____

3. What is the proper way to dispose of used syringes and needles? _____

_____

4. If a needle must be recapped, how should it be done? _____

_____

5. Why must patients be given written information and sign authorization forms before immunizations are administered? _____

_____

_____

6. Explain how to give insulin injections. _____

_____

_____

_____

7. List the various sites for insulin injections. _____

8. List symptoms of anaphylactic shock. _____

_____

9. How long should a patient wait after receiving an injection? And why? _____

_____

10. Explain why you should not rub medications into tissues following a Z-tract injection. _____

_____

11. What is immunity? List the different types. _____

_____

_____

_____

_____

D. BRIEF ANSWER: Refer to Table 18-6 in the text.

1. At what age is the immunization schedule routinely begun? _____

2. What are the first 3 immunizations (vaccines) given to infants? _____

3. How long should the ideal time period be between immunizations in a series? _____

4. Assuming an infant has had a regular routine immunization schedule, at what age will the child be at the completed primary series of DTP, OPV, and Hib? _____

5. What immunization does a child receive at age 18 months? _____

6. At ages 4 to 6 years, what booster immunization should a child receive? _____

7. Td is given to what age group of children? _____

8. How often should adult tetanus and diphtheria toxoids be repeated? _____

E. ESSAY

1. Discuss the drugs that are under federal regulation according to category or Schedules I through V. _____

_____

_____

_____
_____
_____
_____
_____
_____
_____
_____
_____

2. What is the Hib vaccine? Who should receive it? _____
_____

F. TRUE OR FALSE: Place a "T" for True or "F" for False in the space provided.

_____ 1. You should take *only* the medicine which has been prescribed for you by the physician.

_____ 2. Prescribed medicine may be shared with other family members.

_____ 3. Taking more (extra) doses of prescribed medicine will make you get better faster.

_____ 4. Any reaction to or side effect of any medicine must be reported to the physician immediately.

_____ 5. You do not need to instruct patients to tell you of any OTC medications they take on their own.

_____ 6. It is important to advise patients if the physician has prescribed medications that could interfere with their concentration or make them sleepy.

_____ 7. After 6 months, medicines should be thrown away (flushed down the toilet).

_____ 8. Patients should be made aware that generic and brand name products (prescriptions) are the same.

_____ 9. The medical assistant should instruct patients to refrain from taking alcoholic beverages while taking medications.

_____ 10. It is not necessary for female patients to report whether they plan to become pregnant, are pregnant, or are nursing mothers before taking medication.

G. CRITICAL THINKING SITUATIONS

1. One of your adult patients comes in for his first allergy injection. He says to use his left arm because that's the one he always had his allergy shots in before where he used to live. He is also in a hurry and wants to be somewhere in 10 minutes. _____
_____
_____
_____

H. MATCHING: Read the disease in Column I and then find the matching common symptoms in Column II. Place the letter of the correct answer in the space provided.

COLUMN I

_____ 1. Tetanus

_____ 2. Measles

_____ 3. Hepatitis B

_____ 4. Diphtheria

_____ 5. Influenza

_____ 6. Pertussis

_____ 7. Mumps

_____ 8. Haemophilus type B

_____ 9. Pneumonia

_____ 10. Rubella

COLUMN II

a. Headache, malaise, fever, sore throat with yellowish-white or gray membrane

b. Chills, fever, headache, pain and swelling below and in front of ears

c. Begins with fever, malaise, headache, nausea/vomiting, abdominal discomfort, generalized paralysis

d. Abrupt onset-severe chills, high fever, headache, chest pain/dyspnea, rapid pulse, cyanosis, cough/blood stained sputum

e. Slow onset of fever, malaise, no appetite, nausea/vomiting, jaundice

f. Slight fever, sore throat, drowsiness, malaise, swollen glands/lymph nodes, diffuse fine red rash

317

g. Fever, malaise, runny nose, cough, sore throat, Koplik's spots

h. Sudden onset of fever, chills, sore throat, cough, muscle aches/pains, weakness, general malaise

i. Stiffness of jaw/esophageal muscles sometimes neck muscles, fever, painful spasms of all muscles, irritability, headache

j. High WBC count, respiratory drainage, slight fever, irritability, dry cough, whooping inspiration sounds

k. Sudden onset of fever, sore throat, cough, muscle aches, weakness and general malaise

I. MULTIPLE CHOICE

_____ 1. Common flu is a disease that affects the:
   a. kidneys   c. liver
   b. respiratory tract d. spinal column

_____ 2. In addition to bed rest, fluids, analgesics, and antipyretics, pneumonia is sometimes treated with:
   a. muscle relaxants   c. oxygen
   b. vitamins   d. sedatives

_____ 3. Haemophilus influenza type B affects:
   a. infants/small children   c. adolescents
   b. elementary school ages   d. adults
   e. the elderly

_____ 4. Complications of measles can result in deafness, brain damage, and:
   a. paralysis   c. baldness
   b. pneumonia   d. myopia

_____ 5. The incubation period for mumps is:
   a. 14-28 hours   c. 14-28 weeks
   b. 14-28 days   d. 14-28 months

_____ 6. Rubella is a most dangerous disease that can cause severe abnormalities to which of the following:
   a. pregnant female   c. infant
   b. teenager   d. the fetus

_____ 7. A tracheostomy is sometimes necessary to perform in which of these diseases?
   a. tetanus   c. diphtheria
   b. mumps   d. pneumonia

_____ 8. A trace cough may last for several months to 2 years following:
   a. pertussis   c. diphtheria
   b. influenza   d. tetanus

_____ 9. A disease that is commonly transmitted in puncture wounds is:
   a. polio   c. haemophilus
   b. diphtheria   d. tetanus

_____ 10. Alcohol and fats should especially be eliminated from the diet of one who has:
   a. mumps   c. hepatitis
   b. tetanus   d. influenza

_____ 11. An acute infection and inflammation of the gray matter of the spinal cord is:
   a. polio   c. tetanus
   b. hepatitis   d. diphtheria

ACHIEVING SKILL COMPETENCY

Reread the TPO for each procedure and then practice the skills listed below, following the procedure in your textbook.

Obtain and Administer Oral Medication - Procedure 18-1

Withdraw Medication from Ampule - Procedure 18-2

Withdraw Medication from Vial - Procedure 18-3

Administer Intradermal Injection - Procedure 18-4

Administer Subcutaneous Injection - Procedure 18-5

Administer Intramuscular Injection - Procedure 18-6

Administer Intramuscular Injection by Z-Tract Method - Procedure 18-7

When you feel you have mastered the performance of the skill, sign your name on the appropriate evaluation sheet and give it to your instructor to indicate you are prepared to perform the procedure for evaluation.

After your instructor has returned your work to you, make all necessary corrections and place in a 3-ring notebook for future reference.

ASSIGNMENT SHEET

Chapter 19: EMERGENCIES, ACUTE ILLNESS, AND ACCIDENTS
Unit 1: MANAGING EMERGENCIES AT THE MEDICAL OFFICE

MIXED QUIZ

1. What is a universal emergency medical identification symbol and what does it do?

   _____

   _____

2. Identify five medical conditions for which a patient should wear an identification symbol.

   a. _____

   b. _____

   c. _____

   d. _____

   e. _____

3. When is a situation considered to be an emergency? _____

   _____

4. List the 16 items identified in the text which should be included in an emergency kit or cart.

   a. _____

   b. _____

   c. _____

   d. _____

   e. _____

   f. _____

   g. _____

   h. _____

   i. _____

   j. _____

   k. _____

   l. _____

   m. _____

   n. _____

   o. _____

   p. _____

5. True or False

Answer the following statements with "T" for True or "F" for False, where true indicates the data is necessary to document in an emergency situation and false indicates the data is *not* necessary to document in an emergency situation.

- a. _____ Name of injured patient or employee
- b. _____ Date of incident
- c. _____ Social security number of person injured
- d. _____ Time of injury or emergency
- e. _____ Name and phone number of next-of-kin
- f. _____ Identification of location of accident or injury
- g. _____ Description of condition surrounding accident or injury
- h. _____ Description of past like incidences
- i. _____ Employer's name, address, and phone number
- j. _____ Identification of accident or incident witnesses
- k. _____ Signature of examining physician
- l. _____ Description of action taken, including disposition of the patient
- m. _____ Signature of person filing report

6. Enter below the phone number for emergency medical services in your location. (Don't assume the universal 911 number is in effect in your area, be certain)

_____

7. Determine the procedure to follow in your area when an individual dies without benefit of recent medical attention either within a physician's office or at another site.

_____

8. What follow-up record keeping action is necessary following death of a patient?

_____
_____

9. Using the words to know, complete the following puzzle

An emetic	__ __ E __ __ __
Injury	__ __ __ __ M __
Revive	__ E __ __ __ __ __ __ __ __ __ __ __ __
A physician	__ __ R __ __ __ __
A dressing	__ __ __ __ __ G __
Cause vomiting	__ __ E __ __ __
A happening	__ __ __ __ __ __ N __
Unexpected injury	__ __ C __ __ __ __ __
An emblem	__ Y __ __ __ __

10. Unscramble the following terms

_____	EULNRISVA
_____	IANRCOTITFECI
_____	OCRERON
_____	TIDNICNE
_____	OLYSBM
_____	CTICEAND

ASSIGNMENT SHEET

Chapter 19: EMERGENCIES, ACUTE ILLNESS, AND ACCIDENTS
Unit 2: ACUTE ILLNESS

MIXED QUIZ

1. Match the common terms used to describe the severity of illness with the meanings

   COLUMN I   COLUMN II

   _____ Chronic   1. Occurring quickly and without warning
   _____ Insidious   2. Extensive, advanced
   _____ Urgent   3. May cause death
   _____ Sudden   4. Long, drawn out, not acute
   _____ Acute   5. Hidden, not apparent
   _____ Severe   6. Requires intervention as soon as possible
   _____ Life threatening 7. Rapid onset, severe symptoms and short course

2. List the 9 steps or stages which might occur with a major seizure.

   a. _____
   b. _____
   c. _____
   d. _____
   e. _____
   f. _____
   g. _____
   h. _____
   i. _____

3. Listed below are symptoms of diabetic coma and insulin shock. Enter "C" for coma or "S" for shock before the symptom to indicate which condition may be present.

   _____ a. Drooling
   _____ b. Perspiration
   _____ c. Dry mouth
   _____ d. Not hungry
   _____ e. Full bounding pulse
   _____ f. Dry, flushed skin
   _____ g. Fruity odor to breath
   _____ h. Weak, rapid pulse
   _____ i. Intense thirst
   _____ j. Double vision

4. Fill in the blanks

   A temporarily diminished supply of _____ to the _____ may cause _____ .
   The medical term for this condition is _____ . A patient should be positioned with their
   _____ to improve circulation to the _____ . Symptoms of approaching syncope are
   _____ , and complaints of _____ or _____ .
   When using aromatic spirits of ammonia capsules, it is important to _____
   _____ .

5. List the prime symptoms of heart attack.

   a. _____
   b. _____
   c. _____

d. _____

e. _____

f. _____

g. _____

h. _____

i. _____

6. Indicate whether the following symptoms are possible heat stroke (S) or heat exhaustion (E). Place an "S" or "E" in front of the symptoms.

_____ pale, cool skin

_____ profuse perspiration

_____ rapid pulse, possible Cheyne-Stokes respirations

_____ dry, red face

_____ body temperature above average

_____ dilated pupils

_____ hypertension

_____ headache

_____ mental confusion, giddiness

_____ thirst, nausea, vomiting

7. List the six successive symptoms of frostbite and identify the most often damaged body parts.

a. _____

b. _____

c. _____

d. _____

e. _____

f. _____

8. Name the three types of visible bleeding and the characteristics of each type.

a. _____

b. _____

c. _____

9. Identify the pressure points where severe arterial bleeding can be controlled.

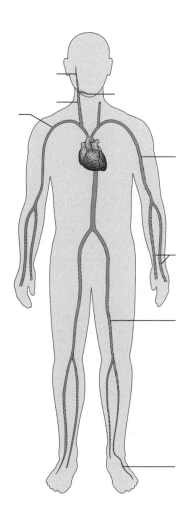

10. What are the symptoms of internal bleeding and how is it initially and eventually treated?

a. _____
b. _____
c. _____
d. _____
e. _____
f. _____
g. _____
h. _____
i. _____

11. Identify six routes by which poison can enter the body.

a. _____
b. _____
c. _____
d. _____
e. _____
f. _____

12. Determine the phone number for your local Poison Control Center. Write it on the line below and add it to the emergency medical service number on your personal reference card.

_____
Poison Control Center Number

13. List the seven most common causes of obstructed airway.

a. _____
b. _____
c. _____
d. _____
e. _____
f. _____
g. _____

14. What are the three names for the method used to relieve an obstructed airway?

a. _____
b. _____
c. _____

15. List six additional conditions which may cause respiratory distress.

a. _____
b. _____
c. _____
d. _____
e. _____
f. _____

16. List the sequence of events required for survival of cardiac arrest.

a. _____
b. _____
c. _____
d. _____
e. _____
f. _____

17. What is the critical concern in cases of cervical spinal injury?

_____

18. Identify the six symptoms of shock.

a. _____
b. _____
c. _____
d. _____
e. _____
f. _____

19. What are the usual causes of shock?

_____

20. What is anaphylactic shock?

_____

21. Name substances which can cause anaphylactic shock.

a. _____
b. _____
c. _____

d. _____
e. _____
f. _____
g. _____
h. _____
i. _____
j. _____

22. What are the symptoms of stroke?

a. _____
b. _____
c. _____
d. _____
e. _____
f. _____
g. _____
h. _____
i. _____

23. Underline the correct spelling in the following lists

asperation	aspirashun	aspiration
diaphoresis	diephoresis	diaforesis
incidious	insidious	insideous
profalatic	profalytic	prophylatic
exhaustion	eghaustion	egaustion
ammonea	ammonia	amoania
seezure	seazure	seizure

ACHIEVING SKILL COMPETENCY

Reread the TPO for the procedures and then practice the skills listed below, following the procedure in your textbook.

Procedure 19 - 1   Give Mouth to Mouth resuscitation
Procedure 19 - 2   Give Cardiopulmonary; Resuscitation (CPR) to Adults
Procedure 19 - 3   Give Cardiopulmonary Resuscitation (CPR) to Infants and Children

When you feel you have mastered the performance of a skill, sign your name on the appropriate evaluation sheet and give it to your instructor to indicate you are prepared to perform the procedure for evaluation.

After your instructor has returned your work to you, make all necessary corrections and place in a 3-ring notebook for future reference.

ASSIGNMENT SHEET

Chapter 19: EMERGENCIES, ACUTE ILLNESS, AND ACCIDENTS
Unit 3: FIRST AID IN ACCIDENTS AND INJURIES

MIXED QUIZ

1. How is a bee stinger removed?

   _____

2. When is anti-rabies serum required following an animal bite?

   _____

3. Name the three types of burns and give examples of each

   a. _____

   _____

   b. _____

   c. _____

4. What is the first priority in the treatment of burns?

   _____

5. Compare the first aid treatment for the three degrees of burns

   _____

   _____

   _____

   _____

   _____

6. Describe the symptoms of a dislocation.

   _____

7. What is the benefit from adding moisture to a heat treatment?

   _____

8. What action does the application of cold treatments have on the body?

   _____

9. What action does the application of heat treatments have on the body?

   _____

   _____

10. Name four types of wounds.

    a. _____

    b. _____

    c. _____

    d. _____

11. Complete the puzzle using the Words to Know

A scrape or scratch   _ _ _ **A** _ _ _ _

Acid or alkaline substance   _ _ _ _ _ **C** _ _

Having a current   _ _ _ **C** _ _ _ _ _ _

Prevent from moving   _ _ _ _ _ **I** _ _ _ _

An injury   _ _ _ _ **D**

A tear   _ _ _ **E** _ _ _ _ _ _

A hole   _ _ **N** _ _ _ _ _

Rub briskly   _ _ _ _ **T** _ _ _

Smooth cut   _ _ _ _ **S** _ _ _

12. Circle the following words in the puzzle.

ANAPHYLACTIC
BANDAGE
BITE
BURN
CHEMICAL
ELECTRICAL
FRICTION
IMMOBILIZE
INCISION
INJURIES
LACERATION
MOLTEN
PUNCTURE
SHOCK
SPLINTER
SPRAIN
STINGS
STRAIN
SUPERFICIAL
THERMAL
WOUND

```
S U P E R F I C I A L E
R I P D J V S H O C K L
L I W N I S P R A I N E
A N A P H Y L A C T I C
C C C H E M I C A L M T
E I P S T I N G S C M R
R S F R I C T I O N O I
A I M O L T E N Q O B C
T O M T H E R M A L I A
I N J U R I E S V X L L
O Q W O U N D B P B I H
N I W S T R A I N U Z P
W R G P U N C T U R E Y
X B A N D A G E P N I U
```

328

ASSIGNMENT SHEET

Chapter 20: PERSONAL BEHAVIORS INFLUENCING HEALTH
Unit 1: NUTRITION, EXERCISE, AND WEIGHT CONTROL

Review the objectives and text for each unit before completing the assignment sheet for that unit in this chapter. When all sheets for the chapter have been completed, remove them from this workbook and give them to the instructor for evaluation.

A. UNSCRAMBLE

1. _ _ _ _ _ _ _   LEACIRO
2. _ _ _ _ _ _ _ _   EPTVOIIS
3. _ _ _ _ _ _   YSRUCV
4. _ _ _ _ _ _ _ _   RAAIOXNE
5. _ _ _ _ _ _ _ _ _   IIANDTCI
6. _ _ _ _ _ _ _   KTRSCIE
7. _ _ _ _ _ _ _ _   ERBBIIRE
8. _ _ _ _ _ _   TONMOI
9. _ _ _ _ _   NREGA
10. _ _ _ _ _ _   ETHALH
11. _ _ _ _ _ _ _ _ _   RIOUNTNTI
12. _ _ _ _ _ _ _ _ _   FNYMIIRTI
13. _ _ _ _ _ _ _ _ _ _ _ _ PHECUTATERI
14. _ _ _ _ _ _ _   LCEBMUI

B. BRIEF ANSWER

1. Explain the significance of diet and exercise to health. _____
_____

2. Name the food groups in the food guide pyramid and the amounts recommended daily for each. _____
_____
_____
_____

3. Name the fat-soluble vitamins. _____

4. Name the water-soluble vitamins. _____

5. Name the essential minerals which are most often missing from the average diet. _____

6. How might you encourage patients to comply in weight control? _____
_____

7. What is the purpose of the flexibility or stretching exercises? _____
_____

8. List four things one can do to improve one's health. _____
_____

9. List the guidelines for promoting good health. _____
_____
_____
_____

10. Why is sleep and a positive outlook important to good health? _____
_____

11. Why is it helpful especially for weight reduction to eat slowly? _____
_____

12. What is the reason for eating several small meals a day instead of the traditional 3 meals a day? _____
_____

13. What is anorexia nervosa? _____
_____
_____

14. Discuss health concerns in regard to adolescents in general. _____
_____
_____

C. LABEL THIS FOOD GUIDE PYRAMID

D. FILL IN THE BLANK: Using Table 20-2 (Principle Micronutrient) complete the following statements.

1. A deficiency of vitamin A could cause _____ .
2. The main source of vitamin D is _____ .
3. Prothrombin formation and normal blood coagulation is the function of _____ .
4. Growth cessation and dermatosis is due to a deficiency of _____ .
5. Vegetable oil, wheat germ, leafy vegetables, egg yolk, margarine, and legumes are the principal sources of the _____ .
6. Carbohydrate metabolism, central and peripheral nerve cell function, and myocardial function are attributed to sufficient amounts of _____ or _____ in the diet.
7. Nicotinic acid, niacinamide, are the other terms for the micronutrient, _____ .
8. The usual therapeutic dosage of folic acid is _____ .
9. Scurvy, hemorrhages, loose teeth, gingivitis, are caused by a deficiency of _____ or
_____ .
10. Some sources of potassium include whole and skim milk, _____ , prunes, and raisins.
11. Magnesium is necessary in bone and _____ formation.

12. One who is diagnosed as having anemia has a(n) _____ .

13. Simple goiter and cretinism are due to a deficiency of _____ .

14. A deficiency in _____ may cause growth retardation.

E. CRITICAL THINKING SITUATIONS: What would you say? What would you do?

1. A female patient in her late 20s calls to tell you that she just read about a diet plan in a new magazine that promises a weight loss of 20 pounds in 2 weeks. She wants to get the physician's permission for her to lose 20pounds before her class reunion in 3 weeks. She has not been seen by the doctor for almost a year.

_____

_____

2. A male patient in his mid 40s is recovering from gall bladder surgery 4 weeks ago. He tells you that he's going to the health spa to work out because he' bored with sitting around. _____

_____

_____

3. A worried mother of 3 grade school children tells you as she is leaving the office that her children aren't eating well at dinner time anymore. She says that they eat so much junk food when they come home from school that they can't finish the meals she prepares. _____

_____

_____

_____

After your instructor has returned your work to you, make all necessary corrections and place in a 3-ring notebook for future reference.

ASSIGNMENT SHEET

Chapter 20: BEHAVIORS INFLUENCING HEALTH
Unit 2: MOBILITY ASSISTANCE

MIXED QUIZ

1. Identify seven situations when the use of some form of device may be indicated to assist patients with mobility.

   _____

   _____

2. Identify six basic benefits from regular exercise. _____

   _____

3. What is range-of-motion exercise? _____

   _____

4. What is flexibility exercise? _____

   _____

5. What two precautions must be observed when applying a sling? _____

   _____

6. Identify two guidelines concerning fitting a cane _____

   _____

7. Explain the proper height for crutches. _____

   _____

8. List four factors which will increase safety for the patient at home. _____

   _____

   _____

   _____

9. **MATCHING: Read the definition in Column II and then find the matching answer in Column I. Place the letter of the correct answer in the space provided.**

COLUMN I	COLUMN II
_____ 1. Ambulate	a. A type of cane
_____ 2. Axilla	b. Manner of walking
_____ 3. Balance	c. Extent of movement
_____ 4. Flexibility	d. To walk
_____ 5. Gait	e. To hold secure
_____ 6. Mobility	f. Area under arm
_____ 7. Quad-base	g. The ability to twist and bend
_____ 8. Range-of-motion	h. Equilibrium
_____ 9. Stabilize	i. Move about freely

10. Using the text, practice the range-of-motion and stretching exercises to become familiar with the movements. See text pages 729 to 731.

After your instructor has returned your work to you, make all necessary corrections and place in a 3-ring notebook for future reference.

ASSIGNMENT SHEET

Chapter 20: BEHAVIORS INFLUENCING HEALTH
Unit 3: HABIT-FORMING SUBSTANCES

A. BRIEF ANSWER

1. List the most commonly abused major groups of drugs and give an example of each. _____

   _____

   _____

2. What are the effects of depressants? _____

3. What are the effects of hallucinogens? _____

4. What are the effects of narcotics? _____

5. What are the effects of stimulants? _____

6. List behaviors that are indicators of drug/alcohol abuse. _____

   _____

   _____

   _____

7. Describe the difference between an alcoholic-dependent drinker and an alcoholic. _____

   _____

8. Describe research efforts into the causes of alcoholism. _____

9. How can the medical assistant be influential in assisting the drug addict or the alcoholic toward rehabilitation?

   _____

   List organizations and facilities that assist in the rehabilitation of drug addicts and alcoholics. _____

   _____

   _____

11. Describe the effect that tar, nicotine, and carbon monoxide have on the body. _____

   _____

   _____

   _____

   _____

12. List ways a person can stop smoking.

   a. _____

   b. _____

   c. _____

   d. _____

   e. _____

   f. _____

   g. _____

h. _____

i. _____

j. _____

k. _____

13. Name the diseases that smokers are more likely to acquire. _____

_____

14. Describe the effects of passive or involuntary smoking. _____

15. What health problems do young children have as a result of being exposed to second-hand smoke of caretakers?

_____

B. MATCHING: Read the definition in Column II and then find the matching answer in Column I. Place the letter of the correct answer in the space provided.

COLUMN I

COLUMN II

_____ 1. Euphoria

_____ 2. Synergism

_____ 3. Addiction

_____ 4. Bizarre

_____ 5. Narcolepsy

_____ 6. Al-Ateen

_____ 7. Barbiturate

_____ 8. Hallucinogen

_____ 9. Al-Anon

_____ 10. Depressant

_____ 11. Amphetamine

_____ 12. Alcoholic

_____ 13. Stimulant

_____ 14. Traumatic

_____ 15. Psychedelics

a. The habitual use of drugs

b. Stimulates the central nervous system

c. Support group for adolescent family members of alcoholics

d. Induce sleep

e. Mixing two or more drugs

f. Refers to a painful emotional experience

g. Exaggerated good feeling

h. A drinker who has become totally dependent on alcohol

i. Referred to as mind-expanding chemicals

j. Support group for family members and close friends of alcoholics

k. Uncontrollable desire to sleep

l. Hallucinogens

m. Strange; odd in manner

n. Used in treatment of patients who need sedation

o. Comprehensive rehabilitation

p. Taken to stay awake, feel more energetic

C. TRUE OR FALSE: Place a "T" for True or "F" for False in the space provided.

_____ 1. Men still have a higher risk of premature death due to smoking cigarettes than women.

_____ 2. Of the 2,000 substances identified in tobacco smoke, most of the harm is done by tar, nicotine, and carbon monoxide.

_____ 3. Nicotine stimulates the appetite.

_____ 4. Approximately 10% of the blood supply in smokers is in the form of carboxyhemoglobin.

_____ 5. Smokers need to become thoroughly educated on the facts about smoking before they can eliminate their habit.

_____ 6. Tobacco contains poisons that could be fatal to toddlers and pets if swallowed.

_____ 7. Cigarette smoking is dangerous to your health.

D. CRITICAL THINKING SITUATIONS: What would you say? What would you do?

1. One of your high-school patients comes in hanging on her mother's shoulder to help her stand up. Her speech is slurred and she is nauseated. The visit, of course, is unexpected. _____

_____

_____

_____

2. A concerned parent has found some strange pills in her son's room and calls to ask you what to do. She says her son's behavior has changed recently and she is worried about him. _____

_____

After your instructor has returned your work to you, make all necessary corrections and place in a 3-ring notebook for future reference.

ASSIGNMENT SHEET

Chapter 20: BEHAVIORS INFLUENCING HEALTH
Unit 4: STRESS AND TIME MANAGEMENT

A. WORD PUZZLE: Complete this puzzle from the list of Words to Know.

```
 1. _ _ _ _ P _ _ _ _ _ _
 2.     _ _ S _ _ _ _
 3.     _ _ Y _ _ _ _ _ _
 4.     _ _ C _ _ _ _ _ _
         H
 5.   _ _ _ O _ _ _ _ _ _
 6     _ _ S _ _ _ _ _ _
 7.     _ O _ _ _ _ _ _
 8.   _ M _ _ _ _ _ _ _
 9.     A _ _ _ _ _ _ _
10.  _ _ _ T _ _ _
11.     I _ _ _ _ _ _ _ _
12.   _ _ C _ _ _ _ _ _
```

B. BRIEF ANSWER
1. Describe the phenomenon of stress. _____
   _____
   _____
   _____

2. List the physical effects of stress. _____
   _____
   _____

3. What is "good stress"? _____

4. What is "bad stress"? _____

5. Describe the Type-A personality. _____
   _____

6. Describe the Type-B personality. _____
   _____

7. List the four basic human physical needs. _____

8. List the four basic human development needs. _____

9. What can be done to eliminate unnecessary stress? _____
   _____

10. List methods for dealing with stress. _____
    _____
    _____

11. List possible mental health resources for patient referrals. _____
    _____

12. List and discuss ways to relax and cope with daily stress. _____
    _____
    _____

13. What is the purpose of time management? _____

14. List some of the benefits of time management. _____

_____

C. MATCHING: **Read the definition in Column II and then find the matching answer in Column I. Place the letter of the correct answer in the space provided.**

COLUMN I

_____ 1. Exercise
_____ 2. Perspective
_____ 3. Implement
_____ 4. Eustress
_____ 5. Psychosomatic
_____ 6. Psychosis
_____ 7. Prioritizing
_____ 8. Flexible
_____ 9. Conflict
_____ 10. Anxiety
_____ 11. Depression

COLUMN II

a. Low spirits; sadness
b. Impairment of normal intellectual and social functioning
c. Arranging in order of importance
d. Constant state of worry
e. Clash, be in opposition
f. To put into effect
g. Support group
h. Real symptoms, not imagined
i. Positive effect in reducing stress
j. Able to bend without breaking
k. Proper evaluation/consideration
l. Planned stress; it motivates

D. BRIEF ANSWER

1. Make a list of the good and bad stress in your life.

_____

_____

_____

_____

E. Use the following words in a complete sentence:

anxiety _____

discretion _____

exemplify _____

flexible _____

nurture _____

perspective _____

prioritize _____

ACHIEVING SKILL COMPETENCY

Reread the TPO for each procedure and then practice the skills listed below, following the procedure in your textbook.

Apply Arm Sling - Procedure 20-1

Use a Cane - Procedure 20-2

Use Crutches - Procedure 20-3

Use a Walker - Procedure 20-4

Assist Patient from Wheelchair to Examination Table - Procedure 20-5

Assist Patient from Examination Table to Wheelchair - Procedure 20-6

When you feel you have mastered the performance of the skill, sign your name on the appropriate evaluation sheet and give it to your instructor to indicate you are prepared to perform the procedure for evaluation.

After your instructor has returned your work to you, make all necessary corrections and place in a 3-ring notebook for future reference.

338

ASSIGNMENT SHEET

Section VI: EMPLOYABILITY SKILLS
Chapter 21: ACHIEVING SATISFACTION IN EMPLOYMENT

Unit 1: THE JOB SEARCH

Review the objectives and text for each unit before completing the assignment sheet for that unit in this chapter. When all sheets for the chapter have been completed, remove them from this workbook and give them to the instructor for evaluation.

A. BRIEF ANSWER

1. What is the purpose of a resume? *The purpose of a resume is to describe a prospective employers your educational, previous back, etc*

2. Why should a cover letter accompany a resume? *It should accompany you resume because it states why you are capable for that particular job*

3. List the different types of resumes and the purpose of each
   a. *traditonal - shows reader background info in organized fashion*
   b. *career objective style - shows career choice, and abilities (qualification)*
   c. *functional type resume - achievements and strength*
   d. *chronological resume - shows prospective to employment history in order*
   e. *targeted resume is used for precise field of employment*

4. Describe the services of an employment agency. *Basically you send them your info, and they look for a job for you.*

5. List three contacts to assist the medical assistant in the job search. _____

6. What is a classified ad? *a classified ad is a request for qualified applications to send info about themselves to a prospective employer.*

7. Where may the medical assistant find additional information abut job opportunities? *you can find additional info for job in computer, newspaper, etc*

B. COMPLETION

1. The job search begins with the _____ to work.
2. The _____ should be complete, accurate, and neatly organized.
3. Preparation of a resume requires you to systematically list experiences which show your valuable _____.
4. In listing your educational background, you should note that a _____ can be furnished upon request.
5. Permission should be obtained from those persons listed as _____.
6. Personal data is _____ on a resume.
7. The resume should be _____ and _____ as needed to document additional employment experience, educational achievements, awards, and personal development.
8. All states offer assistance in locating jobs through the state _____.
9. Many potential jobs are _____ - _____ meaning that the employer pays the agency's fees.
10. The job search takes patience, persistence, and _____.
11. _____ a resume should be done only when an employer requests it.

C. MATCHING: Match the abbreviation in Column I with the corresponding word in Column II.

COLUMN I

_____ 1. SAL
_____ 2. PT
_____ 3. INT
_____ 4. REQ
_____ 5. POS
_____ 6. LIC
_____ 7. FB
_____ 8. BGN
_____ 9. NEG
_____ 10. COL
_____ 11. IMMED
_____ 12. EDUC
_____ 13. NEC
_____ 14. WPM
_____ 15. EXP

COLUMN II

a. Position(s)
b. License
c. Beginning
d. Necessary
e. Negotiable
f. Education
g. Immediate
h. Words per minute
i. Experience
j. Required
k. Interview
l. Part-time
m. Salary
n. College
o. Fringe benefits

D. FILL IN THE BLANK: Grouped below are some of the qualities that employers expect from their employees. After the brief definition of each, place the appropriate quality on the line provided:

initiative	dependability	courteous	responsible
reliability	cooperative	time management skill	
punctuality	enthusiasm	interest	

1. To excite the attention or curiosity of: _____
2. Trustworthy: _____
3. Answerable; accountable: _____
4. The ability to think and act without being urged: _____
5. Organization by priority: _____
6. Intense or eager interest: _____
7. Considerate toward others; well-mannered: _____
8. Working together for a common purpose: _____
9. Being on time: _____
10. Can be depended on: _____

E. ADS/COVER LETTER

In the space below paste a want ad from your local paper for a medical assistant position. Below it respond with the cover letter about yourself that you would send. Show it to your instructor to evaluate when you are finished.

_____

_____

_____

_____

_____

_____

_____

_____

_____

_____

_____

_____

_____

_____

_____

_____

_____

F. CROSSWORD PUZZLE CLUES

ACROSS

2. a quality
5. it's said to be the best teacher
7. abbr/words per minute
10. a wish
11. schooling
12. abbr/salary
14. abbr/high school
15. refers to form or _____of resume
16. abbr/immediately
17. abbr/reference
18. type of letter sent with resume
19. outlined summary of your abilities and experience
21. abbr/equal opportunity employer
22. strong ambition
24. abbr/college
26. capable for position

DOWN

1. abbr/fringe benefit
2. abbr/appointment
3. aimed
4. to hire or _____
5. work
6. employment ads
7. newspaper ad listings that say "help _____"
8. skillful and precise
9. you may furnish on request
13. payment for services
20. abbr/secretary
23. abbr/required
25. abbr/advertisement

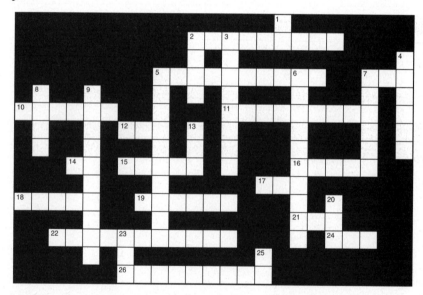

G. CRITICAL THINKING SITUATIONS: What would you say? What would you do?

1. Planning well to allow spare time for traffic, you are on your way to an interview for a position you really want. Traffic is unusually congested because a truck is stalled on the freeway. You realize that you will most likely be late. _____
_____
_____
_____

2. During an interview, the employer asks you if you have ever been late to work. This employer also asks for references. _____
_____
_____

After your instructor has returned your work to you, make all necessary corrections and place in a 3-ring notebook for future reference.

ASSIGNMENT SHEET

Chapter 21
Unit 2: GETTING THE JOB AND KEEPING IT

A. MATCHING: Match the definitions from Column II with the terms in Column I.

COLUMN I

_____ 1. Contemporary
_____ 2. Negate
_____ 3. Demeanor
_____ 4. Competent
_____ 5. Arbitrary
_____ 6. Affiliate
_____ 7. Apprise

COLUMN II

a. Well qualified
b. To connect or associate
c. To inform or notify
d. To discriminate
e. Modern
f. Conduct; outward behavior
g. To make ineffective
h. Not fixed by rules; based on one's preference
i. An attitude or system

B. BRIEF ANSWER

1. What information should you be prepared to provide on an application for employment? _____

   _____

2. What important factor must the medical assistant remember when completing a job application?

   _____

3. Why is appearance so important when interviewing for a job? _____

   _____

4. What is the purpose of a job interview? _____

   _____

5. Why must one be prompt and courteous at a job interview? _____

   _____

6. Explain why it is a good idea to send a follow-up letter to the interviewer after the job interview. _____

   _____

7. What is the best way to close an interview. Why? _____

   _____

8. How may a medical assistant demonstrate price in the profession of medical assisting? _____

   _____

9. How should you dress when applying for a job or when returning an application form and why? _____

   _____

   _____

10. List areas of concern employers have regarding (prospective) employees. _____

    _____

    _____

    _____

    _____

11. What documents are employers required to ask for of prospective employees and why? _____

_____

_____

12. How can time management skills be applied to your work day? _____

_____

13. Explain what "work ethics" is and why it is important regarding your employment. _____

_____

14. What is the value of an employment evaluation review? _____

_____

15. What are some of the subjects you should discuss with your employer during an evaluation review?

_____

_____

_____

_____

16. Discuss the purpose and advantages of a job description. _____

_____

_____

_____

C. COMPLETION

1. An employer will expect you to perform with increasing _____ in your position as you continue to gain experience.
2. One particular quality that the medical assistant must keep in mind is _____ .
3. Your _____ will probably follow you throughout your working life.
4. Advancement will depend largely upon your _____ in performing administrative and clinical tasks.
5. In terminating employment, the employee has the major responsibility giving the employer at least a

   _____ - _____ .
6. The usual cause for termination initiated by the employer is _____ to perform job responsibilities.

D. LETTERS

1. In the space below write a follow-up letter thanking an employer who interviewed you for a job. Show it to your instructor for evaluation.

_____

_____

_____

_____

_____

_____

_____

2. Write a letter of resignation below and show it to your instructor for evaluation.

_____

_____

_____

_____

_____

E. CRITICAL THINKING SITUATIONS: What would you say? What would you do?

1. You have just started to work on some reports, of which you are behind schedule in mailing, when your employer brings the new employee to you for a tour of the clinic. You are also asked to explain the office policy and duties to this person. _____

_____

_____

2. You have been employed at the clinic for almost 3 months. You know that your 3 month (90 day) evaluation is scheduled for next week. Since you have done so well, you feel you will be eligible for a promotion and raise. You have overheard that the supervisor is thinking about hiring a new person for the job. _____

_____

_____

_____

F. WORD SEARCH: Listed below are words from Unit 2 to find in the Word Search Puzzle.

work	ethics	reliability	competent
on time	review	initiative	questions
tact	prompt	cooperation	form
values	goals	grammar	skill
smile	honest	communication	manners
thank	responsibility	advancement	follow up
active	enthusiasm	opportunity	

```
Y T I L I B A I L E R L P T E V O J K T
T C A J N P U T A J E N T H U S I A S M
I A D H O N E S T S S M D A J B S D B R
N R R M I P B M N T P K C N N F L V K B
U T A C T F P K P Y O K I K C G O A L S
T N C Q A R V M S L N G C L K Z M N K M
R O T U R E O B J T S H J F L J S C S I
O C K H E R A G I N I T I A T I V E S L
P C F D P F G J D A B W J B N S M M D E
P R C F O C R C S T I G S C I H T E R Y
O H O R O S A A E C L M A D P S F N A P
J N M C C O M M U N I C A T I O N T M U
A Z P W L B M Y L O T M J N L C R L B W
F W E S C Z A F A I Y B O Y N S W F L O
B Q T A M G R E V I E W T N G E O K V L
J K E R D T L E F W K V Q R A I R I T L
C W N L L F Z I O Q U E S T I O N S V O
O N T I M E A W T W K I A L W R B M A F
```

Name _____

Date _____ Score* _____

PROCEDURE 4–1   Total Charges on Calculator

TERMINAL PERFORMANCE OBJECTIVE - Provided with necessary equipment and materials, calculate a list of 20 charges, performing any necessary mathematical functions, and correctly determine the total amount. The same correct answer must be obtained twice within a maximum of three attempts.

PROCEDURE STEPS	STEP PERFORMED	POINTS POSSIBLE	COMMENTS
EVALUATOR: Place check mark in space following each step performed satisfactorily			
NOTE TIME BEGAN _____			
1. Turned on calculator.	_____	5	
2. Cleared machine.	_____	15	
3. Accurately entered figures from list.	_____	15	
4. Totaled fees.	_____	10	
5. Refigured to see if the same answer was obtained twice.	_____	15	
6. Recorded correct total. _____	_____	15	
EVALUATOR: NOTE TIME COMPLETED _____			

ADD POINTS OF STEPS CHECKED   _____ EARNED
TOTAL POINTS POSSIBLE   75 POSSIBLE

Points assigned reflect importance of step to meeting objective: Important = (5)   Essential = (10)   Critical = (15)
Automatic failure results if any of the critical steps are omitted or performed incorrectly.

DETERMINE SCORE (divide points earned by total points possible, multiply results by 100)   _____ SCORE*

Evaluator's Name (print) _____ Signature _____

Comments _____

Name _____

Date _____ Score* _____

PROCEDURE 4–2   Operate Copy Machine

TERMINAL PERFORMANCE OBJECTIVE - Given access to necessary equipment and supplies, demonstrate adjustment of settings in order to produce the specified copy or copies, while operating the copy machine accurately following the steps in the procedure.

PROCEDURE STEPS	STEP PERFORMED	POINTS POSSIBLE	COMMENTS
EVALUATOR: Place check mark in space following each step performed satisfactorily			
NOTE TIME BEGAN _____			
1. Assembled material to be copied.	_____	10	
2. Determined number of copies needed.	_____	10	
3. Turned on copy machine.	_____	5	
4. Adjusted settings to produce desired copy.			
a. Paper size	_____	15	
b. One/two sided	_____	15	
c. Regular/reduced/enlarged size	_____	15	
d. Number of copies	_____	15	
5. Checked paper supply.	_____	15	
6. Raised lid and placed material to be copied, one sheet at a time, face down on glass, or in feeder.	_____	10	
7. Closed lid, if appropriate.	_____	—	
8. Pressed button or key pad to activate copier.	_____	5	
9. Removed original(s) and copy/copies.	_____	10	
10. Removed special paper, if used, from supply.	_____	10	
11. Returned machine to "standard" settings if changed.	_____	5	
12. Turned off machine (if policy).	_____	5	
EVALUATOR: NOTE TIME COMPLETED _____			

ADD POINTS OF STEPS CHECKED   _____ EARNED
TOTAL POINTS POSSIBLE   145 POSSIBLE

Points assigned reflect importance of step to meeting objective: Important = (5)   Essential = (10)   Critical = (15)
Automatic failure results if any of the critical steps are omitted or performed incorrectly.

DETERMINE SCORE (divide points earned by total points possible, multiply results by 100)   _____ SCORE*

Evaluator's Name (print) _____ Signature _____

Comments _____

Name _____

Date _____ Score* _____

PROCEDURE 4–3   Operate Transcriber

TERMINAL PERFORMANCE OBJECTIVE - Given access to equipment and supplies, operate the transcriber, correctly following all steps in the procedure. Complete an accurate transcription within a specified time period.

PROCEDURE STEPS	STEP PERFORMED	POINTS POSSIBLE	COMMENTS
EVALUATOR: Place check mark in space following each step performed satisfactorily			
NOTE TIME BEGAN _____			
1. Turned on the transcriber.	_____	5	
2. Attached headset with earphones and the foot control to the unit.	_____	10	
3. Selected tape; chose rush reports or oldest dictation first.	_____	10	
4. Adjusted headset with earphones.	_____	5	
5. Inserted tape. Pressed play tab or the pedal to listen for the beginning of the dictation.	_____	10	
6. Adjusted volume, tone, and speed controls for clearest communication reception.	_____	10	
7. Listened for physician's instructions.	_____	15	
8. Set typewriter or computer margins and tabulator stops.	_____	10	
9. Selected appropriate paper for transcription.	_____	10	
10. Inserted paper in typewriter or brought up blank screen on computer.	_____	5	
11. Alternately pressed and released foot pedal to listen and transcribe the recorded message.	_____	10	
12. Turned off the machine and placed accessory items in proper storage space.	_____	5	
13. Completed transcript is accurate copy of recorded message, on appropriate paper, within specified time period.	_____	15	

EVALUATOR: NOTE TIME COMPLETED _____

ADD POINTS OF STEPS CHECKED   _____ EARNED
TOTAL POINTS POSSIBLE   120 POSSIBLE

Points assigned reflect importance of step to meeting objective: Important = (5)   Essential = (10)   Critical = (15)
Automatic failure results if any of the critical steps are omitted or performed incorrectly.

DETERMINE SCORE (divide points earned by total points possible, multiply results by 100)   _____ SCORE*

Evaluator's Name (print) _____ Signature _____

Comments _____

Name _____

Date _____ Score* _____

PROCEDURE 4–4   Operate Office Computer

TERMINAL PERFORMANCE OBJECTIVE - Given access to equipment and material to be entered, operate system following steps in the procedure to produce an accurate print copy of a schedule.

PROCEDURE STEPS	STEP PERFORMED	POINTS POSSIBLE	COMMENTS
EVALUATOR: Place check mark in space following each step performed satisfactorily			
NOTE TIME BEGAN _____			
1. Turned on power to computer.	_____	5	
2. Positioned cursor on appropriate program on main menu, keyed "ENTER" or clicked mouse.	_____	5	
3. Positioned cursor on scheduling software program, keyed "ENTER" or clicked mouse.	_____	5	
4. Positioned cursor or clicked on first cell to be completed.	_____	5	
5. Entered 1:00 P.M. appointment for first patient on list.	_____	10	
6. Entered remaining names at 15-minute intervals.	_____	15	
7. Saved data.	_____	15	
8. Exited scheduling program to main menu.	_____	10	
9. Exited from main menu.	_____	10	
10. Re-entered main menu.	_____	10	
11. Brought up scheduling software.	_____	10	
12. Located cursor at 2:30, entered patient as work-in who was currently scheduled for 1:30.	_____	10	
13. Located cursor at 1:30, canceled appointment.	_____	5	
14. Scrolled through schedule to view and proofread.	_____	10	
15. Turned on printer.	_____	5	
16. Allowed time for test sheet. (If appropriate; subtract 10 points if omitted)	_____	—	
17. Checked paper supply.	_____	5	
18. Keyed or clicked on print.	_____	10	
19. Selected from options.	_____	10	
20. Printed document.	_____	15	
21. Exited program.	_____	10	

PROCEDURE 4–4 Operate Office Computer—continued

PROCEDURE STEPS	STEP PERFORMED	POINTS POSSIBLE	COMMENTS
22. Exited main menu.	_____	10	
23. Turned off power to printer.	_____	5	
24. Turned off power to computer.	_____	5	
EVALUATOR: NOTE TIME COMPLETED _____			

ADD POINTS OF STEPS CHECKED _____ EARNED

TOTAL POINTS POSSIBLE 200 POSSIBLE

Points assigned reflect importance of step to meeting objective: Important = (5)   Essential = (10)   Critical = (15)
Automatic failure results if any of the critical steps are omitted or performed incorrectly.

DETERMINE SCORE (divide points earned by total points possible, multiply results by 100) _____ SCORE*

Evaluator's Name (print) _____ Signature _____

Comments _____

Name _____

Date _____ Score* _____

PROCEDURE 4–5   Open the Office

TERMINAL PERFORMANCE OBJECTIVE - Following all the steps in the procedure, role play the actions necessary to prepare a medical office to see patients. Verbally describe actions while performing.

PROCEDURE STEPS	STEP PERFORMED	POINTS POSSIBLE	COMMENTS
EVALUATOR: Place check mark in space following each step performed satisfactorily			
NOTE TIME BEGAN _____			
1. Unlocked the reception room door.	_____	10	
2. Adjusted heat or air conditioning for the comfort of the patients.	_____	5	
3. Checked for safety hazards in the office.			
a. Checked electrical wires	_____	15	
b. Checked furniture condition	_____	15	
c. Checked floor	_____	15	
4. Checked magazines for condition and date.	_____	5	
5. Checked the telephone answering device or call the answering service for any messages.	_____	10	
6. Pulled the charts of patients to be seen.	_____	15	
7. Wrote or stamped today's date.	_____	15	
8. Checked for previously ordered studies and filed in chart.	_____	15	
9. Checked examining rooms to be sure they were clean and stocked with supplies.	_____	10	
10. If it is the policy of the office, prepared a list of the patients to be seen and the times of their appointments and placed this list on the physician's desk.	_____	5	
EVALUATOR: NOTE TIME COMPLETED _____			

ADD POINTS OF STEPS CHECKED   _____ EARNED
TOTAL POINTS POSSIBLE   135 POSSIBLE

Points assigned reflect importance of step to meeting objective: Important = (5)   Essential = (10)   Critical = (15)
Automatic failure results if any of the critical steps are omitted or performed incorrectly.

DETERMINE SCORE (divide points earned by total points possible, multiply results by 100)   _____ SCORE*

Evaluator's Name (print) _____ Signature _____

Comments _____

Name _____

Date _____ Score* _____

PROCEDURE 4–6 Obtain Preliminary Patient Information

TERMINAL PERFORMANCE OBJECTIVE - In a simulated situation, clearly communicate instructions and complete the steps designated in the procedure within acceptable time limits.

PROCEDURE STEPS	STEP PERFORMED	POINTS POSSIBLE	COMMENTS
EVALUATOR: Place check mark in space following each step performed satisfactorily			
NOTE TIME BEGAN _____			
1. Took new patient to private room to ask preliminary questions.	_____	10	
2. Instructed new patient to complete a data sheet.	_____	10	
a. Provided clipboard and pen	_____	10	
b. Requested return when completed	_____	10	
3. Checked form for completeness.	_____	15	
4. Prepared a patient folder by typing the patient's name on a label and attaching it to the tab of the folder.	_____	5	
5. Transferred information from the data sheet to the chart sheet.	_____	10	
6. Copied the insurance card and returned to patient.	_____	15	
7. Inserted the chart, data sheets, and insurance card copy in folder.	_____	15	
8. Placed any referral material in chart.	_____	15	
9. Prepared charge slip.	_____	10	
10. Placed the folder in the area reserved for charts of patients to be seen.	_____	5	
11. Completed within established time limit.	_____	15	
EVALUATOR: NOTE TIME COMPLETED _____			

ADD POINTS OF STEPS CHECKED   _____ EARNED
TOTAL POINTS POSSIBLE   145 POSSIBLE

Points assigned reflect importance of step to meeting objective: Important = (5) Essential = (10) Critical = (15)
Automatic failure results if any of the critical steps are omitted or performed incorrectly.

DETERMINE SCORE (divide points earned by total points possible, multiply results by 100)   _____ SCORE*

Evaluator's Name (print) _____ Signature _____

Comments _____

Name _____

Date _____ Score* _____

PROCEDURE 4–7   Close the Office

TERMINAL PERFORMANCE OBJECTIVE - Following all the steps in the procedure, role play the actions required to close the office. Actions must be verbally described while performing the procedure.

PROCEDURE STEPS	STEP PERFORMED	POINTS POSSIBLE	COMMENTS
EVALUATOR: Place check mark in space following each step performed satisfactorily			
NOTE TIME BEGAN _____			
1. Checked to see that records were collected and filed in locked cabinets.	_____	15	
2. Placed any money received in safe or took to the bank to be deposited.	_____	15	
3. Turned off all electrical appliances.	_____	15	
4. Checked that rooms were all cleaned and supplied for the next day.	_____	10	
5. Straightened reception room if time allowed.	_____	5	
6. Pulled charts for the next day if time allowed.	_____	5	
7. Activated answering device on phone or called answering service with information about when you would be back in the office.	_____	15	
8. Turned off lights.	_____	10	
9. Activated alarm system.	_____	15	
10. Securely locked doors.	_____	15	
EVALUATOR: NOTE TIME COMPLETED _____			

ADD POINTS OF STEPS CHECKED   _____ EARNED
TOTAL POINTS POSSIBLE   120 POSSIBLE

Points assigned reflect importance of step to meeting objective: Important = (5)   Essential = (10)   Critical = (15)
Automatic failure results if any of the critical steps are omitted or performed incorrectly.

DETERMINE SCORE (divide points earned by total points possible, multiply results by 100)   _____ SCORE*

Evaluator's Name (print) _____ Signature _____

Comments _____

Name _____

Date _____ Score* _____

PROCEDURE 6–1   Answer the Office Phone

TERMINAL PERFORMANCE OBJECTIVE - In a simulated (or actual) situation, using proper grammar, answer the telephone by the third ring, identifying the office and yourself.

PROCEDURE STEPS	STEP PERFORMED	POINTS POSSIBLE	COMMENTS
EVALUATOR: Place check mark in space following each step performed satisfactorily			
NOTE TIME BEGAN _____			
1. Answered the phone promptly (by third ring) in a polite and pleasant manner.	_____	10	
2. Identified the office and yourself by name.	_____	15	
a. Voice clear, distinct, moderate rate of speaking	_____	10	
3. Listened to and recorded the name of the caller.	_____	15	
4. Recorded:			
a. Date	_____	5	
b. Time	_____	5	
c. Reason for call	_____	5	
5. a. Spelled name correctly	_____	10	
b. Processed emergency call immediately	_____	15	
c. Waited for response before placing on hold	_____	15	
d. Checked with caller on hold once each minute	_____	5	
e. Completed interrupted on-hold calls	_____	5	
6. Screened and completed as many calls as possible before adding to the physician's call-back list.	_____	10	
7. Responded to an untimely request to speak to physician by taking a message.	_____	10	
EVALUATOR: NOTE TIME COMPLETED _____			

ADD POINTS OF STEPS CHECKED _____ EARNED
TOTAL POINTS POSSIBLE 135 POSSIBLE

Points assigned reflect importance of step to meeting objective: Important = (5)   Essential = (10)   Critical = (15)
Automatic failure results if any of the critical steps are omitted or performed incorrectly.

DETERMINE SCORE (divide points earned by total points possible, multiply results by 100) _____ SCORE*

Evaluator's Name (print) _____ Signature _____

Comments _____

Name _____

Date _____ Score* _____

PROCEDURE 6–2 Process Phone Message

TERMINAL PERFORMANCE OBJECTIVE - In a simulated situation (or actual situation) receive, evaluate, and document a phone message.

PROCEDURE STEPS	STEP PERFORMED	POINTS POSSIBLE	COMMENTS
EVALUATOR: Place check mark in space following each step performed satisfactorily			
NOTE TIME BEGAN _____			
1. Answered the phone properly.	_____	10	
2. Listened carefully and determined caller's needs.	_____	15	
3. Documented information regarding message (including date/time) on message pad/phone call log—included:			
a. Who the request was for	_____	15	
b. What it concerned	_____	15	
c. When information was needed	_____	15	
d. Where to return call	_____	15	
4. Repeated message to caller to verify the contents.	_____	10	
5. Closed conversation politely.	_____	5	
6. Allowed caller to hang up first.	_____	5	
7. Signed your initials after the message.	_____	5	
8. Pulled patient's chart and recorded or attached message.	_____	10	

EVALUATOR: NOTE TIME COMPLETED _____

ADD POINTS OF STEPS CHECKED   _____ EARNED
TOTAL POINTS POSSIBLE   120 POSSIBLE

Points assigned reflect importance of step to meeting objective: Important = (5)   Essential = (10)   Critical = (15)
Automatic failure results if any of the critical steps are omitted or performed incorrectly.

DETERMINE SCORE (divide points earned by total points possible, multiply results by 100)   _____ SCORE*

Evaluator's Name (print) _____ Signature _____

Comments _____

Name _____

Date _____ Score* _____

PROCEDURE 6–3   Record Telephone Message on Recording Device

TERMINAL PERFORMANCE OBJECTIVE - In a simulated situation (or actual situation) produce, with all necessary information in a pleasant tone of voice, a clear, accurate, and precise phone message on the telephone message device.

PROCEDURE STEPS	STEP PERFORMED	POINTS POSSIBLE	COMMENTS
EVALUATOR: Place check mark in space following each step performed satisfactorily			
NOTE TIME BEGAN _____			
1. Assembled necessary items away from noise and distractions.	_____	10	
a. Determined amount of time allowed on recording device for message before beginning.	_____	10	
2. Wrote out appropriate message			
a. Checked for completeness and accuracy	_____	10	
b. Read and determined the amount of time of message	_____	10	
3. Recorded message following directions of answering device.	_____	15	
a. Spoke in a pleasant, clear, and articulate tone of voice.	_____	5	
b. Sat up straight and projected voice into the speaker.	_____	5	
c. Identified the office	_____	10	
d. Was not too wordy or overly friendly	_____	5	
e. Complete and accurate information	_____	10	
4. Played message back and evaluated quality of message.	_____	5	
a. Listened and determined if the message was of good quality	_____	5	
b. Appropriate for all callers	_____	5	
5. Set the device to play messages when unavailable to answer phone.	_____	15	
EVALUATOR: NOTE TIME COMPLETED _____			

ADD POINTS OF STEPS CHECKED   _____ EARNED

TOTAL POINTS POSSIBLE   120 POSSIBLE

Points assigned reflect importance of step to meeting objective: Important = (5)   Essential = (10)   Critical = (15)
Automatic failure results if any of the critical steps are omitted or performed incorrectly.

DETERMINE SCORE (divide points earned by total points possible, multiply results by 100)   _____ SCORE*

Evaluator's Name (print) _____ Signature _____

Comments _____

Name _____

Date _____ Score* _____

PROCEDURE 6–4   Obtain Telephone Message from Phone Recording Device

TERMINAL PERFORMANCE OBJECTIVE - In a simulated situation (or actual situation) obtain all necessary and pertinent information all phone message from the phone message recording device.

PROCEDURE STEPS	STEP PERFORMED	POINTS POSSIBLE	COMMENTS
EVALUATOR: Place check mark in space following each step performed satisfactorily			
NOTE TIME BEGAN _____			
1. Assembled necessary items in an area away from noise and distractions.	_____	5	
2. Listened to recordings and wrote message(s) accurately.	_____	15	
3. Repeated listening to difficult messages to obtain complete information.	_____	5	
4. Signed initials after message(s).	_____	5	
5. Noted date and time of the message(s).	_____	10	
6. Listed all patients who left messages and pulled their charts.	_____	15	
7. Prioritized messages according to their seriousness.	_____	15	
8. Distributed messages to appropriate staff member/ department to be processed.	_____	10	
EVALUATOR: NOTE TIME COMPLETED _____			

ADD POINTS OF STEPS CHECKED   _____ EARNED

TOTAL POINTS POSSIBLE   80 POSSIBLE

Points assigned reflect importance of step to meeting objective: Important = (5)   Essential = (10)   Critical = (15)

Automatic failure results if any of the critical steps are omitted or performed incorrectly.

DETERMINE SCORE (divide points earned by total points possible, multiply results by 100)   _____ SCORE*

Evaluator's Name (print) _____ Signature _____

Comments _____

Name _____

Date _____ Score* _____

PROCEDURE 6–5   Schedule Appointments

TERMINAL PERFORMANCE OBJECTIVE - In a simulated situation, schedule an appointment for a patient according to accepted medical standards with consideration for the physician, staff, and needs of the patient.

PROCEDURE STEPS	STEP PERFORMED	POINTS POSSIBLE	COMMENTS
EVALUATOR: Place check mark in space following each step performed satisfactorily			
NOTE TIME BEGAN _____			
1. Determined the means of scheduling: appointment book or computer entry.	_____	10	
2. Marked off hours when the physician was unable to see patients.	_____	15	
3. Attempted to give patients two appointment choices.	_____	5	
4. Recorded names in black ink with phone number(s).	_____	10	
5. Asked patient(s) to schedule next appointment before leaving office.	_____	5	
6. Wrote patients' names in the schedule book.	_____	10	
7. Recorded appointment first in appointment book and then on appointment card.	_____	15	
8. Completed appointment card and gave to patient.	_____	15	
9. Left sufficient time for work-ins in appointment book.	_____	10	
10. Allowed time for return phone calls to be made by the doctor.	_____	5	
EVALUATOR: NOTE TIME COMPLETED _____			

ADD POINTS OF STEPS CHECKED   _____ EARNED

TOTAL POINTS POSSIBLE   100 POSSIBLE

Points assigned reflect importance of step to meeting objective: Important = (5)   Essential = (10)   Critical = (15)

Automatic failure results if any of the critical steps are omitted or performed incorrectly.

DETERMINE SCORE (divide points earned by total points possible, multiply results by 100)   _____ SCORE*

Evaluator's Name (print) _____ Signature _____

Comments _____

Name _____

Date _____ Score* _____

PROCEDURE 6–6 Arrange Referral Appointment

TERMINAL PERFORMANCE OBJECTIVE - In a simulated situation, schedule a referral appointment for a patient by phoning the requested medical facility according to accepted medical standards with consideration for the physician, staff, and needs of the patient.

PROCEDURE STEPS	STEP PERFORMED	POINTS POSSIBLE	COMMENTS
EVALUATOR: Place check mark in space following each step performed satisfactorily			
NOTE TIME BEGAN _____			
1. Obtained patient's chart with request for referral to another facility.	_____	15	
2. Used phone directory to obtain phone number and address of referral office.	_____	10	
3. Placed the call to referral office and provided receptionist with:			
a. Your name/physician's name and address	_____	15	
b. Patient's name, address, etc., and reason for appointment	_____	15	
c. Indicated that confirmation letter will be mailed/faxed	_____	5	
d. Recorded appointment information on patient's chart	_____	10	
e. Gave complete information to patient (time, day, date, name, address, etc.)	_____	10	
4. Gave patient printed instructions regarding appointment as appropriate.	_____	5	
a. Initialed patient's chart signifying completion of request	_____	5	
EVALUATOR: NOTE TIME COMPLETED _____			

ADD POINTS OF STEPS CHECKED   _____ EARNED

TOTAL POINTS POSSIBLE   90 POSSIBLE

Points assigned reflect importance of step to meeting objective: Important = (5)   Essential = (10)   Critical = (15)
Automatic failure results if any of the critical steps are omitted or performed incorrectly.

DETERMINE SCORE (divide points earned by total points possible, multiply results by 100)   _____ SCORE*

Evaluator's Name (print) _____   Signature _____

Comments _____

Name _____

Date _____ Score* _____

PROCEDURE 6–7   Make Corrections on Typewritten Copy

TERMINAL PERFORMANCE OBJECTIVE - Given access to all equipment and supplies, make neat, acceptable corrections using the various methods described in the procedure. The corrected copy must be without error and corrections should be difficult to detect.

PROCEDURE STEPS	STEP PERFORMED	POINTS POSSIBLE	COMMENTS
EVALUATOR: Place check mark in space following each step performed satisfactorily			
NOTE TIME BEGAN _____			
1. Proofed copy before removing paper from typewriter.	_____	15	
2. Made corrections with typewriter correcting ribbon.			
a. Positioned over character next to error	_____	10	
b. Pressed correction key	_____	5	
c. Retyped error	_____	5	
d. Typed correct letter	_____	5	
3. Made corrections without correcting ribbon, with erasable paper.			
a. Carefully erased only the error	_____	10	
b. Brushed any eraser crumbs away	_____	5	
c. When using carbon paper, placed a guard between the paper and carbon while erasing. Erased both original and copy	_____	15	
d. Removed the guard before resuming typing	_____	10	
4. Made corrections using correction paper.			
a. Used color to match paper	_____	5	
b. Inserted over error	_____	5	
c. Retyped error	_____	10	
d. Removed paper and typed correct letter(s)	_____	5	
5. Made corrections using correction fluid.			
a. Shook bottle	_____	5	
b. Applied fluid sparingly and smoothly	_____	10	
c. Allowed to dry	_____	15	
d. Retyped letter(s)	_____	5	
6. Made corrections when paper had been removed before error was found.			
a. Studied the relationship of letters on the page to lines on the paper guide	_____	5	
b. Inserted scratch paper in typewriter	_____	5	

PROCEDURE STEPS	STEP PERFORMED	POINTS POSSIBLE	COMMENTS
c. Set typewriter to stencil	_____	10	
d. Cleaned keys by striking scratch paper several times.	_____	5	
e. Reinserted letter. With ribbon still on stencil, realigned and struck missing letters	_____	15	
f. If in alignment, set ribbon on print and typed letters	_____	5	
7. Made corrections using correction tape.			
a. Cut or tore tape to cover error(s)	_____	5	
b. Applied smoothly to paper	_____	10	
c. Typed correct letter(s)	_____	5	

EVALUATOR: NOTE TIME COMPLETED _____

ADD POINTS OF STEPS CHECKED   _____ EARNED
TOTAL POINTS POSSIBLE   205 POSSIBLE

Points assigned reflect importance of step to meeting objective: Important = (5)   Essential = (10)   Critical = (15)
Automatic failure results if any of the critical steps are omitted or performed incorrectly.

DETERMINE SCORE (divide points earned by total points possible, multiply results by 100)   _____ SCORE*

Evaluator's Name (print) _____ Signature _____

Comments _____

Name _____

Date _____ Score* _____

PROCEDURE 6–8   Type Business Letter

TERMINAL PERFORMANCE OBJECTIVE - Given access to equipment and supplies, complete a mailable letter following the steps in the procedure within the number of attempts and time frame specified by the instructor. The final copy must meet mailable standards described in the text.

PROCEDURE STEPS	STEP PERFORMED	POINTS POSSIBLE	COMMENTS
EVALUATOR: Place check mark in space following each step performed satisfactorily			
NOTE TIME BEGAN _____			
1. Moved type down at least three lines below letterhead.	_____	5	
2. Typed the date in appropriate location for letter style.	_____	10	
3. Moved to the fifth line below the date.	_____	5	
4. Typed the inside address in appropriate location for letter style.	_____	5	
a. Typed name as received on letter or listed in a directory	_____	15	
5. Double spaced after the last line of the address.	_____	5	
6. Typed the appropriate salutation followed by a colon.	_____	10	
7. Double spaced.	_____	5	
8. a. Entered the reference line in the location appropriate for letter style	_____	5	
b. Typed RE: Entered patient's name or person about whom the letter was written	_____	10	
9. Double spaced.	_____	5	
10. Typed the body of letter.			
a. Paragraph style appropriate to the style of the letter.	_____	5	
b. Double spaced between paragraphs.	_____	5	
11. (If second page)—			
a. When typewritten—proofed page one and corrected before removing	_____	—	
b. Typed second page heading at 7th line	_____	—	
c. Typed name, page number, date	_____	—	
d. At least two lines of paragraph were on first page	_____	—	
e. Last word on first page not divided	_____	—	
(Note: Subtract 10 points for each step a–e if omitted)			
12. Continued body of letter	_____	—	

PROCEDURE STEPS	STEP PERFORMED	POINTS POSSIBLE	COMMENTS
13. Complimentary closing typed in letter style format.	_____	10	
14. Four spaces entered.	_____	5	
15. Sender's name typed in letter style format exactly as printed on letterhead;	_____	15	
a. Title followed name after comma or			
b. Title typed below name			
16. Double space.	_____	5	
17. Typed reference initials to indicate typist.	_____	15	
18. Single or double spaced if enclosed materials.	_____	—	
19. "cc" and recipient's name typed	_____	—	
a. Numbered and identified if more than one.	_____	—	
20. Double spaced (if needed)	_____	—	
(Subtract 10 points if omitted in error)			
21. PS for postscript if applicable	_____	—	
(Subtract 10 points if omitted in error)			
EVALUATOR: NOTE TIME COMPLETED _____			
Completed within specified time		15	
Meets mailable standard		15	

ADD POINTS OF STEPS CHECKED   _____ EARNED
TOTAL POINTS POSSIBLE   170 POSSIBLE

Points assigned reflect importance of step to meeting objective: Important = (5)   Essential = (10)   Critical = (15)
Automatic failure results if any of the critical steps are omitted or performed incorrectly.

DETERMINE SCORE (divide points earned by total points possible, multiply results by 100)   _____ SCORE*

Evaluator's Name (print) _____ Signature _____

Comments _____

Name _____

Date _____ Score* _____

PROCEDURE 7–1   File Item(s) Alphabetically

TERMINAL PERFORMANCE OBJECTIVE - In a simulated situation, given the patient's file or other items, accurately file and store the file(s) and/or other items within acceptable time limit according to acceptable medical standards.

PROCEDURE STEPS	STEP PERFORMED	POINTS POSSIBLE	COMMENTS
EVALUATOR: Place check mark in space following each step performed satisfactorily			
NOTE TIME BEGAN _____			
1. Used rules for filing items alphabetically.	_____	10	
a. Double-checked spelling of name for accuracy when using cross-reference file	_____	15	
2. Determined appropriate storage file.	_____	10	
3. For new material, scanned guides for area nearest to letters of name(s) on items to file.	_____	10	
4. Placed folder in correct alphabetical order between two files.	_____	15	
a. Inserted new file *between* two other folders and *not* within another folder, where it could be lost	_____	15	
5. In filing material previously in file, scanned for the out-guide.			
a. Removed out-guide after you have removed file	_____	5	
b. Checked to be sure it was marking the space for the file you just returned and not another	_____	5	
EVALUATOR: NOTE TIME COMPLETED _____			

ADD POINTS OF STEPS CHECKED   _____ EARNED

TOTAL POINTS POSSIBLE   85 POSSIBLE

Points assigned reflect importance of step to meeting objective: Important = (5)   Essential = (10)   Critical = (15)
Automatic failure results if any of the critical steps are omitted or performed incorrectly.

DETERMINE SCORE (divide points earned by total points possible, multiply results by 100)   _____ SCORE*

Evaluator's Name (print) _____ Signature _____

Comments _____

PROCEDURE 7–2   File Item(s) Numerically

TERMINAL PERFORMANCE OBJECTIVE - In a simulated situation, given the patient's file or other items, accurately file and store the file(s) and/or other items within acceptable time limit according to accepted medical standards.

PROCEDURE STEPS	STEP PERFORMED	POINTS POSSIBLE	COMMENTS
EVALUATOR: Place check mark in space following each step performed satisfactorily			
NOTE TIME BEGAN _____			
1. Used rules for numerical filing.	_____	15	
a. Double-checked spelling of name for accuracy using cross-reference file	_____	15	
2. Determined appropriate storage file.	_____	5	
3. Matched the first two or three numbers with those already in the file.	_____	15	
4. Matched remaining numbers with those in the file.	_____	15	
EVALUATOR: NOTE TIME COMPLETED _____			

ADD POINTS OF STEPS CHECKED   _____ EARNED

TOTAL POINTS POSSIBLE   35 POSSIBLE

Points assigned reflect importance of step to meeting objective: Important = (5)   Essential = (10)   Critical = (15)
Automatic failure results if any of the critical steps are omitted or performed incorrectly.

DETERMINE SCORE (divide points earned by total points possible, multiply results by 100)   _____ SCORE*

Evaluator's Name (print) _____ Signature _____

Comments _____

Name _____

Date _____ Score* _____

PROCEDURE 7–3 Pull File Folder From Alphabetical Files

TERMINAL PERFORMANCE OBJECTIVE - In a simulated situation, given the patient's name, accurately prepare the out-guide and pull the file, replacing the file with the out-guide within acceptable time limit according to accepted medical standards.

PROCEDURE STEPS	STEP PERFORMED	POINTS POSSIBLE	COMMENTS
EVALUATOR: Place check mark in space following each step performed satisfactorily			
NOTE TIME BEGAN _____			
1. Found name of patient in alphabetical file.	_____	15	
a. Double-checked the spelling of the name for accuracy	_____	15	
2. Completed out-guide with date and your name.	_____	5	
3. Pulled file(s) needed and replaced with out-guide(s).	_____	5	

EVALUATOR: NOTE TIME COMPLETED _____

ADD POINTS OF STEPS CHECKED   _____ EARNED
TOTAL POINTS POSSIBLE   40 POSSIBLE

Points assigned reflect importance of step to meeting objective: Important = (5)   Essential = (10)   Critical = (15)
Automatic failure results if any of the critical steps are omitted or performed incorrectly.

DETERMINE SCORE (divide points earned by total points possible, multiply results by 100)   _____ SCORE*

Evaluator's Name (print) _____ Signature _____

Comments _____

Name _____

Date _____ Score* _____

PROCEDURE 7–4   Pull File Folder From Numerical Files

TERMINAL PERFORMANCE OBJECTIVE - In a simulated situation, given the patient's name or account number, accurately prepare the out-guide and pull the file, replacing the file with the out-guide within acceptable time limit according to accepted medical standards.

PROCEDURE STEPS	STEP PERFORMED	POINTS POSSIBLE	COMMENTS
EVALUATOR: Place check mark in space following each step performed satisfactorily			
NOTE TIME BEGAN _____			
1. Found name of patient in card file and obtained account number.	_____	10	
a. Double-checked the spelling of name for accuracy	_____	10	
2. Completed out-guide with date and your name.	_____	5	
3. Located corresponding section of numerical file.	_____	10	
4. Scanned the files for the number.	_____	15	
5. Pulled requested file and replaced with prepared out-guide.	_____	15	

EVALUATOR: NOTE TIME COMPLETED _____

ADD POINTS OF STEPS CHECKED   _____ EARNED
TOTAL POINTS POSSIBLE   65 POSSIBLE

Points assigned reflect importance of step to meeting objective: Important = (5)   Essential = (10)   Critical = (15)
Automatic failure results if any of the critical steps are omitted or performed incorrectly.

DETERMINE SCORE (divide points earned by total points possible, multiply results by 100)   _____ SCORE*

Evaluator's Name (print) _____ Signature _____

Comments _____

Name _____

Date _____ Score* _____

PROCEDURE 8–1   Prepare Patient Ledger Card

TERMINAL PERFORMANCE OBJECTIVE - In a simulated medical office situation, prepare a patient ledger card following the steps in the procedure.

PROCEDURE STEPS	STEP PERFORMED	POINTS POSSIBLE	COMMENTS
EVALUATOR: Place check mark in space following each step performed satisfactorily			
NOTE TIME BEGAN _____			
1. Typed the name of patient, last name first.	_____	15	
2. Typed complete address with zip code.	_____	10	
3. Typed name and address of person responsible for charges if different from patient.	_____	5	
4. Typed telephone number of patient.	_____	10	
5. Typed name of insurance company.	_____	15	
6. Typed referring individual.	_____	5	
7. Typed balance due amount.	_____	10	
EVALUATOR: NOTE TIME COMPLETED _____			

ADD POINTS OF STEPS CHECKED   _____ EARNED

TOTAL POINTS POSSIBLE   70 POSSIBLE

Points assigned reflect importance of step to meeting objective: Important = (5)   Essential = (10)   Critical = (15)

Automatic failure results if any of the critical steps are omitted or performed incorrectly.

DETERMINE SCORE (divide points earned by total points possible, multiply results by 100)   _____ SCORE*

Evaluator's Name (print) _____ Signature _____

Comments _____

Name _____

Date _____ Score* _____

PROCEDURE 8–2   Record Charges and Credits

TERMINAL PERFORMANCE OBJECTIVE - In a simulated medical office situation, record charges and credits following the steps in the procedure.

PROCEDURE STEPS	STEP PERFORMED	POINTS POSSIBLE	COMMENTS
EVALUATOR: Place check mark in space following each step performed satisfactorily			
NOTE TIME BEGAN _____			
1. Pulled patients' ledger cards.	_____	10	
2. Posted charges and credits on ledger cards.	_____	15	
a. Used small, neat figures	_____	5	
3. Checked each off on day sheet	_____	5	
4. Posted charges in debit column	_____	15	
a. Added balance and new debit for new balance	_____	10	
5. Posted payments in credit column	_____	15	
a. Subtracted payments from balance due	_____	10	
b. Showed credits in red	_____	5	
EVALUATOR: NOTE TIME COMPLETED _____			

ADD POINTS OF STEPS CHECKED   _____ EARNED
TOTAL POINTS POSSIBLE   90 POSSIBLE

Points assigned reflect importance of step to meeting objective: Important = (5)   Essential = (10)   Critical = (15)
Automatic failure results if any of the critical steps are omitted or performed incorrectly.

DETERMINE SCORE (divide points earned by total points possible, multiply results by 100)   _____ SCORE*

Evaluator's Name (print) _____ Signature _____

Comments _____

Name _____

Date _____ Score* _____

PROCEDURE 8–3   Type Itemized Statement

TERMINAL PERFORMANCE OBJECTIVE - In a simulated medical office situation, type itemized statement(s) with 100 percent accuracy following the steps in the procedure.

PROCEDURE STEPS	STEP PERFORMED	POINTS POSSIBLE	COMMENTS
EVALUATOR: Place check mark in space following each step performed satisfactorily			
NOTE TIME BEGAN _____			
1. Stacked ledger cards beside typewriter.	_____	5	
2. Assembled statement forms and window envelopes.	_____	5	
3. Stamped ledger card on line below last entry with date stamp.	_____	5	
4. Typed name and complete address in area that shows in window of envelope.	_____	15	
5. Listed balance first under services.	_____	10	
6. Typed each service charge and payment for current month.	_____	15	
7. Folded and placed form in envelope	_____	5	
a. Address shown in window	_____	15	
b. Only one form in envelope	_____	15	
8. Fanned and exposed several envelope flaps.	_____	5	
9. Dampened flaps sufficiently.	_____	5	
10. Folded flaps of envelopes down to seal.	_____	10	
EVALUATOR: NOTE TIME COMPLETED _____			

ADD POINTS OF STEPS CHECKED   _____ EARNED

TOTAL POINTS POSSIBLE   110 POSSIBLE

Points assigned reflect importance of step to meeting objective: Important = (5)   Essential = (10)   Critical = (15)
Automatic failure results if any of the critical steps are omitted or performed incorrectly.

DETERMINE SCORE (divide points earned by total points possible, multiply results by 100)   _____ SCORE*

Evaluator's Name (print) _____ Signature _____

Comments _____

Name _____

Date _____ Score* _____

PROCEDURE 8–4   Compose Collection Letter

TERMINAL PERFORMANCE OBJECTIVE - In a simulated medical office situation, compose and type appropriate collection letters for assigned accounts to be collected following the procedure.

PROCEDURE STEPS	STEP PERFORMED	POINTS POSSIBLE	COMMENTS
EVALUATOR: Place check mark in space following each step performed satisfactorily			
NOTE TIME BEGAN _____			
1. Identified patients to whom an initial collection letter should be sent.	_____	10	
2. Composed a rough draft	_____	10	
a. First paragraph stated reason for letter	_____	10	
3. Second paragraph indicated expected response.	_____	10	
4. Reread rough draft	_____	5	
a. Had clear message	_____	10	
b. Contained correctly spelled words	_____	5	
c. Had correct punctuation	_____	5	
5. Typed letter according to standard form.	_____	5	
a. Proofread letter	_____	10	
b. Signed letter	_____	10	
6. Typed envelope.	_____	5	
7. Folded letter properly.	_____	5	
a. Sealed envelope	_____	5	
b. Stamped and mailed letter	_____	10	
EVALUATOR: NOTE TIME COMPLETED _____			

ADD POINTS OF STEPS CHECKED _____ EARNED

TOTAL POINTS POSSIBLE 115 POSSIBLE

Points assigned reflect importance of step to meeting objective: Important = (5)   Essential = (10)   Critical = (15)
Automatic failure results if any of the critical steps are omitted or performed incorrectly.

DETERMINE SCORE (divide points earned by total points possible, multiply results by 100) _____ SCORE*

Evaluator's Name (print) _____ Signature _____

Comments _____

Name _____

Date _____ Score* _____

PROCEDURE 9–1   Complete a Claim Form

TERMINAL PERFORMANCE OBJECTIVE - Given access to all necessary equipment and information, follow the procedure to complete the HCFA 1500 claim form without error within the instructor's prescribed time limit.

PROCEDURE STEPS	STEP PERFORMED	POINTS POSSIBLE	COMMENTS
EVALUATOR: Place check mark in space following each step performed satisfactorily			
NOTE TIME BEGAN _____			
1. Checked for a photocopy of the patient's insurance card.	_____	10	
2. Checked the chart to see if the patient signature was on file for release of information and assignment of benefits.	_____	15	
3. Explained procedure to obtain signature when not on file.	_____	10	
4. Using Figure 9–8 as an example, completed the HCFA 1500 claim form.			
a. Checked appropriate box at top of form	_____	5	
b. Entered name of patient	_____	10	
c. Entered birthdate using digits *and*	_____	10	
d. Checked box for male or female			
5. Entered insured's name.	_____	5	
6. Entered patient's full address and telephone number.	_____	5	
7. Entered patient's relationship to insured.	_____	5	
8. Entered insured's full address and telephone number.	_____	5	
9. Entered patient's status.	_____	5	
10. Entered other insured's name, if applicable.	_____	—	
a. Other insured's policy or group number	_____	—	
b. Other insured's birthdate and box for male or female	_____	—	
c. Employer's name or school name	_____	—	
d. Insurance plan name or program name	_____	—	
11. Checked appropriate box regarding employment and/or accident.	_____	5	
12. Entered insured's policy number			
a. Insured's birthdate and box for male or female	_____	5	
b. Employer or school name	_____	5	
c. Insurance plan name or program name	_____	5	
d. Was there another health benefit plan?	_____	5	
13. Obtained signature or indicated "on file."	_____	15	

PROCEDURE 9–1 Complete a Claim Form—continued

PROCEDURE STEPS	STEP PERFORMED	POINTS POSSIBLE	COMMENTS
14. Obtained insured's or authorized signature.	_____	10	
15. Entered current illness date, accident, or pregnancy.	_____	10	
16. Entered date patient first treated for same or similar illness.	_____	5	
17. Entered dates unable to work or stated N/A.	_____	—	
18. Entered referring physician or other.	_____	5	
a. Physician's ID number	_____	5	
19. Entered hospital dates or stated N/A.	_____	—	
20. Left blank.	_____	—	
21. Completed outside lab as appropriate.	_____	—	
22. Entered ICN codes.	_____	15	
23. Completed Medicaid resubmission if applicable.	_____	—	
24. Entered prior authorization number.	_____	—	
25. Completed Section 24 A–E with dates, appropriate codes, and charges for services.	_____	15	
26. Entered physician's Social Security number or practice tax identification number.	_____	10	
27. Entered patient's account number if applicable.	_____	—	
28. Checked appropriate box for assignment.	_____	10	
29. Totaled charges.	_____	15	
30. Entered amount paid.	_____	15	
31. Entered balance due.	_____	15	
32. Obtained physician's signature and date.	_____	15	
33. Completed name and address where services given.	_____	5	
34. Completed physician's information.	_____	5	
35. Completed within time specified.	_____	15	

EVALUATOR: NOTE TIME COMPLETED _____

Note: Subtract 10 points each for steps 9, 16, 18, 19, 20, 23, and 26 if applicable and not entered.

ADD POINTS OF STEPS CHECKED   _____ EARNED

TOTAL POINTS POSSIBLE   295 POSSIBLE

Points assigned reflect importance of step to meeting objective: Important = (5)   Essential = (10)   Critical = (15)
Automatic failure results if any of the critical steps are omitted or performed incorrectly.

DETERMINE SCORE (divide points earned by total points possible, multiply results by 100)   _____ SCORE*

Evaluator's Name (print) _____ Signature _____

Comments _____

Name _____

Date _____ Score* _____

PROCEDURE 10–1   Write a Check

TERMINAL PERFORMANCE OBJECTIVE - Prepare a check following the steps of the procedure. The check must be dated, accurately identify the payer, the correct numerical and written amount, and have appropriate signature. The register must accurately reflect the check.

PROCEDURE STEPS	STEP PERFORMED	POINTS POSSIBLE	COMMENTS
EVALUATOR: Place check mark in space following each step performed satisfactorily			
NOTE TIME BEGAN _____			
1. Filled out check register using black or blue ink.			
a. Check number	_____	5	
b. Date	_____	10	
c. Payee information	_____	10	
d. Amount	_____	15	
e. Previous balance	_____	10	
f. Entered new balance	_____	10	
2. Entered date on check.	_____	5	
3. Entered payee.	_____	15	
4. Entered numerically the amount of check.	_____	10	
5. Wrote out amount of check.			
a. Began as far left as possible	_____	10	
b. Wrote out amount	_____	15	
c. Made straight line to fill space	_____	10	
6. Obtained signature; must agree with authorization card.	_____	15	
EVALUATOR: NOTE TIME COMPLETED _____			

ADD POINTS OF STEPS CHECKED   _____ EARNED
TOTAL POINTS POSSIBLE   140 POSSIBLE

Points assigned reflect importance of step to meeting objective: Important = (5)   Essential = (10)   Critical = (15)
Automatic failure results if any of the critical steps are omitted or performed incorrectly.

DETERMINE SCORE (divide points earned by total points possible, multiply results by 100)   _____ SCORE*

Evaluator's Name (print) _____ Signature _____

Comments _____

Name _____

Date _____ Score* _____

PROCEDURE 10–2   Prepare Deposit Slip

TERMINAL PERFORMANCE OBJECTIVE - Prepare a bank deposit slip following the steps in the procedure. The slip will correctly reflect the currency, coin, and checks to be deposited, and be totaled accurately.

PROCEDURE STEPS	STEP PERFORMED	POINTS POSSIBLE	COMMENTS
EVALUATOR: Place check mark in space following each step performed satisfactorily			
NOTE TIME BEGAN _____			
1. Separated money to be deposited, by check, currency, and coin.	_____	5	
2. Listed currency.			
a. Sorted bills by denomination	_____	5	
b. Portrait side up	_____	5	
c. Highest denomination to lowest	_____	5	
d. Totaled currency accurately	_____	15	
e. Recorded accurately on deposit slip	_____	10	
3. Listed coin.			
a. Sorted by denomination	_____	5	
b. Totaled coin accurately	_____	15	
c. Recorded accurately on deposit slip	_____	10	
4. Listed checks.			
a. Checked for endorsement	_____	10	
b. Listed by number, maker, amount	_____	5	
c. Listed from largest to smallest amount	_____	5	
d. Listed money orders with MO and name	_____	5	
e. Accurately totaled and entered on slip	_____	15	
5. Accurately totaled currency, coin, and checks to be deposited.	_____	15	
6. Made copy of deposit slip for files.	_____	5	
7. Entered deposit total in checkbook.	_____	10	
8. Made deposit at bank and kept record.	_____	10	
EVALUATOR: NOTE TIME COMPLETED _____			

ADD POINTS OF STEPS CHECKED   _____ EARNED

TOTAL POINTS POSSIBLE   155 POSSIBLE

Points assigned reflect importance of step to meeting objective: Important = (5)   Essential = (10)   Critical = (15)
Automatic failure results if any of the critical steps are omitted or performed incorrectly.

DETERMINE SCORE (divide points earned by total points possible, multiply results by 100)   _____ SCORE*

Evaluator's Name (print) _____ Signature _____

Comments _____

Name _____

Date _____ Score* _____

PROCEDURE 10–3   Reconcile a Bank Statement

TERMINAL PERFORMANCE OBJECTIVE - Follow the steps in the procedure "Reconcile a Bank Statement;" after performing mathematical calculations, the checkbook and bank statement balance should agree.

PROCEDURE STEPS	STEP PERFORMED	POINTS POSSIBLE	COMMENTS
EVALUATOR: Place check mark in space following each step performed satisfactorily			
NOTE TIME BEGAN _____			
1. Compared the opening balance on the new statement with the closing balance on the previous statement.	_____	10	
2. Listed the bank balance in the appropriate space on the reconciliation worksheet.	_____	5	
3. Compared the check entries on the statement with the returned checks.	_____	10	
4. Determined if any outstanding checks.			
a. Marked stub or entry on register if check returned	_____	5	
b. Listed ones not checked on worksheet	_____	15	
c. Totaled outstanding checks	_____	10	
5. Subtracted from checkbook balance items such as withdrawals, automatic payments or service charges that appeared on the statement but not in the checkbook.	_____	15	
6. Added to checkbook any interest earned as indicated on statement.	_____	15	
7. Added to the bank statement balance any deposits not shown on the bank statement.	_____	15	
8. The balance in the checkbook and the bank statement agreed.	_____	15	
EVALUATOR: NOTE TIME COMPLETED _____			

ADD POINTS OF STEPS CHECKED   _____ EARNED
TOTAL POINTS POSSIBLE   115 POSSIBLE

Points assigned reflect importance of step to meeting objective: Important = (5)   Essential = (10)   Critical = (15)
Automatic failure results if any of the critical steps are omitted or performed incorrectly.

DETERMINE SCORE (divide points earned by total points possible, multiply results by 100)   _____ SCORE*

Evaluator's Name (print) _____ Signature _____

Comments _____

Name _____

Date _____ Score* _____

PROCEDURE 12–1   Hand Washing

TERMINAL PERFORMANCE OBJECTIVE - Provided with liquid hand soap in a dispenser, cuticle stick, nail brush, paper towels, and a waste receptacle, the student will stand at a sink with hot and cold faucets and demonstrate each step in the hand washing procedure as specified in the procedure sheet.

PROCEDURE STEPS	STEP PERFORMED	POINTS POSSIBLE	COMMENTS
EVALUATOR: Place check mark in space following each step performed satisfactorily			
NOTE TIME BEGAN _____			
1. Removed jewelry.	_____	5	
2. a. Stood, not touching sink	_____	10	
b. Used paper towel to turn on faucets	_____	5	
c. Adjusted water temperature	_____	5	
d. Discarded paper towel	_____	5	
3. a. Wet hands	_____	10	
b. Dispensed 1 tsp soap into palm	_____	10	
c. Distributed soap into lather on both hands	_____	15	
d. Washed, in circular motion, for two minutes	_____	15	
4. a. Used nail brush/1 dozen circular motions	_____	5	
b. Used cuticle stick under nails	_____	5	
5. a. Rinsed thoroughly	_____	10	
b. Wet arms to elbow	_____	5	
c. Re-applied soap (1 tsp) to palm	_____	5	
d. Did not touch inside of sink or faucets	_____	10	
e. Used brush in one dozen circular motions to elbow	_____	5	
f. Rinsed thoroughly	_____	5	
6 a. Let water continue to run	_____	5	
b. Got paper towels	_____	5	
c. Dried hands and arms to elbow	_____	5	
d. Turned water off with paper towel	_____	5	
e. Discarded paper towel in proper receptacle			
EVALUATOR: NOTE TIME COMPLETED _____			

ADD POINTS OF STEPS CHECKED   _____ EARNED

TOTAL POINTS POSSIBLE   155 POSSIBLE

Points assigned reflect importance of step to meeting objective: Important = (5)   Essential = (10)   Critical = (15)

Automatic failure results if any of the critical steps are omitted or performed incorrectly.

DETERMINE SCORE (divide points earned by total points possible, multiply results by 100)   _____ SCORE*

Evaluator's Name (print) _____ Signature _____

Comments _____

Name _____

Date _____ Score* _____

PROCEDURE 12–2 Wrap Items for Autoclave

TERMINAL PERFORMANCE OBJECTIVE - Provided with several items to be autoclaved or sterilized, the student will wrap each in autoclave paper in preparation for the sterilization process. Each item must be wrapped neatly and snugly but not too tightly. After the paper wrapping procedure is demonstrated and checked, the paper should be removed and discarded. This procedure should be performed with both paper and muslin wrap.

PROCEDURE STEPS	STEP PERFORMED	POINTS POSSIBLE	COMMENTS
EVALUATOR: Place check mark in space following each step performed satisfactorily			
NOTE TIME BEGAN _____			
Wrapping Items			
1. Washed hands.	_____	10	
a. Assembled all necessary items	_____	10	
b. Worked in a clean area	_____	5	
c. Allowed for sufficient work space	_____	5	
2. Checked items for flaws.	_____	15	
a. Checked items for proper functioning	_____	15	
b. Made sure items were sanitized before wrapping	_____	15	
3. Wrapped items in double thickness paper wrap.	_____	10	
a. Made sure of no opening	_____	10	
b. Sealed with autoclave tape	_____	5	
c. Wrapped items snugly	_____	10	
d. Did not wrap items too tight	_____	10	
4. Made tab with tape for ease in opening following sterilization.	_____	5	
5. Labeled contents.	_____	15	
a. Wrote date on package	_____	10	
b. Wrote your initials on package	_____	5	_____ EARNED
6. Returned all items to proper storage.	_____	5	160 POSSIBLE
Envelope Type			
Repeated steps 1–2	_____	65	
3. Placed item in envelope and	_____	15	
a. Sealed	_____	5	
b. Labeled contents	_____	15	
c. Dated label	_____	10	
d. Initialed label	_____	5	_____ EARNED
4. Returned items to proper storage.	_____	5	120 POSSIBLE

PROCEDURE 12–2   Wrap Items for Autoclave—continued

PROCEDURE STEPS	STEP PERFORMED	POINTS POSSIBLE	COMMENTS
Spinal needle(s), small items			
Repeated steps 1–2.	_____	65	
3. Placed cotton/gauze in bottom of glass test tube.	_____	10	
4. Wrapped autoclave tape around top of test tube to seal.	_____	15	
a. Made pull tab with tape	_____	5	
5. Labeled contents on piece of tape, secured to glass and	_____	15	
a. Dated label	_____	15	
b. Initialed	_____	5	
6. Returned items to storage.	_____	5	
EVALUATOR: NOTE TIME COMPLETED _____			_____ EARNED
			135 POSSIBLE

ADD POINTS OF STEPS CHECKED
TOTAL POINTS POSSIBLE

Points assigned reflect importance of step to meeting objective: Important = (5)   Essential = (10)   Critical = (15)
Automatic failure results if any of the critical steps are omitted or performed incorrectly.

DETERMINE SCORE (divide points earned by total points possible, multiply results by 100)   _____ SCORE*

Evaluator's Name (print) _____ Signature _____

Comments _____

Name _____

Date _____ Score* _____

PROCEDURE 13–1   Interview Patient to Complete Medical History Form

TERMINAL PERFORMANCE OBJECTIVE - Using copies of the medical history forms included in the text and a blue or black ink pen, obtain and record a medical history from a patient within a set time specified by the instructor.

PROCEDURE STEPS	STEP PERFORMED	POINTS POSSIBLE	COMMENTS
EVALUATOR: Place check mark in space following each step performed satisfactorily			
NOTE TIME BEGAN _____			
1. Assembled necessary items.	_____	15	
2. Courteously escorted patient to private area.	_____	5	
3. Sat opposite patient.	_____	5	
4. Explained procedure to patient and put them at ease.	_____	15	
5. Maintained eye contact with patient throughout procedure.	_____	10	
6. Asked questions clearly and distinctly.	_____	15	
7. Gave patient sufficient time to answer.	_____	10	
8. Recorded information neatly and accurately.	_____	15	
9. Avoided getting off subject.	_____	5	
10. Made necessary comments.	_____	5	
11. Highlighted in red ink when necessary (example: allergies).	_____	10	
12. Clearly stated patient's chief complaint.	_____	15	
13. Thanked patient for cooperation.	_____	5	
14. Explained next procedure to patient.	_____	5	
15. Made patient comfortable.	_____	5	
16. Placed patient's history form in chart.	_____	10	
17. Placed chart in appropriate area for physician.	_____	10	
EVALUATOR: NOTE TIME COMPLETED _____			

ADD POINTS OF STEPS CHECKED   _____ EARNED
TOTAL POINTS POSSIBLE   160 POSSIBLE

Points assigned reflect importance of step to meeting objective: Important = (5)   Essential = (10)   Critical = (15)
Automatic failure results if any of the critical steps are omitted or performed incorrectly.

DETERMINE SCORE (divide points earned by total points possible, multiply results by 100)   _____ SCORE*

Evaluator's Name (print) _____ Signature _____

Comments _____

Name _____

Date _____ Score* _____

PROCEDURE 13–2 Measure Height

TERMINAL PERFORMANCE OBJECTIVE - Demonstrate each step of the height measurement procedure to determine the precise height of five students who have been measured previously by the instructor. Measurements should be recorded and agree with instructor by ± ⅛ inch.

PROCEDURE STEPS	STEP PERFORMED	POINTS POSSIBLE	COMMENTS
EVALUATOR: Place check mark in space following each step performed satisfactorily			
NOTE TIME BEGAN _____			
1. Raised measuring bar higher than patient.	_____	15	
2. Aware of patient's safety.	_____	10	
3. Asked patient to remove shoes.	_____	5	
4. Placed paper towel on platform.	_____	5	
5. Helped patient onto scale.	_____	10	
6. Moved measuring bar slowly and carefully to rest on top of patient's head.	_____	10	
7. Gently compressed hair.	_____	15	
8. Read measurement correctly.	_____	15	
9. Told patient the reading.	_____	5	
10. Helped patient down from scale.	_____	10	
11. Asked patient to put shoes back on.	_____	5	
12. Placed measuring extension bar back.	_____	5	
13. Discarded paper towel.	_____	5	
14. Recorded measurement accurately on patient's chart.	_____	15	
EVALUATOR: NOTE TIME COMPLETED _____			

ADD POINTS OF STEPS CHECKED   _____ EARNED
TOTAL POINTS POSSIBLE   130 POSSIBLE

Points assigned reflect importance of step to meeting objective: Important = (5)   Essential = (10)   Critical = (15)
Automatic failure results if any of the critical steps are omitted or performed incorrectly.

DETERMINE SCORE (divide points earned by total points possible, multiply results by 100)   _____ SCORE*

Evaluator's Name (print) _____ Signature _____

Comments _____

DOCUMENTATION

Chart the procedure in the patient's medical record.

Date: _____

Charting: _____

_____

_____

_____

Student's Initials: _____

Name _____

Date _____ Score* _____

PROCEDURE 13–3   Measure Recumbent Length of Infant

TERMINAL PERFORMANCE OBJECTIVE - Demonstrate each step required in measuring the recumbent length of an infant and record; measurement should agree with instructor by ± ⅛ inch.

PROCEDURE STEPS	STEP PERFORMED	POINTS POSSIBLE	COMMENTS
EVALUATOR: Place check mark in space following each step performed satisfactorily			
NOTE TIME BEGAN _____			
1. Washed hands.	_____	15	
2. Asked parent to place infant on exam table and explained procedure.	_____	5	
3. Instructed parent to remove shoes, socks/booties from infant.	_____	5	
4. Moved infant to end of table so that infant's head was at the zero mark of the ruler.	_____	15	
5. Asked parent to hold infant's head against the end of the table.	_____	15	
6. Straightened (gently) infant's back and legs to line up along ruler.	_____	10	
7. Placed infant's heels against footboard.	_____	10	
8. Read length of infant in inches or centimeters from ruler accurately.	_____	15	
9. Returned infant to parent.	_____	5	
10. Recorded measurement on			
a. Growth chart	_____	10	
b. Patient's chart	_____	10	
c. Parent's booklet	_____	5	
d. Initialed all	_____	5	

EVALUATOR: NOTE TIME COMPLETED _____

ADD POINTS OF STEPS CHECKED   _____ EARNED
TOTAL POINTS POSSIBLE   125 POSSIBLE

Points assigned reflect importance of step to meeting objective: Important = (5)   Essential = (10)   Critical = (15)
Automatic failure results if any of the critical steps are omitted or performed incorrectly.

DETERMINE SCORE (divide points earned by total points possible, multiply results by 100)   _____ SCORE*

Evaluator's Name (print) _____ Signature _____

Comments _____

DOCUMENTATION

Chart the procedure in the patient's medical record.

Date: _____

Charting: _____

_____

_____

_____

Student's Initials: _____

Name _____

Date _____ Score* _____

PROCEDURE 13–4   Weigh Patient on Upright Scale

TERMINAL PERFORMANCE OBJECTIVE - Demonstrate each step of the procedure of weighing a patient on an upright scale and record; weight measurement should agree with instructor by ± ¼ lb.

PROCEDURE STEPS	STEP PERFORMED	POINTS POSSIBLE	COMMENTS
EVALUATOR: Place check mark in space following each step performed satisfactorily			
NOTE TIME BEGAN _____			
1. Washed hands.	_____	5	
2. Balanced scales.	_____	15	
3. Asked patient to remove shoes.	_____	5	
4. Placed paper towel on scale.	_____	5	
5. Helped patient onto scale.	_____	5	
6. Asked patient to stand in center of platform.	_____	10	
7. Asked patient to stand still.	_____	10	
8. Adjusted balance.	_____	10	
9. Read weight accurately.	_____	15	
10. Told patient the reading.	_____	5	
11. Helped patient from scales.	_____	5	
12. Discarded paper towel.	_____	5	
13. Recorded weight accurately on patient's chart.	_____	15	
a. Noted what patient was wearing	_____	10	
14. Returned scales to balance at zero.	_____	5	
EVALUATOR: NOTE TIME COMPLETED _____			

ADD POINTS OF STEPS CHECKED   _____ EARNED

TOTAL POINTS POSSIBLE   125 POSSIBLE

Points assigned reflect importance of step to meeting objective: Important = (5)   Essential = (10)   Critical = (15)
Automatic failure results if any of the critical steps are omitted or performed incorrectly.

DETERMINE SCORE (divide points earned by total points possible, multiply results by 100)   _____ SCORE*

Evaluator's Name (print) _____ Signature _____

Comments _____

DOCUMENTATION

Chart the procedure in the patient's medical record.

Date: _____

Charting: _____

_____

_____

_____

Student's Initials: _____

Name _____

Date _____ Score* _____

PROCEDURE 13–5   Weigh Infant

TERMINAL PERFORMANCE OBJECTIVE - Demonstrate each step of the procedure of weighing infants and record; weight must agree with instructor by ± ⅛ lb.

PROCEDURE STEPS	STEP PERFORMED	POINTS POSSIBLE	COMMENTS
EVALUATOR: Place check mark in space following each step performed satisfactorily			
NOTE TIME BEGAN _____			
1. Washed hands.	_____	15	
2. Asked parent to remove infant's clothes.	_____	5	
3. Placed towel on scale.	_____	5	
4. Balanced scale at zero with towel in place.	_____	15	
5. Placed infant gently on scale.	_____	5	
6. Held hand over infant—not touching.	_____	5	
7. Talked to infant in quiet tone.	_____	5	
8. Kept diaper over genital area.	_____	5	
9. Slid weight easily.	_____	10	
10. Returned infant to parent.	_____	5	
11. Read weight accurately.	_____	15	
12. Removed towel from scale.	_____	5	
13. Placed towel in proper receptacle.	_____	5	
14. Balanced scale at zero.	_____	10	
15. Recorded weight accurately on:			
a. Growth chart	_____	15	
b. Patient's chart	_____	15	
c. Parent's booklet	_____	5	
d. Initialed all	_____	5	
EVALUATOR: NOTE TIME COMPLETED _____			

ADD POINTS OF STEPS CHECKED   _____ EARNED

TOTAL POINTS POSSIBLE   150 POSSIBLE

Points assigned reflect importance of step to meeting objective: Important = (5)   Essential = (10)   Critical = (15)
Automatic failure results if any of the critical steps are omitted or performed incorrectly.

DETERMINE SCORE (divide points earned by total points possible, multiply results by 100)   _____ SCORE*

Evaluator's Name (print) _____   Signature _____

Comments _____

DOCUMENTATION

Chart the procedure in the patient's medical record.

Date: _____

Charting: _____

_____

_____

_____

Student's Initials: _____

Name _____

Date _____ Score* _____

PROCEDURE 13–6   Measure Head Circumference

TERMINAL PERFORMANCE OBJECTIVE - Demonstrate each step of the procedure for measuring head circumference of infants and record; measurement must agree with instructor by ± ½ inch or 0.1 cm.

PROCEDURE STEPS	STEP PERFORMED	POINTS POSSIBLE	COMMENTS
EVALUATOR: Place check mark in space following each step performed satisfactorily			
NOTE TIME BEGAN _____			
1. Washed hands.	_____	15	
2. Talked to infant.	_____	5	
3. Asked parent for assistance.	_____	5	
4. Used thumb to hold tape measure at zero mark against forehead over the eyebrows.	_____	15	
5. Brought tape measure around infant's head over the ears to meet in front.	_____	15	
6. Pulled tape measure snugly to compress hair.	_____	10	
7. Read measurement to nearest 0.1 cm or 0.5 inch.	_____	15	
8. Recorded measurement accurately on:			
a. Growth chart	_____	15	
b. Patient's chart	_____	15	
c. Parent's booklet	_____	5	
d. Initialed all	_____	5	
EVALUATOR: NOTE TIME COMPLETED _____			

ADD POINTS OF STEPS CHECKED   _____ EARNED

TOTAL POINTS POSSIBLE   120 POSSIBLE

Points assigned reflect importance of step to meeting objective: Important = (5)   Essential = (10)   Critical = (15)
Automatic failure results if any of the critical steps are omitted or performed incorrectly.

DETERMINE SCORE (divide points earned by total points possible, multiply results by 100)   _____ SCORE*

Evaluator's Name (print) _____ Signature _____

Comments _____

DOCUMENTATION

Chart the procedure in the patient's medical record.

Date: _____

Charting: _____

_____

_____

_____

Student's Initials: _____

Name _____

Date _____ Score* _____

PROCEDURE 13–7   Measure Infant's Chest

TERMINAL PERFORMANCE OBJECTIVE - Provided with a lifelike clinical infant doll and a flexible tape measure, demonstrate each step required in obtaining the chest measurement and record; the chest measurement must agree with instructor by ± ⅛ inch (0.3 cm).

PROCEDURE STEPS	STEP PERFORMED	POINTS POSSIBLE	COMMENTS
EVALUATOR: Place check mark in space following each step performed satisfactorily			
NOTE TIME BEGAN _____			
1. Washed hands.	_____	15	
2. Talked to infant/gained cooperation.	_____	5	
3. Asked parent for assistance.	_____	5	
4. Held tape at zero with thumb at mid-sternal area of chest.	_____	15	
5. Brought tape around child's back to meet in front at zero mark under axillary region.	_____	15	
6. Made tape snug against chest.	_____	10	
7. Read measurement to nearest 0.1 cm or ½ inch.	_____	15	
8. Recorded measurement accurately on:			
a. Patient's chart	_____	15	
b. Parent's booklet	_____	15	
c. Initialed both	_____	5	
EVALUATOR: NOTE TIME COMPLETED _____			

ADD POINTS OF STEPS CHECKED _____ EARNED

TOTAL POINTS POSSIBLE 115 POSSIBLE

Points assigned reflect importance of step to meeting objective: Important = (5)   Essential = (10)   Critical = (15)

Automatic failure results if any of the critical steps are omitted or performed incorrectly.

DETERMINE SCORE (divide points earned by total points possible, multiply results by 100) _____ SCORE*

Evaluator's Name (print) _____ Signature _____

Comments _____

DOCUMENTATION

Chart the procedure in the patient's medical record.

Date: _____

Charting: _____

_____

_____

_____

Student's Initials: _____

Name _____

Date _____ Score* _____

PROCEDURE 13–8   Clean and Store Mercury Thermometers

TERMINAL PERFORMANCE OBJECTIVE - Given soiled mercury thermometers and access to all necessary equipment and supplies, clean, inspect, disinfect, and store the thermometers aseptically, in accordance with procedure technique and observing aseptic and safety precautions.

PROCEDURE STEPS	STEP PERFORMED	POINTS POSSIBLE	COMMENTS
EVALUATOR: Place check mark in space following each step performed satisfactorily. Check to see if oral and rectal are separated. Subtract 15 pts if not.			
NOTE TIME BEGAN _____			
1. Washed hands, assembled equipment, and put on gloves.	_____	15	
2. Took soiled thermometers to sink.	_____	—	
3. Applied soap, or other cleanser to cotton ball and added water to make solution.	_____	10	
4. While holding thermometer by stem, rotated and wiped it from stem to bulb with soapy solution.	_____	5	
5. Discarded cotton ball in biohazardous waste container.	_____	5	
6. While holding by stem with bulb pointed downward, rinsed thermometer in cool running water.	_____	5	
7. Inspected for cleanliness and condition, discarded damaged thermometer.	_____	15	
8. Grasped stem firmly between thumb and index finger.	_____	5	
9. Shook mercury down to 95.0° or below.	_____	15	
10. Placed thermometers in gauze-lined container filled with disinfectant.	_____	10	
11. Using correct procedure, removed and discarded gloves.	_____	10	
12. Washed hands.	_____	5	
13. Noted time or set timer for at least 20 minutes.	_____	15	
14. After allowing time for disinfection, washed hands.	_____	5	
15. Rinsed, inspected, and placed clean thermometers in individual envelopes, individual dry holders, or storage container.	_____	15	

PROCEDURE 13–8   Clean and Store Mercury Thermometers—continued

PROCEDURE STEPS	STEP PERFORMED	POINTS POSSIBLE	COMMENTS
16. Cleaned area and equipment. Returned thermometers to appropriate locations.	_____	5	
EVALUATOR: NOTE TIME COMPLETED _____			

ADD POINTS OF STEPS CHECKED   _____ EARNED

TOTAL POINTS POSSIBLE   140 POSSIBLE

Points assigned reflect importance of step to meeting objective: Important = (5)   Essential = (10)   Critical = (15)
Automatic failure results if any of the critical steps are omitted or performed incorrectly.

DETERMINE SCORE (divide points earned by total points possible, multiply results by 100)   _____ SCORE*

Evaluator's Name (print) _____ Signature _____

Comments _____

PROCEDURE 13–9   Measure Oral Temperature with Mercury Thermometer

TERMINAL PERFORMANCE OBJECTIVE - In a simulated or actual situation and given access to all necessary equipment and supplies, measure and record a patient's oral temperature. The procedure will be done within six minutes, following correct procedural technique, and observing aseptic and safety precautions. The recorded findings must agree with the instructor's reading.

PROCEDURE STEPS	STEP PERFORMED	POINTS POSSIBLE	COMMENTS
EVALUATOR: Place check mark in space following each step performed satisfactorily			
NOTE TIME BEGAN _____			
1. Washed hands, assembled equipment, and put on gloves.	_____	15	
2. Identified patient.	_____	5	
3. Explained procedure.	_____	5	
4. Determined if patient had recently had a hot or cold drink or smoked.	_____	15	
5. Removed thermometer from holder or envelope. Avoid touching bulb end with fingers.	_____	5	
6. Inspected thermometer. Discarded a chipped or cracked thermometer.	_____	15	
7. Read thermometer and shook down to 95° or below if necessary.	_____	15	
8. Put plastic sheath on thermometer and ensured it is intact.	_____	10	
9. Placed bulb sublingually in patient's mouth.	_____	10	
10. Told patient how to maintain proper position of thermometer: to keep lips closed, breathe through nose, and avoid biting.	_____	5	
11. Left thermometer in position a minimum of three minutes.	_____	15	
12. Removed and read thermometer. Reinserted for one minute if less than 97°.	_____	10	
13. Reread thermometer, if appropriate.	_____	—	
14. Holding by stem, pulled off plastic sheath and discarded in biohazardous waste container.	_____	5	
EVALUATOR: NOTE TIME COMPLETED _____			
Completed within six minutes	_____	15	
EVALUATOR: Read thermometer and record temperature: _____			

PROCEDURE STEPS	STEP PERFORMED	POINTS POSSIBLE	COMMENTS
15. Followed procedure for soiled thermometers.	_____	5	
16. Removed gloves and discarded in biohazardous waste container.	_____	5	
17. Washed hands.	_____	5	
18. Accurately recorded temperature.	_____	15	

ADD POINTS OF STEPS CHECKED   _____ EARNED

TOTAL POINTS POSSIBLE   175 POSSIBLE

Points assigned reflect importance of step to meeting objective: Important = (5)   Essential = (10)   Critical = (15)
Automatic failure results if any of the critical steps are omitted or performed incorrectly.

DETERMINE SCORE (divide points earned by total points possible, multiply results by 100)   _____ SCORE*

Evaluator's Name (print) _____ Signature _____

Comments _____

DOCUMENTATION

Chart the procedure in the patient's medical record.

Date: _____

Charting: _____

_____

_____

_____

Student's Initials: _____

Name _____

Date _____ Score* _____

PROCEDURE 13–10   Measure Rectal Temperature with Mercury Thermometer

TERMINAL PERFORMANCE OBJECTIVE - In a simulated or actual situation and given access to all necessary equipment and supplies, measure and record a patient's rectal temperature within eight minutes, following correct procedural technique, and observing aseptic and safety precautions. The recorded findings must agree with the instructor's reading.

PROCEDURE STEPS	STEP PERFORMED	POINTS POSSIBLE	COMMENTS
EVALUATOR: Place check mark in space following each step performed satisfactorily			
NOTE TIME BEGAN _____			
1. Washed hands, assembled equipment, and put on gloves.	_____	15	
2. Identified patient.	_____	5	
3. Explained procedure.	_____	5	
4. Placed a small amount of lubricant on a tissue.	_____	5	
5. Removed thermometer from holder or envelope.	_____	5	
6. Inspected thermometer. Discarded a chipped or cracked thermometer.	_____	15	
7. Read thermometer and shook down to 95°, or below.	_____	15	
8. Placed thermometer in plastic sheath. Checked that sheath is intact.	_____	15	
9. Rotated thermometer bulb in lubricant on tissue and placed in convenient location.	_____	5	
10. Instructed patient to remove appropriate clothing, assisting as needed.	_____	5	
11. Provided privacy.	_____	5	
12. Assisted adult patient onto examining table and covered with drape. Avoided overexposure.	_____	5	
13. Positioned patient on side. Ensured patient's comfort and safety.	_____	5	
14. Arranged drape to expose buttocks.	_____	5	
15. With one hand raised upper buttock to expose anus.	_____	5	
16. With other hand, carefully inserted lubricated thermometer into anal canal approximately 1½ ″.	_____	5	
a. Did not force thermometer. Rotated if necessary to facilitate insertion.	_____	10	
b. If opening was not apparent, requested patient to bear down slightly.	_____	5	
17. Held thermometer in place for a minimum of three minutes.	_____	15	

PROCEDURE STEPS	STEP PERFORMED	POINTS POSSIBLE	COMMENTS
18. Withdrew thermometer. Carefully removed plastic sheath and discarded it in biohazardous waste container.	_____	10	
19. Read thermometer.	_____	5	
20. Reread to check temperature.	_____	5	
21. Placed thermometer on tissue.	_____	5	
EVALUATOR: NOTE TIME COMPLETED _____			
Completed within eight minutes	_____	15	
EVALUATOR: Read thermometer and record temperature: _____			
22. Removed any excess lubricant from anal area with tissue; wiped from front to back.	_____	5	
23. Assisted adult patient from examining table and instructed to redress.	_____	5	
24. Followed procedure for soiled thermometer.	_____	5	
25. Removed and discarded gloves in biohazardous waste container.	_____	5	
26. Accurately recorded temperature.	_____	15	

ADD POINTS OF STEPS CHECKED   _____ EARNED
TOTAL POINTS POSSIBLE   225 POSSIBLE

Points assigned reflect importance of step to meeting objective: Important = (5)   Essential = (10)   Critical = (15)
Automatic failure results if any of the critical steps are omitted or performed incorrectly.

DETERMINE SCORE (divide points earned by total points possible, multiply results by 100)   _____ SCORE*

Evaluator's Name (print) _____ Signature _____

Comments _____

DOCUMENTATION

Chart the procedure in the patient's medical record.

Date: _____

Charting: _____
_____
_____
_____

Student's Initials: _____

Name _____

Date _____ Score* _____

PROCEDURE 13–11   Measure Axillary Temperature with Mercury Thermometer

TERMINAL PERFORMANCE OBJECTIVE - In a simulated or actual situation and given access to all necessary equipment and supplies, measure and record axillary temperature within fourteen minutes, following correct procedural technique, and observing aseptic and safety precautions. Recorded findings must agree with the instructor's reading.

PROCEDURE STEPS	STEP PERFORMED	POINTS POSSIBLE	COMMENTS
EVALUATOR: Place check mark in space following each step performed satisfactorily			
NOTE TIME BEGAN _____			
1. Washed hands, assembled equipment.	_____	5	
2. Identified patient.	_____	5	
3. Explained procedure.	_____	5	
4. Removed thermometer from holder or envelope.	_____	5	
5. Inspected thermometer. Discarded a chipped or cracked thermometer.	_____	15	
6. Read thermometer and shook down to 95° or below.	_____	15	
7. Placed thermometer on tissue or in envelope in convenient location.	_____	5	
8. Assisted patient, as necessary, to expose axilla, provided privacy.	_____	5	
9. Patted axillary space with tissue to remove perspiration.	_____	10	
10. Placed thermometer deep in the axillary space.	_____	10	
a. Bulb at top of axillary space	_____	5	
b. Stem projecting anteriorly or posteriorly	_____	5	
11. Instructed patient to hold arm tightly against body and to maintain position for a minimum of ten minutes.	_____	15	
12. Removed thermometer and wiped with tissue from stem to bulb.	_____	5	
13. Read and recorded findings accurately.	_____	15	
14. Reread and checked recording.	_____	5	
EVALUATOR: NOTE TIME COMPLETED _____ Completed within fourteen minutes.		15	
EVALUATOR: Read thermometer and record temperature: _____			

PROCEDURE STEPS	STEP PERFORMED	POINTS POSSIBLE	COMMENTS
15. Helped patient replace clothing.	_____	5	
16. Followed procedure for soiled thermometer.	_____	5	
17. Washed hands.	_____	5	

ADD POINTS OF STEPS CHECKED _____ EARNED

TOTAL POINTS POSSIBLE 160 POSSIBLE

Points assigned reflect importance of step to meeting objective: Important = (5)   Essential = (10)   Critical = (15)
Automatic failure results if any of the critical steps are omitted or performed incorrectly.

DETERMINE SCORE (divide points earned by total points possible, multiply results by 100) _____ SCORE*

Evaluator's Name (print) _____ Signature _____

Comments _____

DOCUMENTATION

Chart the procedure in the patient's medical record.

Date: _____

Charting: _____

_____

_____

_____

Student's Initials: _____

Name _____

Date _____ Score* _____

PROCEDURE 13–12   Measure Oral Temperature with Disposable Plastic Thermometer

TERMINAL PERFORMANCE OBJECTIVE - In a simulated or actual situation and given access to all necessary equipment and supplies, measure and record oral temperature within four minutes, following correct procedural technique and observing aseptic and safety precautions. Recorded findings must agree with the instructor's reading.

PROCEDURE STEPS	STEP PERFORMED	POINTS POSSIBLE	COMMENTS
EVALUATOR: Place check mark in space following each step performed satisfactorily			
NOTE TIME BEGAN _____			
1. Washed hands, assembled equipment.	_____	5	
2. Identified patient.	_____	5	
3. Explained procedure.	_____	5	
4. Determined if patient had recently had a hot or cold drink or smoked.	_____	15	
5. Opened package by peeling back top of wrapper to expose handle end of thermometer.	_____	5	
6. Grasped handle and removed from wrapper without touching matrix section.	_____	15	
7. Inserted thermometer into patient's mouth as far back as possible into one of the heat pockets.	_____	10	
8. Instructed patient to press tongue down on thermometer and keep mouth closed.	_____	10	
9. Instructed patient to maintain position for sixty seconds; timed by watch.	_____	15	
10. Removed thermometer and waited ten seconds for dots to stabilize. Did not touch dots.	_____	15	
11. Read thermometer.	_____	—	
EVALUATOR: NOTE TIME COMPLETED _____			
Completed within four minutes.		15	
EVALUATOR: Read thermometer and record temperature: _____			
12. Discarded in biohazardous waste container.	_____	10	
13. Washed hands.	_____	5	
14. Accurately recorded temperature.	_____	15	

ADD POINTS OF STEPS CHECKED   _____ EARNED

TOTAL POINTS POSSIBLE   145 POSSIBLE

Points assigned reflect importance of step to meeting objective: Important = (5)   Essential = (10)   Critical = (15)
Automatic failure results if any of the critical steps are omitted or performed incorrectly.

DETERMINE SCORE (divide points earned by total points possible, multiply results by 100)   _____ SCORE*

Evaluator's Name (print) _____ Signature _____

Comments _____

DOCUMENTATION

Chart the procedure in the patient's medical record.

Date: _____

Charting: _____

_____

_____

_____

Student's Initials: _____

Name _____

Date _____ Score* _____

PROCEDURE 13–13   Measure Oral Temperature Electronically

TERMINAL PERFORMANCE OBJECTIVE - In a simulated or actual situation and given access to all necessary equipment and supplies, measure the patient's temperature electronically. The temperature will be read and recorded in two minutes, following correct procedural technique, and observing aseptic and safety precautions. Recorded findings must agree with instructor's reading.

PROCEDURE STEPS	STEP PERFORMED	POINTS POSSIBLE	COMMENTS
EVALUATOR: Place check mark in space following each step performed satisfactorily			
NOTE TIME BEGAN _____			
1. Washed hands; assembled equipment.	_____	5	
2. Identified patient.	_____	5	
3. Explained procedure.	_____	5	
4. Placed probe connector in receptacle of unit base and checked to make sure it was properly seated.	_____	10	
5. Holding it by the collar, removed appropriate probe from stored position.	_____	5	
6. Inserted probe firmly into probe cover to ensure that it was properly seated.	_____	5	
7. Inserted covered probe into mouth, and provided support.	_____	15	
8. Maintained covered probe in position until unit signals.	_____	10	
9. Removed probe; avoided touching cover.	_____	15	
10. Accurately read and recorded temperature measurement.	_____	15	
11. Rechecked reading and recording.	_____	5	
12. Pressed the eject button and discarded used probe cover into biohazardous waste container.	_____	10	
13. Returned probe to stored position in unit. Thermometer display read zero and shut off.	_____	5	
14. Stored unit in charging stand.	_____	5	
EVALUATOR: NOTE TIME COMPLETED _____			
Completed within two minutes	_____	15	
EVALUATOR: Read thermometer and record temperature: _____			

ADD POINTS OF STEPS CHECKED   _____ EARNED

TOTAL POINTS POSSIBLE   130 POSSIBLE

Points assigned reflect importance of step to meeting objective: Important = (5)   Essential = (10)   Critical = (15)
Automatic failure results if any of the critical steps are omitted or performed incorrectly.

DETERMINE SCORE (divide points earned by total points possible, multiply results by 100)   _____ SCORE*

Evaluator's Name (print) _____ Signature _____

Comments _____

DOCUMENTATION

Chart the procedure in the patient's medical record.

Date: _____

Charting: _____

_____

_____

_____

Student's Initials: _____

Name _____

Date _____ Score* _____

PROCEDURE 13–14   Measure Core Body Temperature
with an Infrared Tympanic Thermometer

TERMINAL PERFORMANCE OBJECTIVE - In a simulated or actual situation and given access to all necessary equipment and supplies, measure and record core body temperature within three minutes, following correct procedural technique and observing aseptic and safety precautions. Recorded findings must agree with instructor's reading.

PROCEDURE STEPS	STEP PERFORMED	POINTS POSSIBLE	COMMENTS
EVALUATOR: Place check mark in space following each step performed satisfactorily			
NOTE TIME BEGAN _____			
1. Washed hands, assembled equipment.	_____	5	
2. Identified patient.	_____	5	
3. Explained procedure.	_____	5	
4. Removed thermometer from base.	_____	5	
5. Attached a disposable probe cover to the ear piece.	_____	10	
6. Inserted covered probe into ear canal, sealing opening.	_____	15	
7. Pressed the scan button to activate the thermometer.	_____	5	
8. Withdrew the thermometer.	_____	—	
9. Observed the display window, noting the temperature.	_____	5	
10. Pressed the release button on the thermometer and ejected probe cover into a wastebasket.	_____	5	
11. Accurately read and recorded temperature.	_____	15	
12. Returned thermometer to base.	_____	5	
EVALUATOR: NOTE TIME COMPLETED _____			
Completed within three minutes.	_____	15	
EVALUATOR: Read thermometer and record temperature: _____			

ADD POINTS OF STEPS CHECKED _____ EARNED

TOTAL POINTS POSSIBLE 95 POSSIBLE

Points assigned reflect importance of step to meeting objective: Important = (5)   Essential = (10)   Critical = (15)

Automatic failure results if any of the critical steps are omitted or performed incorrectly.

DETERMINE SCORE (divide points earned by total points possible, multiply results by 100) _____ SCORE*

Evaluator's Name (print) _____ Signature _____

Comments _____

DOCUMENTATION

Chart the procedure in the patient's medical record.

Date: _____

Charting: _____

_____

_____

_____

Student's Initials: _____

Name _____

Date _____ Score* _____

PROCEDURE 13–15 Measure Radial Pulse

TERMINAL PERFORMANCE OBJECTIVE - In a simulated or actual situation and given access to all necessary equipment and supplies, within four minutes, assess and record the quality, and measure and record the rate of a patient's radial pulse following correct procedural technique. Recorded rate findings must be within two beats per minute of instructor's measurement and agree as to rhythm and quality characteristics.

PROCEDURE STEPS	STEP PERFORMED	POINTS POSSIBLE	COMMENTS
EVALUATOR: Place check mark in space following each step performed satisfactorily			
NOTE TIME BEGAN _____			
1. Washed hands, assembled equipment.	_____	5	
2. Identified patient.	_____	5	
3. Explained procedure.	_____	5	
4. Determined patient's recent activity.	_____	10	
5. Had patient assume a comfortable position.	_____	5	
6. Located radial artery.	_____	15	
7. Observed quality of pulse before beginning to count.	_____	15	
8. Counted pulse.	_____	15	
a. Regular for 30 seconds—*or*—			
b. Irregular for one minute			
9. Accurately recorded pulse rate	_____	15	
10. Described characteristics	_____	15	
EVALUATOR: NOTE TIME COMPLETED _____			
Completed within four minutes.	_____	15	
EVALUATOR: Record pulse rate _____			
Characteristics _____			
_____			
_____			

ADD POINTS OF STEPS CHECKED   _____ EARNED

TOTAL POINTS POSSIBLE   120 POSSIBLE

Points assigned reflect importance of step to meeting objective: Important = (5) Essential = (10) Critical = (15)

Automatic failure results if any of the critical steps are omitted or performed incorrectly.

DETERMINE SCORE (divide points earned by total points possible, multiply results by 100)   _____ SCORE*

Evaluator's Name (print) _____ Signature _____

Comments _____

DOCUMENTATION

Chart the procedure in the patient's medical record.

Date: _____

Charting: _____

_____

_____

_____

Student's Initials: _____

Name _____

Date _____ Score* _____

PROCEDURE 13–16 Measure Apical Pulse

TERMINAL PERFORMANCE OBJECTIVE - In a simulated or actual situation and given access to all necessary equipment and supplies, within five minutes, locate the apex of the heart, assess and record the quality and measure and record the rate of a patient's apical pulse, following correct technique, and observing aseptic precautions. Recorded rate findings must be within one beat per minute of instructor's measurement and agree as to rhythm and quality characteristics.

PROCEDURE STEPS	STEP PERFORMED	POINTS POSSIBLE	COMMENTS
EVALUATOR: Place check mark in space following each step performed satisfactorily			
NOTE TIME BEGAN _____			
1. Washed hands; assembled equipment.	_____	5	
2. Prepared stethoscope by wiping earpieces and chestpiece with germicidal solution to prevent transfer of organisms.	_____	10	
3. Identified patient.	_____	5	
4. Explained procedure. If patient is an infant or small child, explained to parent.	_____	5	
5. Provided privacy and a gown or drape if indicated.	_____	5	
6. Uncovered left side of chest.	_____	10	
7. Placed earpieces in ears. Openings in tips should be forward, entering auditory canal: held chestpiece in hand.	_____	10	
8. Located apex.	_____	15	
9. Placed chestpiece of stethoscope at apex.	_____	5	
10. Determined quality of heart sounds.	_____	15	
11. Counted beats for a full minute.	_____	15	
12. Removed earpieces from ears.	_____	5	
13. Accurately recorded rate of heart sounds.	_____	15	
14. Accurately recorded quality of heart sounds.	_____	15	
15. Assisted patient as necessary to redress.	_____	—	
16. Wiped earpieces and chestpiece of stethoscope with disinfectant. Returned to storage.	_____	5	
17. Washed hands.	_____	5	
EVALUATOR: NOTE TIME COMPLETED _____			
Completed within five minutes.	_____	15	
EVALUATOR: Record rate _____			
Characteristics _____			
_____			

ADD POINTS OF STEPS CHECKED   _____ EARNED
TOTAL POINTS POSSIBLE   160 POSSIBLE

Points assigned reflect importance of step to meeting objective: Important = (5)   Essential = (10)   Critical = (15)
Automatic failure results if any of the critical steps are omitted or performed incorrectly.

DETERMINE SCORE (divide points earned by total points possible, multiply results by 100)   _____ SCORE*

Evaluator's Name (print) _____ Signature _____

Comments _____

DOCUMENTATION

Chart the procedure in the patient's medical record.

Date: _____

Charting: _____

_____

_____

_____

Student's Initials: _____

Name _____

Date _____ Score* _____

PROCEDURE 13–17   Measure Respirations

TERMINAL PERFORMANCE OBJECTIVE - In a simulated or actual situation and given access to all necessary equipment and supplies, assess and record the quality and rate of a patient's respirations within three minutes, following the correct procedural technique. Recorded rate findings must be within two breaths per minute of instructor's measurement and agree as to rhythm, sound, and depth quality characteristics.

PROCEDURE STEPS	STEP PERFORMED	POINTS POSSIBLE	COMMENTS
EVALUATOR: Place check mark in space following each step performed satisfactorily			
NOTE TIME BEGAN _____			
1. Washed hands; assembled equipment.	_____	5	
2. Identified patient.	_____	5	
3. Asked about recent activity level.	_____	10	
4. Avoided identifying respiration evaluation.	_____	10	
5. Placed patient in comfortable position.	_____	5	
6. Assumed pulse measurement position.	_____	10	
7. Assessed respiration quality.	_____	15	
8. Accurately counted respirations for thirty seconds.	_____	15	
9. Accurately recorded rate.	_____	15	
10. Recorded characteristics.	_____	15	
EVALUATOR: NOTE TIME COMPLETED _____			
Completed within three minutes.	_____	15	
EVALUATOR: Record rate _____			
Characteristics _____			

ADD POINTS OF STEPS CHECKED   _____ EARNED
TOTAL POINTS POSSIBLE   120 POSSIBLE

Points assigned reflect importance of step to meeting objective: Important = (5)   Essential = (10)   Critical = (15)
Automatic failure results if any of the critical steps are omitted or performed incorrectly.

DETERMINE SCORE (divide points earned by total points possible, multiply results by 100)   _____ SCORE*

Evaluator's Name (print) _____ Signature _____

Comments _____

DOCUMENTATION

Chart the procedure in the patient's medical record.

Date: _____

Charting: _____

_____

_____

_____

Student's Initials: _____

PROCEDURE 13–18   Measure Blood Pressure

TERMINAL PERFORMANCE OBJECTIVE - In a simulated or actual situation and given access to all equipment and supplies, within a four-minute period of time, measure palpatory and auscultatory blood pressure and record findings, following correct procedural technique and observing safety and aseptic precautions. Recorded findings must be within 4 mmHg of instructor's measurement using teaching stethoscope.

PROCEDURE STEPS	STEP PERFORMED	POINTS POSSIBLE	COMMENTS
EVALUATOR: Place check mark in space following each step performed satisfactorily			
NOTE TIME BEGAN _____			
1. Washed hands.	_____	5	
2. Assembled equipment.	_____	5	
3. Cleaned earpieces and head of stethoscope with antiseptic.	_____	5	
4. Identified patient.	_____	5	
5. Explained procedure.	_____	5	
6. Placed a mercury manometer on a flat, level surface near patient. Put aneroid type within easy reach.	_____	5	
7. Placed patient in a relaxed and comfortable sitting or lying position.	_____	5	
8. a. Positioned arm, palm up.	_____	5	
b. Clothing appropriately managed	_____	10	
9. a. Opened valve, deflated bladder completely	_____	5	
b. Located center of bladder; assured adequate cuff size	_____	15	
c. Applied cuff to upper arm, bladder centered over brachial artery; 1″ to 2″ above elbow	_____	15	
d. Attached tubing if appropriate	_____	—	
10. Assured manometer in proper view.	_____	5	
11. Closed valve with one hand.	_____	5	
12. Positioned other hand to palpate radial pulse.	_____	5	
13. Observing manometer, rapidly inflated cuff to 30 mm above level where radial pulse disappears.	_____	10	
14. Opened valve, slowly releasing air until radial pulse was detected.	_____	10	
15. Observed mercury or dial reading.	_____	10	
16. Deflated cuff rapidly and completely. Squeezed cuff with hands to empty.	_____	5	
17. Positioned earpieces of stethoscope in ears with openings entering ear canal; held head of scope in one hand.	_____	5	
18. Palpated brachial artery at medial antecubital space with fingertips.	_____	15	
19. Placed head of stethoscope directly over palpated pulse.	_____	5	
20. Closed valve on bulb and rapidly inflated cuff to 30 mm above palpated systolic pressure.	_____	10	

PROCEDURE STEPS	STEP PERFORMED	POINTS POSSIBLE	COMMENTS
21. Opened valve, slowly deflating cuff.	_____	10	
22. With eyes at level of descending meniscus or directly in line with dial, noted reading at which systolic pressure heard.	_____	10	
23. Allowed pressure to lower steadily.	_____	5	
24. Continued to release pressure until all sound disappears.	_____	5	
25. Released remaining air. Squeezed cuff between hands.	_____	5	
26. Recorded accurate systolic and whichever diastolic instructed to read.	_____	15	
27. Reevaluated if indicated after a minimum of fifteen seconds.	_____	—	
28. Removed stethoscope from ears.	_____	—	
29. Removed cuff from patient's arm.	_____	—	
EVALUATOR: NOTE TIME COMPLETED _____			
Completed within four minutes.	_____	15	
EVALUATOR: Record B/P _____			
30. Assisted patient with clothing, if necessary.	_____	—	
31. Cleaned tips and head of stethoscope with alcohol to disinfect.	_____	10	
32. Folded cuff properly and placed with manometer and stethoscope in storage.	_____	5	
33. Washed hands.	_____	5	

ADD POINTS OF STEPS CHECKED   _____ EARNED
TOTAL POINTS POSSIBLE   255 POSSIBLE

Points assigned reflect importance of step to meeting objective: Important = (5)   Essential = (10)   Critical = (15)
Automatic failure results if any of the critical steps are omitted or performed incorrectly.

DETERMINE SCORE (divide points earned by total points possible, multiply results by 100)   _____ SCORE*

Evaluator's Name (print) _____ Signature _____

Comments _____

DOCUMENTATION

Chart the procedure in the patient's medical record.

Date: _____

Charting: _____

_____

_____

_____

Student's Initials: _____

Name _____

Date _____ Score* _____

PROCEDURE 14–1   Irrigate the Eye

TERMINAL PERFORMANCE OBJECTIVE - Provided with a mannequin and all equipment required for eye irrigation, demonstrate the steps of the procedure in proper order.

PROCEDURE STEPS	STEP PERFORMED	POINTS POSSIBLE	COMMENTS
EVALUATOR: Place check mark in space following each step performed satisfactorily			
NOTE TIME BEGAN _____			
1. Assembled necessary items.	_____	10	
2. Washed hands and put on gloves.	_____	15	
3. Prepared solution.	_____	10	
4. Identified patient, called by name.	_____	5	
5. Explained procedure to patient.	_____	5	
6. Positioned patient comfortably.	_____	5	
7. Draped patient.	_____	5	
8. Asked patient to turn head to side then back.	_____	10	
9. Placed emesis basin against head to catch solution, gave tissues.	_____	10	
10. Wiped eye with gauze square from bridge of nose out.	_____	10	
11. Filled bulb syringe with solution.	_____	10	
12. Held eye open with thumb and index finger.	_____	15	
13. Released solution over eye gently from inner canthus to outer canthus.	_____	15	
14. Used sterile gauze square to blot area dry.	_____	5	
15. Attended to patient's comfort.	_____	5	
16. Removed gloves and washed hands.	_____	10	
17. Provided patient education.	_____	5	
18. Recorded procedure in patient's chart.	_____	10	
19. Initialed procedure.	_____	5	
20. Noted observations during procedure.	_____	5	
21. Washed items and returned to storage.	_____	5	

EVALUATOR: NOTE TIME COMPLETED _____

ADD POINTS OF STEPS CHECKED   _____ EARNED

TOTAL POINTS POSSIBLE   175 POSSIBLE

Points assigned reflect importance of step to meeting objective: Important = (5)   Essential = (10)   Critical = (15)
Automatic failure results if any of the critical steps are omitted or performed incorrectly.

DETERMINE SCORE (divide points earned by total points possible, multiply results by 100)   _____ SCORE*

Evaluator's Name (print) _____ Signature _____

Comments _____

DOCUMENTATION

Chart the procedure in the patient's medical record.

Date: _____

Charting: _____

_____

_____

_____

Student's Initials: _____

Name _____

Date _____ Score* _____

PROCEDURE 14–2 Irrigate the Ear

TERMINAL PERFORMANCE OBJECTIVE - Provided with anatomical model of the ear, and all equipment required for ear irrigation, demonstrate the steps of the procedure in proper order.

PROCEDURE STEPS	STEP PERFORMED	POINTS POSSIBLE	COMMENTS
EVALUATOR: Place check mark in space following each step performed satisfactorily			
NOTE TIME BEGAN _____			
1. Washed hands and put on gloves.	_____	10	
2. Assembled necessary items.	_____	15	
3. Prepared solution between 100 and 105°F as directed by the physician.	_____	15	
4. a. Identified patient, called by name.	_____	10	
b. Explained procedure to patient.	_____	5	
5. Viewed affected area with otoscope.	_____	10	
6. Asked patient to turn head to side and back.	_____	10	
7. Placed ear basin under ear.	_____	5	
8. Placed towel over patient's shoulder.	_____	5	
9. Used gauze square to wipe ear.	_____	5	
10. Filled syringe with solution.	_____	10	
11. Pulled auricle up and back for adult or down and back for child.	_____	15	
12. Placed tip of syringe into side of ear canal.	_____	5	
13. Irrigated ear with solution to desired results.	_____	15	
14. Used gauze square to wipe excess solution from outside of patient's ear.	_____	5	
15. Instructed patient to tilt head to allow drainage, give tissues.	_____	5	
16. Inspected ear canal with otoscope to determine results of irrigation. Repeat irrigation PRN.	_____	5	
17. Provided patient education.	_____	5	
18. a. Recorded procedure in patient's chart	_____	10	
b. Initialed chart	_____	5	
c. Wrote observations	_____	5	

PROCEDURE 14–2   Irrigate the Ear—continued

PROCEDURE STEPS	STEP PERFORMED	POINTS POSSIBLE	COMMENTS
19. Washed equipment.	_____	5	
20. Removed gloves and washed hands.	_____	5	
21. Returned equipment to proper storage area.	_____	5	
EVALUATOR: NOTE TIME COMPLETED _____			

ADD POINTS OF STEPS CHECKED   _____ EARNED
TOTAL POINTS POSSIBLE   190 POSSIBLE

Points assigned reflect importance of step to meeting objective: Important = (5)   Essential = (10)   Critical = (15)
Automatic failure results if any of the critical steps are omitted or performed incorrectly.

DETERMINE SCORE (divide points earned by total points possible, multiply results by 100)   _____ SCORE*

Evaluator's Name (print) _____ Signature _____

Comments _____

DOCUMENTATION

Chart the procedure in the patient's medical record.

Date: _____

Charting: _____

_____

_____

_____

Student's Initials: _____

Name _____

Date _____ Score* _____

PROCEDURE 14–3   Instill Eardrops

TERMINAL PERFORMANCE OBJECTIVE - Provided with a mannequin or anatomical model of the ear, and all necessary equipment, demonstrate each step of the procedure for instilling eardrops in proper order.

PROCEDURE STEPS	STEP PERFORMED	POINTS POSSIBLE	COMMENTS
EVALUATOR: Place check mark in space following each step performed satisfactorily			
NOTE TIME BEGAN _____			
1. Verified medication ordered.	_____	15	
a. Assembled items	_____	5	
2. Washed hands and put on gloves.	_____	10	
3. Called patient by name.	_____	10	
a. Explained procedure	_____	10	
4. Opened medication container/drew up ordered amount in dropper.	_____	15	
5. Positioned patient/tilt head to instill left for right ear (right for left).	_____	10	
6. Asked for assistance if necessary.	_____	5	
7. Gave patient tissues.	_____	5	
8. Instilled drops in ear (without touching ear tissues).	_____	15	
9. Advised patient to remain in position for drops to settle in ear.	_____	10	
10. Provided patient education.	_____	5	
11. Repeated for other ear if ordered.	_____	10	
12. Closed medication container without touching outside of the container.	_____	15	
13. Removed gloves and washed hands.	_____	10	
14. Recorded procedure on patient's chart.	_____	5	
a. Noted observations	_____	5	
b. Initialed	_____	10	
15. Returned items to proper storage area.	_____	5	
EVALUATOR: NOTE TIME COMPLETED _____			

ADD POINTS OF STEPS CHECKED   _____ EARNED

TOTAL POINTS POSSIBLE   175 POSSIBLE

Points assigned reflect importance of step to meeting objective: Important = (5)   Essential = (10)   Critical = (15)
Automatic failure results if any of the critical steps are omitted or performed incorrectly.

DETERMINE SCORE (divide points earned by total points possible, multiply results by 100)   _____ SCORE*

Evaluator's Name (print) _____ Signature _____

Comments _____

DOCUMENTATION

Chart the procedure in the patient's medical record.

Date: _____

Charting: _____

_____

_____

_____

Student's Initials: _____

Name _____

Date _____ Score* _____

PROCEDURE 14–4   Instill Eyedrops

TERMINAL PERFORMANCE OBJECTIVE - Provided with a mannequin or anatomical model of the eye, and all necessary equipment, demonstrate each step of the procedure for instilling eyedrops in proper order.

PROCEDURE STEPS	STEP PERFORMED	POINTS POSSIBLE	COMMENTS
EVALUATOR: Place check mark in space following each step performed satisfactorily			
NOTE TIME BEGAN _____			
1. Verified medication ordered.	_____	15	
a. Assembled items	_____	5	
2. Washed hands and put on gloves.	_____	10	
3. Called patient by name.	_____	10	
a. Explained procedure	_____	10	
4. Opened medication container/drew up ordered amount in dropper.	_____	15	
5. Positioned patient/asked for assistance if necessary.	_____	10	
6. Used gauze to touch area just under eyelid to form pocket.	_____	10	
7. Instilled drops into pocket of eye **without** touching tissues.	_____	15	
8. Asked patient to blink to distribute medication.	_____	15	
a. Repeated for other eye	_____	10	
9. Advised patient **not** to rub eyes.	_____	10	
10. Offered patient tissues to blot excess medication gently.	_____	5	
11. Provided patient education.	_____	5	
12. Closed medication container without touching cap to the outside of the container.	_____	10	
13. Removed gloves and washed hands.	_____	5	
14. Recorded procedure on patient's chart.	_____	10	
a. Noted observations	_____	5	
b. Initialed	_____	5	
15. Returned items to proper storage area.	_____	5	
EVALUATOR: NOTE TIME COMPLETED _____			

ADD POINTS OF STEPS CHECKED   _____ EARNED

TOTAL POINTS POSSIBLE   185 POSSIBLE

Points assigned reflect importance of step to meeting objective: Important = (5)   Essential = (10)   Critical = (15)

Automatic failure results if any of the critical steps are omitted or performed incorrectly.

DETERMINE SCORE (divide points earned by total points possible, multiply results by 100)   _____ SCORE*

Evaluator's Name (print) _____ Signature _____

Comments _____

DOCUMENTATION

Chart the procedure in the patient's medical record.

Date: _____

Charting: _____

_____

_____

_____

Student's Initials: _____

Name _____

Date _____ Score* _____

PROCEDURE 14–5   Screen Visual Acuity with Snellen Chart

TERMINAL PERFORMANCE OBJECTIVE - Measure the visual acuity of a patient by demonstrating each step of the vision screening procedure using the Snellen chart; record the results accurately on the patient's chart.

PROCEDURE STEPS	STEP PERFORMED	POINTS POSSIBLE	COMMENTS
EVALUATOR: Place check mark in space following each step performed satisfactorily			
NOTE TIME BEGAN _____			
1. Identified patient.	_____	10	
2. Explained the procedure to the patient.	_____	10	
3. Instructed patient to stand 20 feet from chart.	_____	10	
a. Adjusted eye chart to patient's eye level	_____	10	
4. Told patient to keep both eyes open.	_____	10	
a. Instructed patient to keep corrective lenses on/in during the first part of the screening	_____	10	
5. Instructed patient to read lines as you point to them.	_____	5	
6. Asked patient to read chart with both eyes.	_____	5	
7. Recorded smallest line patient could read (without making a mistake).	_____	15	
8. Asked patient to cover left eye.	_____	10	
a. Instructed patient to leave both eyes open	_____	10	
b. Recorded smallest line patient could read (without making a mistake)	_____	15	
9. Asked patient to cover right eye.	_____	10	
a. Instructed patient to leave both eyes open	_____	10	
10. Recorded smallest line patient could read (without making a mistake).	_____	15	
11. Recorded observations of patient during screening.	_____	5	

EVALUATOR: NOTE TIME COMPLETED _____

ADD POINTS OF STEPS CHECKED   _____ EARNED

TOTAL POINTS POSSIBLE   160 POSSIBLE

Points assigned reflect importance of step to meeting objective: Important = (5)   Essential = (10)   Critical = (15)
Automatic failure results if any of the critical steps are omitted or performed incorrectly.

DETERMINE SCORE (divide points earned by total points possible, multiply results by 100)   _____ SCORE*

Evaluator's Name (print) _____ Signature _____

Comments _____

DOCUMENTATION

Chart the procedure in the patient's medical record.

Date: _____

Charting: _____

_____

_____

_____

Student's Initials: _____

Name _____

Date _____ Score* _____

PROCEDURE 14–6   Screen Visual Acuity with Jaeger System

TERMINAL PERFORMANCE OBJECTIVE - Determine the near distance visual acuity of a patient using the Jaeger near vision acuity chart by demonstrating each step of the visual acuity procedure; record results accurately in patient's chart.

PROCEDURE STEPS	STEP PERFORMED	POINTS POSSIBLE	COMMENTS
EVALUATOR: Place check mark in space following each step performed satisfactorily			
NOTE TIME BEGAN _____			
1. Identified patient.	_____	10	
2. Positioned patient for procedure.	_____	10	
3. Instructed patient to hold Jaeger chart between 14″ and 16″ from eyes.	_____	15	
4. Instructed patient to read various paragraphs/both eyes open first without corrective lenses.	_____	10	
a. With corrective lenses	_____	10	
5. Instructed patient to cover left eye and read.	_____	10	
6. Instructed patient to cover right eye and read.	_____	10	
7. Observed patient during procedure.	_____	5	
8. Listened to remarks made by patient during procedure.	_____	5	
9. Recorded results on patient's chart listing the smallest print patient could read (without making a mistake).	_____	15	
10. Initialed patient's chart.	_____	5	
11. Thanked patient for cooperation.	_____	5	
12. Answered patient's questions.	_____	5	
13. Returned Jaeger chart to proper storage.	_____	5	

EVALUATOR: NOTE TIME COMPLETED _____

ADD POINTS OF STEPS CHECKED   _____ EARNED

TOTAL POINTS POSSIBLE   120 POSSIBLE

Points assigned reflect importance of step to meeting objective: Important = (5)   Essential = (10)   Critical = (15)

Automatic failure results if any of the critical steps are omitted or performed incorrectly.

DETERMINE SCORE (divide points earned by total points possible, multiply results by 100)   _____ SCORE*

Evaluator's Name (print) _____ Signature _____

Comments _____

DOCUMENTATION

Chart the procedure in the patient's medical record.

Date: _____

Charting: _____

_____

_____

_____

Student's Initials: _____

Name _____

Date _____ Score* _____

PROCEDURE 14–7 Determine Color Vision Acuity by Ishihara Method

TERMINAL PERFORMANCE OBJECTIVE - In a well-lighted area, determine the color vision acuity of a patient using the Ishihara method demonstrating each step of the procedure and accurately recording the results in the patient's chart.

PROCEDURE STEPS	STEP PERFORMED	POINTS POSSIBLE	COMMENTS
EVALUATOR: Place check mark in space following each step performed satisfactorily			
NOTE TIME BEGAN _____			
1. Identified patient.	_____	10	
a. Explained procedure to patient	_____	10	
2. Obtained chart from back of Ishihara book.	_____	10	
a. Worked in well-lighted area	_____	10	
3. Instructed patient to wear corrective lenses during procedure.	_____	10	
4. Asked patient to read plates with both eyes.	_____	10	
5. Instructed patient to trace the letters/numbers, etc. with their finger.	_____	5	
6. Asked patient to cover left eye	_____	5	
a. Repeated steps 3–5	_____	25	
7. Asked patient to cover right eye	_____	5	
a. Repeated steps 3–5	_____	25	
8. Recorded any difficulty/complaints on patient's chart.	_____	5	
9. Compared answers of patient with Ishihara chart.	_____	10	
10. Recorded frames patient missed.	_____	10	
11. Recorded what patient reports.	_____	5	
12. Initialed procedure on patient's chart.	_____	5	
EVALUATOR: NOTE TIME COMPLETED _____			

ADD POINTS OF STEPS CHECKED   _____ EARNED

TOTAL POINTS POSSIBLE   160 POSSIBLE

Points assigned reflect importance of step to meeting objective: Important = (5)   Essential = (10)   Critical = (15)
Automatic failure results if any of the critical steps are omitted or performed incorrectly.

DETERMINE SCORE (divide points earned by total points possible, multiply results by 100)   _____ SCORE*

Evaluator's Name (print) _____ Signature _____

Comments _____

DOCUMENTATION

Chart the procedure in the patient's medical record.

Date: _____

Charting: _____

_____

_____

_____

Student's Initials: _____

Name _____

Date _____ Score* _____

PROCEDURE 14–8   Assist Patient to Horizontal Recumbent Position

TERMINAL PERFORMANCE OBJECTIVE - Assist patient to assume the horizontal recumbent position while providing for safety and privacy according to the standards identified in the procedure.

PROCEDURE STEPS	STEP PERFORMED	POINTS POSSIBLE	COMMENTS
EVALUATOR: Place check mark in space following each step performed satisfactorily			
NOTE TIME BEGAN _____			
1. Checked examination room for cleanliness.	_____	5	
a. Provided clean table paper	_____	5	
b. Provided clean pillow cover	_____	5	
2. Identified patient	_____	15	
3. Instructed patient to remove appropriate clothing.	_____	10	
a. Instructed patient where to put belongings	_____	5	
4. Instructed patient in putting on gown.	_____	5	
5. Assisted patient as necessary.	_____	5	
6. Instructed patient to sit on side of exam table.	_____	5	
7. Instructed patient to lie flat on table with legs together.	_____	15	
8. Pulled out extension of table for leg support.	_____	5	
9. Provided pillow under patient's head.	_____	5	
10. Asked patient to put arms at her side or crossed over chest.	_____	5	
11. Placed drape sheet over patient.	_____	5	
12. Assisted with examination as necessary.	_____	5	
13. Assisted patient from table as necessary.	_____	5	
14. Cleaned up examination room as needed.	_____	5	
a. Replaced supplies as needed (Glove PRN)	_____	5	

EVALUATOR: NOTE TIME COMPLETED _____

ADD POINTS OF STEPS CHECKED   _____ EARNED
TOTAL POINTS POSSIBLE   115 POSSIBLE

Points assigned reflect importance of step to meeting objective: Important = (5)   Essential = (10)   Critical = (15)
Automatic failure results if any of the critical steps are omitted or performed incorrectly.

DETERMINE SCORE (divide points earned by total points possible, multiply results by 100)   _____ SCORE*

Evaluator's Name (print) _____ Signature _____

Comments _____

Name _____

Date _____ Score* _____

PROCEDURE 14–9   Assist Patient to Prone Position

TERMINAL PERFORMANCE OBJECTIVE - Assist patient to assume the prone position while providing for safety and privacy according to the standards identified in the procedure.

PROCEDURE STEPS	STEP PERFORMED	POINTS POSSIBLE	COMMENTS
EVALUATOR: Place check mark in space following each step performed satisfactorily			
NOTE TIME BEGAN _____			
1. Checked examination room for cleanliness.	_____	5	
a. Provided clean table paper	_____	5	
b. Provided clean pillow cover	_____	5	
2. Identified patient.	_____	15	
3. Instructed patient to remove appropriate clothing.	_____	10	
a. Instructed patient where to put belongings	_____	5	
4. Instructed patient in putting on gown.	_____	5	
5. Assisted patient as necessary.	_____	5	
6. Instructed patient to sit on side of exam table.	_____	5	
7. Instructed patient to lie flat on table with legs together.	_____	10	
8. Pulled out extension of table for leg support.	_____	5	
9. Placed drape sheet over patient.	_____	5	
10. Asked patient to turn toward you onto her stomach.	_____	15	
a. Cautioned patient to stay in center of table to avoid falling	_____	5	
11. Instructed patient to turn her head to one side.	_____	5	
12. Instructed patient to flex arms at elbows with her hands at side or under head.	_____	5	
13. Adjusted drape sheet evenly and loosely on all sides.	_____	5	
14. Assisted with examination as necessary.	_____	5	
15. Instructed patient to turn on back.	_____	5	
a. Reminded her to stay in center of table	_____	5	
16. Assisted patient in sitting up.	_____	5	
17. Advised patient to regain balance before standing.	_____	5	

PROCEDURE 14–9   Assist Patient to Prone Position—continued

PROCEDURE STEPS	STEP PERFORMED	POINTS POSSIBLE	COMMENTS
18. Assisted patient from table as necessary.	_____	5	
19. Cleaned up examination room as needed.	_____	5	
a. Replaced supplies as needed (Glove PRN)	_____	5	
EVALUATOR: NOTE TIME COMPLETED _____			

ADD POINTS OF STEPS CHECKED   _____ EARNED
TOTAL POINTS POSSIBLE   155 POSSIBLE

Points assigned reflect importance of step to meeting objective: Important = (5)   Essential = (10)   Critical = (15)
Automatic failure results if any of the critical steps are omitted or performed incorrectly.

DETERMINE SCORE (divide points earned by total points possible, multiply results by 100)   _____ SCORE*

Evaluator's Name (print) _____ Signature _____

Comments _____

Name _____

Date _____ Score* _____

PROCEDURE 14–10 Assist Patient to Sims' Position

TERMINAL PERFORMANCE OBJECTIVE - Assist patient to assume the Sims' position while providing for safety and privacy according to the standards identified in the procedure.

PROCEDURE STEPS	STEP PERFORMED	POINTS POSSIBLE	COMMENTS
EVALUATOR: Place check mark in space following each step performed satisfactorily			
NOTE TIME BEGAN _____			
1. Checked examination room for cleanliness.	_____	5	
a. Provided clean table paper	_____	5	
b. Provided clean pillow cover	_____	5	
2. Identified patient	_____	15	
3. Instructed patient to remove appropriate clothing.	_____	10	
a. Instructed patient where to put belongings	_____	5	
4. Instructed patient in putting on gown.	_____	5	
5. Assisted patient as necessary.	_____	5	
6. Instructed patient to sit on side of exam table.	_____	5	
7. Instructed patient to lie on left side.	_____	10	
8. Provided pillow under patient's head.	_____	5	
9. Asked patient to put left arm and shoulder behind body.	_____	5	
10. Asked patient to flex right arm with hand toward head.	_____	5	
11. Asked patient to flex left leg slightly.	_____	5	
12. Asked patient to move buttocks near side of table.	_____	5	
13. Instruct patient to flex right leg sharply toward chest.	_____	15	
14. Placed fenestrated drape sheet over patient.	_____	5	
15. Assisted with examination as necessary.	_____	5	
16. Assisted patient from table as necessary.	_____	5	
17. Cleaned up examination room as needed.	_____	5	
a. Replaced supplies as needed (Glove PRN)	_____	5	

EVALUATOR: NOTE TIME COMPLETED _____

ADD POINTS OF STEPS CHECKED _____ EARNED

TOTAL POINTS POSSIBLE 135 POSSIBLE

Points assigned reflect importance of step to meeting objective: Important = (5) Essential = (10) Critical = (15)
Automatic failure results if any of the critical steps are omitted or performed incorrectly.

DETERMINE SCORE (divide points earned by total points possible, multiply results by 100) _____ SCORE*

Evaluator's Name (print) _____ Signature _____

Comments _____

Name _____

Date _____ Score* _____

PROCEDURE 14–11   Assist Patient to Knee-Chest Position

TERMINAL PERFORMANCE OBJECTIVE - Assist patient to assume the knee-chest position while providing for safety and privacy according to the standards identified in the procedure.

PROCEDURE STEPS	STEP PERFORMED	POINTS POSSIBLE	COMMENTS
EVALUATOR: Place check mark in space following each step performed satisfactorily			
NOTE TIME BEGAN _____			
1. Checked examination room for cleanliness.	_____	5	
a. Provided clean table paper	_____	5	
b. Provided clean pillow cover	_____	5	
2. Prepared examination equipment on tray.	_____	5	
3. Identified patient.	_____	15	
4. Instructed patient to remove appropriate clothing.	_____	15	
a. Instructed patient where to put belongings	_____	5	
5. Instructed patient in putting on gown.	_____	5	
6. Assisted patient as necessary.	_____	5	
7. Instructed patient to sit on side of exam table.	_____	5	
8. Instructed patient to lie down on table.	_____	5	
9. Placed drape sheet over patient.	_____	5	
10. Instructed patient to turn toward you onto stomach.	_____	5	
a. Guided patient to center of table	_____	5	
11. Instructed patient to get on hands and knees.	_____	10	
12. Instructed patient to flex arms and fold under head.	_____	5	
13. Asked patient to separate knees slightly and keep thighs at right angle to table.	_____	15	
14. Adjusted drape sheet as needed.	_____	5	
15. Called physician to begin exam.	_____	5	
16. Assisted with examination as necessary.	_____	5	
17. Instructed patient to lie flat on stomach.	_____	5	
a. Assisted patient to turn over on back	_____	5	

PROCEDURE 14–11   Assist Patient to Knee-Chest Position—continued

PROCEDURE STEPS	STEP PERFORMED	POINTS POSSIBLE	COMMENTS
18. Assisted patient to sit up.	_____	5	
19. Assisted patient from table as necessary.	_____	5	
20. Cleaned up examination room as needed.	_____	5	
a. Replaced supplies as needed (Glove PRN)	_____	5	
EVALUATOR: NOTE TIME COMPLETED _____			

ADD POINTS OF STEPS CHECKED   _____ EARNED

TOTAL POINTS POSSIBLE   165 POSSIBLE

Points assigned reflect importance of step to meeting objective: Important = (5)   Essential = (10)   Critical = (15)
Automatic failure results if any of the critical steps are omitted or performed incorrectly.

DETERMINE SCORE (divide points earned by total points possible, multiply results by 100)   _____ SCORE*

Evaluator's Name (print) _____ Signature _____

Comments _____

Name _____

Date _____ Score* _____

PROCEDURE 14–12   Assist Patient to Semi-Fowler's Position

TERMINAL PERFORMANCE OBJECTIVE - Assist patient to assume the semi-Fowler's position while providing for safety and privacy according to the standards identified in the procedure.

PROCEDURE STEPS	STEP PERFORMED	POINTS POSSIBLE	COMMENTS
EVALUATOR: Place check mark in space following each step performed satisfactorily			
NOTE TIME BEGAN _____			
1. Checked examination room for cleanliness.	_____	5	
a. Provided clean table paper	_____	5	
b. Provided clean pillow cover	_____	5	
2. Identified patient.	_____	15	
3. Instructed patient to remove appropriate clothing.	_____	15	
a. Instructed patient where to put belongings	_____	5	
4. Instructed patient in putting on gown.	_____	5	
5. Assisted patient as necessary.	_____	5	
6. Instructed patient to sit at end of exam table.	_____	10	
a. Asked patient to scoot back toward center of table	_____	10	
7. Raised head of table to desired height—45° angle for semi-Fowler's (90° angle for Fowler's)	_____	15	
8. Instructed patient to lie flat on table with legs together.	_____	5	
9. Asked patient to lean back for comfort.	_____	5	
10. Pulled out extension of table for leg support.	_____	5	
11. Placed drape sheet over patient.	_____	5	
12. Assisted patient as necessary.	_____	5	
13. Assisted patient in sitting up.	_____	5	
14. Advised patient to regain balance before standing.	_____	5	
15. Assisted patient from table as necessary.	_____	5	
16. Cleaned up examination room as needed.	_____	5	
a. Replaced supplies as needed (Glove PRN)	_____	5	
EVALUATOR: NOTE TIME COMPLETED _____			

ADD POINTS OF STEPS CHECKED _____ EARNED
TOTAL POINTS POSSIBLE 145 POSSIBLE

Points assigned reflect importance of step to meeting objective: Important = (5)   Essential = (10)   Critical = (15)
Automatic failure results if any of the critical steps are omitted or performed incorrectly.

DETERMINE SCORE (divide points earned by total points possible, multiply results by 100) _____ SCORE*

Evaluator's Name (print) _____ Signature _____

Comments _____

Name _____

Date _____ Score* _____

PROCEDURE 14–13 Assist Patient to Lithotomy Position

TERMINAL PERFORMANCE OBJECTIVE - Assist patient to assume the lithotomy position while providing for safety and privacy according to the standards identified in the procedure.

PROCEDURE STEPS	STEP PERFORMED	POINTS POSSIBLE	COMMENTS
EVALUATOR: Place check mark in space following each step performed satisfactorily			
NOTE TIME BEGAN _____			
1. Checked examination room for cleanliness.	_____	5	
a. Provided clean table paper	_____	5	
b. Provided clean pillow cover	_____	5	
2. Assembled necessary equipment.	_____	5	
3. Identified patient.	_____	15	
4. Instructed patient to remove appropriate clothing.	_____	10	
a. Instructed patient where to put belongings	_____	5	
5. Instructed patient in putting on gown.	_____	5	
6. Assisted patient as necessary.	_____	5	
7. Instructed patient to sit at end of exam table.	_____	10	
8. Instructed patient to lie back on table.	_____	10	
9. Pulled out extension of table for leg support.	_____	5	
10. Positioned stirrups away from table.	_____	5	
a. Adjusted height of stirrups	_____	5	
b. Secured stirrups in place	_____	5	
11. Asked patient to move buttocks toward end of table.	_____	10	
a. Placed the back of your hand at end of table to guide patient	_____	5	
b. Assisted patient's feet into stirrups	_____	15	
12. Pushed table extension in.	_____	5	
a. Positioned examination stool for physician	_____	5	
b. Positioned examination light for physician	_____	5	
13. Placed drape sheet over patient.	_____	5	
14. Assisted with examination as necessary.	_____	5	

PROCEDURE 14–13   Assist Patient to Lithotomy Position—continued

PROCEDURE STEPS	STEP PERFORMED	POINTS POSSIBLE	COMMENTS
15. Assisted patient from table as necessary.	_____	5	
16. Cleaned up examination room as needed.	_____	5	
a. Replaced supplies as needed (Glove RPN)	_____	5	
EVALUATOR: NOTE TIME COMPLETED _____			

ADD POINTS OF STEPS CHECKED   _____ EARNED

TOTAL POINTS POSSIBLE   170 POSSIBLE

Points assigned reflect importance of step to meeting objective: Important = (5)   Essential = (10)   Critical = (15)
Automatic failure results if any of the critical steps are omitted or performed incorrectly.

DETERMINE SCORE (divide points earned by total points possible, multiply results by 100)   _____ SCORE*

Evaluator's Name (print) _____ Signature _____

Comments _____

Name _____

Date _____ Score* _____

PROCEDURE 14–14   Assist with a Gynecological Examination and Pap Test

TERMINAL PERFORMANCE OBJECTIVE - Demonstrate each of the steps required in assisting with the gynecological (GYN) examination and Pap test.

PROCEDURE STEPS	STEP PERFORMED	POINTS POSSIBLE	COMMENTS
EVALUATOR: Place check mark in space following each step performed satisfactorily			
NOTE TIME BEGAN _____			
1. Stated purpose of procedure.	_____	10	
2. Washed hands.	_____	5	
3. Assembled all needed items on Mayo table.	_____	10	
4. Asked patient to empty her bladder.	_____	5	
(Instructed patient to leave urine specimen if ordered by physician).	_____	—	
5. Printed patient's name in pencil on frosted end of slide(s).	_____	10	
6. Explained procedure to patient.	_____	5	
7. Gave gown/drape sheet to patient and instructed her how to put it on.	_____	10	
a. Assisted patient PRN	_____	5	
b. Instructed patient to sit at end of table when ready and left door unlocked	_____	5	
8. Assisted patient to horizontal recumbent position.	_____	10	
9. Assisted patient into lithotomy position and draped.	_____	15	
10. Encouraged patient to breathe slowly and deeply through the mouth during exam.	_____	10	
11. Put on gloves.	_____	5	
12. Warmed vaginal speculum with warm water.	_____	5	
13. Handed speculum and spatula to physician.	_____	10	
14. Held slide for physician to apply smear.	_____	10	
15. Marked smear(s) accordingly.	_____	15	
16. Applied fixative or placed in alcohol-ether solution bottle.	_____	10	
17. Placed lubricant on physician's fingers for bimanual exam.	_____	5	
18. Discarded disposables in biohazardous container.	_____	10	
19. Removed gloves and washed hands.	_____	5	

PROCEDURE STEPS	STEP PERFORMED	POINTS POSSIBLE	COMMENTS
20. Helped patient to sit up.	_____	5	
a. Pushed foot rest in	_____	5	
21. Helped patient down from exam table.	_____	5	
22. Returned items to proper storage area.	_____	5	
a. If metal speculum was used—placed in cool water to soak	_____	5	
23. Regloved PRN.	_____	5	
24. Instructed patient to dress.	_____	5	
25. Placed Pap smear slide(s) with completed request form in lab pick-up area.	_____	10	

EVALUATOR: NOTE TIME COMPLETED _____

ADD POINTS OF STEPS CHECKED   _____ EARNED
TOTAL POINTS POSSIBLE   220 POSSIBLE

Points assigned reflect importance of step to meeting objective: Important = (5)   Essential = (10)   Critical = (15)
Automatic failure results if any of the critical steps are omitted or performed incorrectly.

DETERMINE SCORE (divide points earned by total points possible, multiply results by 100)   _____ SCORE*

Evaluator's Name (print) _____ Signature _____

Comments _____

DOCUMENTATION

Chart the procedure in the patient's medical record.

Date: _____

Charting: _____

_____

_____

_____

Student's Initials: _____

Name _____

Date _____ Score* _____

PROCEDURE 14–15 Assist with Sigmoidoscopy

TERMINAL PERFORMANCE OBJECTIVE - Demonstrate each of the steps required in assisting with the sigmoidoscopy procedure.

PROCEDURE STEPS	STEP PERFORMED	POINTS POSSIBLE	COMMENTS
EVALUATOR: Place check mark in space following each step performed satisfactorily			
NOTE TIME BEGAN _____			
1. Stated purpose of procedure.	_____	10	
2. Explained procedure to patient.	_____	5	
3. Asked patient to empty bladder.	_____	10	
4. Assembled all needed items on Mayo table at end of exam table.	_____	10	
a. Completed lab request form for biopsy if requested; labeled container	_____	10	
5. Checked light source.	_____	5	
6. Instructed patient to disrobe from waist down.	_____	5	
a. Assisted patient to sit at end of exam table	_____	5	
b. Covered patient with drape	_____	5	
7. Assisted patient with knee-chest or Sims' position just before exam.	_____	15	
8. Applied approximately two tablespoons of lubricant on gauze square for physician to use during exam.	_____	5	
9. Plugged in light source of sigmoidoscope.	_____	5	
a. Secured air inflation tubing	_____	5	
10. Washed hands and put on gloves.	_____	10	
11. Handed sigmoidoscope to physician.	_____	10	
a. Assisted as needed	_____	5	
12. Cleaned patient's anal area with tissues.	_____	5	
13. Removed gloves and washed hands.	_____	5	
14. Assisted patient to resting prone position.	_____	5	
15. Assisted patient to sitting position.	_____	5	
a. Then from table to dress	_____	5	
16. Regloved.	_____	5	
17. Cleaned up exam area.	_____	5	
a. Placed used instruments in basin of detergent solution to soak	_____	5	

PROCEDURE STEPS	STEP PERFORMED	POINTS POSSIBLE	COMMENTS
18. Removed gloves and washed hands.	_____	5	
19. Scheduled patient for further appointment(s).	_____	5	
20. Recorded procedure on patient's chart.	_____	5	
a. Initialed	_____	5	
21. Cleaned exam room; readied instruments for autoclave (regloved as necessary).	_____	5	
EVALUATOR: NOTE TIME COMPLETED _____			

ADD POINTS OF STEPS CHECKED   _____ EARNED

TOTAL POINTS POSSIBLE   185 POSSIBLE

Points assigned reflect importance of step to meeting objective: Important = (5)   Essential = (10)   Critical = (15)
Automatic failure results if any of the critical steps are omitted or performed incorrectly.

DETERMINE SCORE (divide points earned by total points possible, multiply results by 100)   _____ SCORE*

Evaluator's Name (print) _____ Signature _____

Comments _____

DOCUMENTATION

Chart the procedure in the patient's medical record.

Date: _____

Charting: _____

_____

_____

_____

Student's Initials: _____

Name _____

Date _____ Score* _____

PROCEDURE 14–16   Administer Disposable Cleansing Enema

TERMINAL PERFORMANCE OBJECTIVE - Demonstrate each of the steps required in administering a cleansing enema.

PROCEDURE STEPS	STEP PERFORMED	POINTS POSSIBLE	COMMENTS
EVALUATOR: Place check mark in space following each step performed satisfactorily			
NOTE TIME BEGAN _____			
1. Identified patient.	_____	5	
a. Explained procedure to patient	_____	5	
2. Instructed patient to disrobe from waist down.	_____	5	
a. Provided drape sheet	_____	5	
b. Assisted patient on to exam table	_____	5	
3. Helped patient into Sims' position:	_____	10	
a. Instructed patient to lie on left side	_____	10	
b. Asked patient to bring right knee up to waist level	_____	15	
c. Adjusted drape sheet over patient	_____	5	
4. Washed hands.	_____	5	
a. Put on gloves	_____	5	
5. Removed protective covering from tip of enema container.	_____	10	
a. Applied small amount of lubricant to the tip	_____	5	
6. Separated buttocks to expose anus.	_____	10	
7. Inserted tip of bottle into anus.	_____	10	
a. Advised patient to breathe deeply and slowly through the mouth	_____	5	
8. Expressed entire contents into the anus	_____	15	
a. Advised patient to retain contents for as long as possible	_____	15	
9. Withdrew enema tip slowly.	_____	5	
a. Provided tissues to patient	_____	5	
b. Disposed of used tissues in biohazardous container	_____	5	
10. Directed patient to rest room.	_____	5	
a. Asked patient to let you check results before flushing	_____	15	
11. Reported results to physician.	_____	10	

PROCEDURE 14–16 Administer Disposable Cleansing Enema—continued

PROCEDURE STEPS	STEP PERFORMED	POINTS POSSIBLE	COMMENTS
12. Cleaned room	_____	5	
a. Discarded disposables in appropriate waste containers	_____	5	
13. Removed gloves	_____	10	
a. Washed hands	_____	10	
14. Initialed chart.	_____	5	

EVALUATOR: NOTE TIME COMPLETED _____

ADD POINTS OF STEPS CHECKED   _____ EARNED
TOTAL POINTS POSSIBLE   225 POSSIBLE

Points assigned reflect importance of step to meeting objective: Important = (5)   Essential = (10)   Critical = (15)
Automatic failure results if any of the critical steps are omitted or performed incorrectly.

DETERMINE SCORE (divide points earned by total points possible, multiply results by 100)   _____ SCORE*

Evaluator's Name (print) _____ Signature _____

Comments _____

DOCUMENTATION

Chart the procedure in the patient's medical record.

Date: _____

Charting: _____

_____

_____

_____

Student's Initials: _____

Name _____

Date _____ Score* _____

PROCEDURE 15–1   Using the Microscope

TERMINAL PERFORMANCE OBJECTIVE - Provided with all necessary equipment and supplies, demonstrate the use of the microscope following the steps in the procedure with the instructor observing each step.

PROCEDURE STEPS	STEP PERFORMED	POINTS POSSIBLE	COMMENTS
EVALUATOR: Place check mark in space following each step performed satisfactorily			
NOTE TIME BEGAN _____			
1. Washed hands and put on gloves.	_____	5	
2. Assembled necessary equipment.	_____	5	
3. Labeled specimen on frosted end of slide with pencil.	_____	10	
4. Cleaned ocular lens with lens cleaning tissue.	_____	10	
5. Plugged light source into electrical outlet.	_____	15	
6. Turned light source on.	_____	10	
7. Placed specimen slide on stage with frosted side up between clips.	_____	10	
8. Secured slide over opening of stage.	_____	5	
9. Raised substage carefully.	_____	5	
10. Turned revolving nosepiece to 1pf (10X).	_____	5	
11. Began to focus until specimen was in view.	_____	10	
12. Turned fine adjustment until specimen was seen in detail.	_____	10	
13. Adjusted substage diaphragm lever for proper lighting.	_____	5	
14. Turned revolving nosepiece to intermediate (40X).	_____	5	
15. Adjusted fine focus for detail in viewing specimen.	_____	10	
16. Use hpf:			
a. Use cover slide	_____	10	
b. Clean lens after use	_____	5	
c. Adjust diaphragm lever	_____	5	
17. Identified specimen.	_____	5	
18. Turned light off.	_____	5	
19. Cleaned microscopic stage.	_____	5	
20. Disposed of clean slide(s).	_____	5	
21. Removed gloves and washed hands.	_____	5	

PROCEDURE STEPS	STEP PERFORMED	POINTS POSSIBLE	COMMENTS
22. Recorded findings of microscopic examination on chart	_____	15	
a. Initialed	_____	5	

EVALUATOR: NOTE TIME COMPLETED _____

ADD POINTS OF STEPS CHECKED   _____ EARNED
TOTAL POINTS POSSIBLE   185 POSSIBLE

Points assigned reflect importance of step to meeting objective: Important = (5)   Essential = (10)   Critical = (15)
Automatic failure results if any of the critical steps are omitted or performed incorrectly.

DETERMINE SCORE (divide points earned by total points possible, multiply results by 100)   _____ SCORE*

Evaluator's Name (print) _____ Signature _____

Comments _____

Name _____

Date _____ Score* _____

PROCEDURE 15–2   Puncture Skin with Sterile Lancet

TERMINAL PERFORMANCE OBJECTIVE - Demonstrate skin puncture procedure following all steps to obtain capillary blood for
test(s) specified by physician/instructor.

PROCEDURE STEPS	STEP PERFORMED	POINTS POSSIBLE	COMMENTS
EVALUATOR: Place check mark in space following each step performed satisfactorily			
NOTE TIME BEGAN _____			
1. Identified patient.	_____	5	
2. Explained procedure to patient.	_____	5	
3. Inspected patient's finger and selected puncture site.	_____	5	
4. Washed hands and put on gloves.	_____	5	
5. Assembled needed items next to patient.	_____	5	
6. Cleaned site with alcohol pad.	_____	5	
7. Allowed site to air dry.	_____	5	
8. Removed sterile lancet from package without contaminating it.	_____	10	
9. Secured puncture site between thumb and great finger.	_____	5	
10. Held lancet pointed downward between thumb and great finger of other hand.	_____	5	
11. Punctured site with a quick, firm, steady down-and-up motion.	_____	10	
a. Approximately 2mm deep	_____	5	
b. Control entry and exit of lancet to avoid ripping skin	_____	5	
12. Discarded first drop of blood by blotting with gauze square.	_____	10	
13. Applied gentle pressure on either side of puncture site to obtain desired amount of blood.	_____	15	
14. Wiped site with cotton ball/gauze square.	_____	10	
15. Asked patient to apply gentle pressure with gauze square over site to control bleeding.	_____	10	
16. Checked site and attended to patient.	_____	5	
17. Discarded disposable in proper receptacles.	_____	5	

PROCEDURE STEPS	STEP PERFORMED	POINTS POSSIBLE	COMMENTS
18. Removed gloves.	_____	5	
19. Washed hands.	_____	5	
EVALUATOR: NOTE TIME COMPLETED _____			

ADD POINTS OF STEPS CHECKED   _____ EARNED
TOTAL POINTS POSSIBLE   140 POSSIBLE

Points assigned reflect importance of step to meeting objective: Important = (5)   Essential = (10)   Critical = (15)
Automatic failure results if any of the critical steps are omitted or performed incorrectly.

DETERMINE SCORE (divide points earned by total points possible, multiply results by 100)   _____ SCORE*

Evaluator's Name (print) _____ Signature _____

Comments _____

DOCUMENTATION

Chart the procedure in the patient's medical record.

Date: _____

Charting: _____

_____

_____

_____

Student's Initials: _____

Name _____

Date _____ Score* _____

PROCEDURE 15–3   Obtain Blood for PKU Test

TERMINAL PERFORMANCE OBJECTIVE - Demonstrate the steps of the procedure for obtaining a blood specimen for determination of phenylketonuria level in the blood.

PROCEDURE STEPS	STEP PERFORMED	POINTS POSSIBLE	COMMENTS
EVALUATOR: Place check mark in space following each step performed satisfactorily			
NOTE TIME BEGAN _____			
1. Identified patient.	_____	5	
2. Explained procedure to patient.	_____	5	
3. Washed hands.	_____	5	
a. Put on gloves	_____	5	
4. Assembled all needed items.	_____	10	
5. Explained procedure to parent of patient.	_____	5	
6. Asked all necessary information.	_____	10	
7. Completed form.	_____	10	
8. Asked assistance of parent.	_____	5	
9. Performed skin puncture adequately.	_____	10	
10. Wiped first drop of blood from site.	_____	5	
11. Secured site between great finger and thumb.	_____	5	
12. Applied gentle pressure to produce large drop of blood.	_____	10	
13. Applied blood to the circles on the back of the form, saturating each circle completely.	_____	15	
14. Repeated steps 11 and 12 until all circles have been saturated.	_____	15	
15. Wiped puncture site with dry gauze square.	_____	5	
a. Asked patient to hold gently	_____	5	
b. Placed small round bandage over area	_____	5	
16. Placed completed PKU test form in protective paper envelope.	_____	10	
a. Then, into addressed envelope to health dept.	_____	10	
17. Discarded used items properly.	_____	5	
18. Removed gloves.	_____	5	
a. Washed hands	_____	5	

PROCEDURE STEPS	STEP PERFORMED	POINTS POSSIBLE	COMMENTS
19. Returned items to proper storage.	_____	5	
20. Recorded procedure on patient's chart.	_____	10	
a. Initialed	_____	5	

EVALUATOR: NOTE TIME COMPLETED _____

ADD POINTS OF STEPS CHECKED   _____ EARNED

TOTAL POINTS POSSIBLE   190 POSSIBLE

Points assigned reflect importance of step to meeting objective: Important = (5)   Essential = (10)   Critical = (15)

Automatic failure results if any of the critical steps are omitted or performed incorrectly.

DETERMINE SCORE (divide points earned by total points possible, multiply results by 100)   _____ SCORE*

Evaluator's Name (print) _____ Signature _____

Comments _____

DOCUMENTATION

Chart the procedure in the patient's medical record.

Date: _____

Charting: _____

_____

_____

_____

Student's Initials: _____

PERFORMANCE EVALUATION CHECKLIST

Name _____

Date _____ Score* _____

PROCEDURE 15–4   Determine Hematocrit Hct Using Microhematocrit Centrifuge

TERMINAL PERFORMANCE OBJECTIVE - Demonstrate the steps of the procedure for determining hematocrit (Hct) readings using the microhematocrit centrifuge.

PROCEDURE STEPS	STEP PERFORMED	POINTS POSSIBLE	COMMENTS
EVALUATOR: Place check mark in space following each step performed satisfactorily			
NOTE TIME BEGAN _____			
1. Identified patient.	_____	5	
2. Explained procedure to patient.	_____	5	
3. Washed hands.	_____	5	
a. Put on gloves	_____	5	
4. Assembled necessary items.	_____	5	
5. Followed desired skin puncture procedure.	_____	5	
6. Held microhematocrit tube horizontally. (There should be no bubbles in tube. Subtract points if bubbles are present.)	_____	10	
7. Filled tube(s) to line.	_____	15	
8. Wiped puncture site with cotton ball.	_____	5	
9. Wiped outside end of glass tube while holding horizontally.	_____	5	
10. Placed carefully into clay tray to seal end of tube.	_____	10	
11. Instructed patient to hold dry gauze over site gently.	_____	5	
a. Make sure bleeding has stopped	_____	5	
12. Secured sealed end of tube against rubber padding of centrifuge.	_____	10	
13. Balanced centrifuge.	_____	10	
14. Noted number of placed tube in centrifuge.	_____	10	
15. Closed inside cover and locked by turning clockwise.	_____	10	
16. Closed and locked outside cover.	_____	10	
17. Listened for click to assure locking.	_____	5	
18. Turned timer switch past desired time and then to three minutes to set automatic timer.	_____	5	
19. Waited until completely stopped to unlock cover.	_____	15	
20. Placed bottom line of packed red cells up to buffy coat against calibrated chart (in centrifuge).	_____	15	
21. Used magnifying glass to read results.	_____	10	
22. Reclosed cover of centrifuge.	_____	5	

PROCEDURE STEPS	STEP PERFORMED	POINTS POSSIBLE	COMMENTS
23. Discarded used items in proper receptacle.	_____	5	
24. Removed gloves.	_____	5	
a. Washed hands	_____	5	
25. Returned items to proper storage.	_____	5	
26. Recorded reading in patient's chart as %	_____	15	
a. Initialed	_____	5	

EVALUATOR: NOTE TIME COMPLETED _____

ADD POINTS OF STEPS CHECKED   _____ EARNED
TOTAL POINTS POSSIBLE   230 POSSIBLE

Points assigned reflect importance of step to meeting objective: Important = (5)   Essential = (10)   Critical = (15)
Automatic failure results if any of the critical steps are omitted or performed incorrectly.

DETERMINE SCORE (divide points earned by total points possible, multiply results by 100)   _____ SCORE*

Evaluator's Name (print) _____ Signature _____

Comments _____

DOCUMENTATION

Chart the procedure in the patient's medical record.

Date: _____

Charting: _____

_____

_____

_____

Student's Initials: _____

Name _____

Date _____ Score* _____

PROCEDURE 15–5   Hemoglobin (Hb) Determination Using the Hemoglobinometer

TERMINAL PERFORMANCE OBJECTIVE - Demonstrate the steps of the procedure for determining hemoglobin (Hb) using the hemoglobinometer.

PROCEDURE STEPS	STEP PERFORMED	POINTS POSSIBLE	COMMENTS
EVALUATOR: Place check mark in space following each step performed satisfactorily			
NOTE TIME BEGAN _____			
1. Identified patient.	_____	5	
2. Washed hands.	_____	5	
a. Put on gloves	_____	5	
3. Assembled all necessary items.	_____	5	
4. Checked batteries and light bulb in hemoglobinometer.	_____	10	
5. Explained procedure to patient.	_____	5	
6. Followed desired skin puncture procedure.	_____	15	
7. Pulled glass chamber out of hemoglobinometer and fixed lower part of slide so that it was slightly offset.	_____	5	
8. Placed large drop of blood directly onto offset glass chamber.	_____	10	
9. Gave patient dry gauze to place over site gently.	_____	5	
10. Mixed blood on slide with hemolysis applicator.	_____	15	
11. Pushed chamber into clip and into slot on left side of hemoglobinometer.	_____	10	
12. Held hemoglobinometer in left hand at eye level.	_____	10	
13. Depressed light button on bottom of instrument.	_____	10	
14. Looked into hemoglobinometer to view green field.	_____	10	
15. Slid button on right of meter to match green field.	_____	15	
16. Left sliding scale lever where fields match.	_____	5	
17. Read hemoglobin level at top of calibrator scale.	_____	15	
18. Recorded reading on patient's chart.	_____	10	
a. Initialed	_____	5	
19. Washed chambers, rinsed, dried and returned to hemoglobinometer	_____	5	

PROCEDURE STEPS	STEP PERFORMED	POINTS POSSIBLE	COMMENTS
20. Removed gloves.	_____	5	
a. Washed hands.	_____	5	
21. Discarded disposable items.	_____	5	
22. Returned items to proper storage.	_____	5	

EVALUATOR: NOTE TIME COMPLETED _____

ADD POINTS OF STEPS CHECKED   _____ EARNED

TOTAL POINTS POSSIBLE   200 POSSIBLE

Points assigned reflect importance of step to meeting objective: Important = (5)   Essential = (10)   Critical = (15)
Automatic failure results if any of the critical steps are omitted or performed incorrectly.

DETERMINE SCORE (divide points earned by total points possible, multiply results by 100)   _____ SCORE*

Evaluator's Name (print) _____ Signature _____

Comments _____

DOCUMENTATION

Chart the procedure in the patient's medical record.

Date: _____

Charting: _____

_____

_____

_____

Student's Initials: _____

Name _____

Date _____ Score* _____

PROCEDURE 15–6   Screen Blood Sugar (Glucose) Level

TERMINAL PERFORMANCE OBJECTIVE - Demonstrate the steps required in the procedure for determining blood glucose level.

PROCEDURE STEPS	STEP PERFORMED	POINTS POSSIBLE	COMMENTS
EVALUATOR: Place check mark in space following each step performed satisfactorily			
NOTE TIME BEGAN _____			
1. Identified patient.	_____	10	
2. Washed hands.	_____	5	
a. Put on gloves	_____	5	
3. Assembled all necessary items.	_____	5	
4. Calibrated instrument to be used (dextrometer).	_____	15	
5. Explained procedure to patient.	_____	5	
6. Followed desired skin puncture procedure.	_____	10	
7. Removed reagent strip from bottle without contaminating it.	_____	5	
8. Closed bottle.	_____	5	
9. Applied large drop of blood onto entire chemically treated surface of reagent strip.	_____	15	
10. Began timing immediately.	_____	15	
11. Wiped puncture site with cotton ball.	_____	5	
12. Gave patient dry gauze square to hold over site.	_____	5	
13. Blotted reagent strip after timing precisely.	_____	10	
14. Moved strip to clean area of tissue and blotted again.	_____	10	
15. Read strip by matching with color chart to determine glucose level of blood.	_____	15	
16. Recorded reading in patient's chart.	_____	15	
a. Initialed	_____	5	
17. Discarded used items.	_____	5	
18. Removed gloves.	_____	5	
a. Washed hands	_____	5	
19. Returned items to proper storage area.	_____	5	
EVALUATOR: NOTE TIME COMPLETED _____			

ADD POINTS OF STEPS CHECKED   _____ EARNED

TOTAL POINTS POSSIBLE   180 POSSIBLE

Points assigned reflect importance of step to meeting objective: Important = (5)   Essential = (10)   Critical = (15)

Automatic failure results if any of the critical steps are omitted or performed incorrectly.

DETERMINE SCORE (divide points earned by total points possible, multiply results by 100)   _____ SCORE*

Evaluator's Name (print) _____ Signature _____

Comments _____

DOCUMENTATION

Chart the procedure in the patient's medical record.

Date: _____

Charting: _____

_____

_____

_____

Student's Initials: _____

Name _____

Date _____ Score* _____

PROCEDURE 15–7   Count Erythrocytes (RBCs) Manually

TERMINAL PERFORMANCE OBJECTIVE - Demonstrate each of the steps required to perform a manual RBC count.

PROCEDURE STEPS	STEP PERFORMED	POINTS POSSIBLE	COMMENTS
EVALUATOR: Place check mark in space following each step performed satisfactorily			
NOTE TIME BEGAN _____			
1. Washed hands.	_____	5	
a. Put on gloves	_____	5	
2. Assembled all needed items near patient.	_____	5	
a. Explained procedure	_____	5	
3. Identified patient.	_____	5	
4. Performed skin puncture.	_____	5	
5. Filled RBC unopette pipette and reservoir:	_____	10	
a. Punctured diaphragm of reservoir	_____	10	
b. Removed shield from pipette assembly with a twist	_____	5	
c. Held pipette almost horizontally to touch tip of pipette to sample	_____	5	
d. Wiped excess sample from pipette	_____	5	
e. Squeezed reservoir slightly	_____	5	
f. Covered opening of overflow chamber with index finger and seated pipette securely in reservoir neck	_____	5	
g. Released pressure on reservoir	_____	5	
h. Squeezed reservoir gently 2 to 3 times to rinse capillary bore	_____	5	
i. Placed index finger over upper opening and gently inverted several times to mix well	_____	5	
6. Converted to dropper assembly:			
a. Withdrew pipette from reservoir and reseated securely in reverse position	_____	5	
b. Inverted reservoir and gently squeezed sides to discard first 3 to 4 drops	_____	5	
7. Positioned cover glass onto hemocytometer.	_____	5	
8. Placed tip of pipette almost touching the "V" on the slide's chamber.	_____	10	
9. Released moderate drop of solution onto both sides of chamber.	_____	10	
10. Waited 2 to 3 minutes for cells to settle.	_____	5	
11. Placed slide on microscope stage.	_____	5	
a. Turned light on	_____	5	

PROCEDURE STEPS	STEP PERFORMED	POINTS POSSIBLE	COMMENTS
b. Moved nosepiece to low-power objective	_____	5	
12. Scanned for even distribution of cells.	_____	5	
a. Checked both sides	_____	5	
13. Turned nosepiece to high-power objective.	_____	5	
14. Focused first at top left square of RBC counting area.	_____	15	
a. Adjusted light and fine focus as necessary	_____	10	
15. Counted only RBCs within the squares and those touching the top and left lines.	_____	15	
16. Counted cells in proper pattern.	_____	15	
a. Recorded number of cells counted	_____	10	
17. Repeated counting of squares in same pattern for B, C, D, and E.	_____	15	
a. Recorded number of cells counted in each	_____	10	
18. Added total number of cells counted in all squares (A–E) correctly.	_____	15	
19. Multiplied by 10,000 to get number of RBCs.	_____	15	
20. Recorded RBC count on patient's chart.	_____	15	
a. Initialed	_____	5	
21. Washed hemocytometer.	_____	5	
a. Rinsed	_____	5	
b. Dried on paper towels	_____	5	
22. Returned items to proper storage.	_____	5	
23. Removed gloves	_____	5	
a. Washed hands	_____	5	

EVALUATOR: NOTE TIME COMPLETED _____

ADD POINTS OF STEPS CHECKED   _____ EARNED
TOTAL POINTS POSSIBLE   330 POSSIBLE

Points assigned reflect importance of step to meeting objective: Important = (5)   Essential = (10)   Critical = (15)
Automatic failure results if any of the critical steps are omitted or performed incorrectly.

DETERMINE SCORE (divide points earned by total points possible, multiply results by 100)   _____ SCORE*

Evaluator's Name (print) _____ Signature _____

Comments _____

DOCUMENTATION

Chart the procedure in the patient's medical record.

Date: _____

Charting: _____

_____

_____

_____

Student's Initials: _____

PROCEDURE 15–8   Count Leukocytes (WBCs) Manually

TERMINAL PERFORMANCE OBJECTIVE - Demonstrate the steps required to perform a manual WBC count.

PROCEDURE STEPS	STEP PERFORMED	POINTS POSSIBLE	COMMENTS
EVALUATOR: Place check mark in space following each step performed satisfactorily			
NOTE TIME BEGAN _____			
1. Washed hands.	_____	5	
a. Put on gloves	_____	5	
2. Assembled all needed items near patient.	_____	5	
. a. Explained procedure	_____	5	
3. Identified patient.	_____	5	
4. Performed skin puncture.	_____	10	
5. Filled WBC unopette and reservoir:	_____	10	
a. Punctured diaphragm of reservoir (performed before finger puncture)	_____	5	
b. Removed shield from pipette assembly with a twist	_____	5	
c. Held pipette almost horizontally to touch tip of pipette to sample	_____	5	
d. Wiped excess sample from pipette	_____	5	
e. Squeezed reservoir slightly	_____	5	
f. Covered opening of overflow chamber with index finger and seated pipette securely in reservoir neck	_____	5	
g. Released pressure on reservoir	_____	5	
h. Squeezed reservoir gently 2 to 3 times to rinse capillary bore	_____	5	
i. Placed index finger over upper opening and gently inverted several times to mix well	_____	5	
6. Converted to dropper assembly:			
a. Withdrew pipette from reservoir and reseated securely in reverse position	_____	5	
b. Inverted reservoir and gently squeezed sides to discard first 3 to 4 drops	_____	5	
7. Positioned cover glass onto hemocytometer.	_____	5	
8. Placed tip of pipette almost touching the "V" on the slide's chamber.	_____	10	
9. Released moderate drop of solution onto both sides of chamber.	_____	10	
10. Waited 2 to 3 minutes for cells to settle.	_____	5	
11. Placed slide on microscope stage.	_____	5	

PROCEDURE STEPS	STEP PERFORMED	POINTS POSSIBLE	COMMENTS
a. Turned light on	_____	5	
b. Moved nosepiece to low-power objective	_____	5	
12. Scanned for even distribution of cells.	_____	5	
a. Checked both sides	_____	5	
13. Focused low-power objective at top left square	_____	15	
a. Adjusted fine focus	_____	10	
14. Counted only WBCs within the squares	_____	15	
a. Counted WBCs on top and left lines	_____	15	
15. Counted cells in pattern	_____	15	
a. Recorded number of cells counted	_____	5	
16. Repeated counting of cells in squares of 2, 3, and 4, in same pattern.	_____	10	
17. Added total number of cells counted in all 4 squares correctly.	_____	15	
18. Multiplied total by 50 correctly.	_____	15	
19. Recorded WBC count on patient's chart.	_____	15	
a. Initialed	_____	5	
20. Washed hemocytometer.	_____	5	
a. Rinsed	_____	5	
b. Dried on paper towels	_____	5	
21. Returned items to proper storage.	_____	5	
22. Removed gloves.	_____	5	
a. Washed hands	_____	5	

EVALUATOR: NOTE TIME COMPLETED _____

ADD POINTS OF STEPS CHECKED _____ EARNED
TOTAL POINTS POSSIBLE 320 POSSIBLE

Points assigned reflect importance of step to meeting objective: Important = (5)   Essential = (10)   Critical = (15)
Automatic failure results if any of the critical steps are omitted or performed incorrectly.

DETERMINE SCORE (divide points earned by total points possible, multiply results by 100) _____ SCORE*

Evaluator's Name (print) _____ Signature _____

Comments _____

DOCUMENTATION

Chart the procedure in the patient's medical record.

Date: _____

Charting: _____

_____

_____

_____

Student's Initials: _____

Name _____

Date _____ Score* _____

PROCEDURE 15–9   Making a Blood Smear

TERMINAL PERFORMANCE OBJECTIVE - Demonstrate the steps required to make an adequate blood smear for a differential white blood cell count.

PROCEDURE STEPS	STEP PERFORMED	POINTS POSSIBLE	COMMENTS
EVALUATOR: Place check mark in space following each step performed satisfactorily			
NOTE TIME BEGAN _____			
1. Identified patient.	_____	10	
2. Explained procedure to patient.	_____	5	
3. Completed lab request form.	_____	5	
4. Printed patient's name on frosted end of slide(s).	_____	10	
5. Assembled necessary items near patient.	_____	5	
6. Washed hands.	_____	5	
a. Put on gloves	_____	5	
7. Performed desired method of obtaining blood specimen.	_____	10	
8. Placed a small drop of blood on end of slide	_____	5	
a. ¼" from frosted end	_____	10	
b. Approximately ⅛" in diameter	_____	10	
9. Held corners of frosted end of glass slide down on flat surface.	_____	10	
a. Held second slide at 45° angle	_____	10	
10. Rested spreader slide against frosted slide.	_____	10	
a. Moved slide back carefully into the blood	_____	10	
b. Allowed blood to flow to edge of slide	_____	15	
c. Moved angled slide toward frosted end quickly and gently	_____	15	
d. Made feathered edge	_____	15	
11. Allowed smear to air dry/fan dry.	_____	5	
12. Placed blood smear in lab container.	_____	5	
a. Attached lab request form	_____	5	

PROCEDURE STEPS	STEP PERFORMED	POINTS POSSIBLE	COMMENTS
13. Removed gloves.	_____	5	
a. Washed hands	_____	5	
14. Discarded waste in appropriate containers.	_____	5	
15. Initialed procedure in patient's chart.	_____	5	

EVALUATOR: NOTE TIME COMPLETED _____

ADD POINTS OF STEPS CHECKED   _____ EARNED

TOTAL POINTS POSSIBLE   200 POSSIBLE

Points assigned reflect importance of step to meeting objective: Important = (5)   Essential = (10)   Critical = (15)
Automatic failure results if any of the critical steps are omitted or performed incorrectly.

DETERMINE SCORE (divide points earned by total points possible, multiply results by 100)   _____ SCORE*

Evaluator's Name (print) _____ Signature _____

Comments _____

DOCUMENTATION

Chart the procedure in the patient's medical record.

Date: _____

Charting: _____

_____

_____

_____

Student's Initials: _____

Name _____

Date _____ Score* _____

PROCEDURE 15–10   Obtain Venous Blood with Butterfly Needle Method

TERMINAL PERFORMANCE OBJECTIVE - Demonstrate the steps necessary for obtaining blood specimens using the butterfly needle method.

PROCEDURE STEPS	STEP PERFORMED	POINTS POSSIBLE	COMMENTS
EVALUATOR: Place check mark in space following each step performed satisfactorily			
NOTE TIME BEGAN _____			
1. Identified patient.	_____	5	
2. Explained procedure to patient.	_____	5	
3. Completed lab request form.	_____	5	
4. Assembled necessary items near patient.	_____	5	
5. Attached butterfly needle to syringe.	_____	10	
6. Put on gloves.	_____	5	
7. Palpated vein.	_____	5	
a. Cleaned skin with alcohol	_____	5	
b. Dried excess alcohol with cottonball	_____	5	
8. Applied tourniquet properly.	_____	10	
9. Asked patient to make fist and hold.	_____	10	
10. Removed needle guard.	_____	5	
a. Pushed air out of syringe	_____	5	
b. Quickly inserted needle into vein	_____	5	
c. Pulled back on plunger slowly	_____	10	
d. Obtained sufficient amount of blood	_____	15	
e. Removed tourniquet	_____	5	
f. Withdrew needle quickly	_____	5	
11. Filled appropriate blood tubes.	_____	15	
a. Filled in correct order	_____	15	
12. Applied gentle pressure to site with cottonball.	_____	5	
a. Advised patient to hold arm slightly upward	_____	5	
13. Applied bandaid to puncture site.	_____	5	
a. Asked if patient is allergic to adhesive	_____	5	
14. Placed used needle in biohazard sharps container.	_____	5	
15. Placed used disposables in biohazard bag.	_____	5	
16. Removed gloves and placed in biohazard bag.	_____	5	
17. Washed hands.	_____	5	

PROCEDURE STEPS	STEP PERFORMED	POINTS POSSIBLE	COMMENTS
18. Recorded procedure in patient's chart.	_____	5	
a. Initialed	_____	5	

EVALUATOR: NOTE TIME COMPLETED _____

ADD POINTS OF STEPS CHECKED   _____ EARNED
TOTAL POINTS POSSIBLE   200 POSSIBLE

Points assigned reflect importance of step to meeting objective: Important = (5)   Essential = (10)   Critical = (15)
Automatic failure results if any of the critical steps are omitted or performed incorrectly.

DETERMINE SCORE (divide points earned by total points possible, multiply results by 100)   _____ SCORE*

Evaluator's Name (print) _____ Signature _____

Comments _____

DOCUMENTATION

Chart the procedure in the patient's medical record.

Date: _____

Charting: _____

_____

_____

_____

Student's Initials: _____

Name _____

Date _____ Score* _____

PROCEDURE 15–11   Obtain Venous Blood with Sterile Needle and Syringe

TERMINAL PERFORMANCE OBJECTIVE - Demonstrate the steps necessary for obtaining venous blood using the sterile needle and syringe method.

PROCEDURE STEPS	STEP PERFORMED	POINTS POSSIBLE	COMMENTS
EVALUATOR: Place check mark in space following each step performed satisfactorily			
NOTE TIME BEGAN _____			
1. Identified patient.	_____	10	
2. Washed hands.	_____	5	
a. Put on gloves	_____	5	
3. Assembled necessary items near patient.	_____	5	
4. Completed lab request form.	_____	5	
a. Labeled specimen tube(s)	_____	5	
5. Explained procedure to patient.	_____	5	
a. Asked patient for preferred venipuncture site	_____	5	
6. Positioned patient appropriately.	_____	5	
7. Secured needle into syringe.	_____	10	
a. Pushed in plunger to expel air from barrel	_____	10	
8. Applied tourniquet to patient's upper arm.	_____	5	
a. Placed 3″ above elbow	_____	10	
9. Cleansed site lightly with alcohol/cottonball.	_____	5	
a. Allowed alcohol to air dry/dried with cottonball	_____	5	
10. Asked patient to clench fist to make vein stand up.	_____	5	
11. Took needle guard off.	_____	5	
a. Pointed bevel of needle up	_____	10	
b. Inserted needle tip into vein with quick and steady motion	_____	10	
c. Inserted needle into vein at 15° angle	_____	10	
d. Held skin taut for easier insertion	_____	5	
e. Inserted needle between ¼″ and ½″	_____	15	
12. Held barrel of syringe in one hand.	_____	5	
a. Pulled plunger back with other hand	_____	5	
b. Pulled plunger slowly/steadily	_____	5	
c. Allowed sufficient blood collection for specimen tube(s)	_____	15	
d. Asked patient to release clenched fist slowly	_____	5	
e. Released tourniquet within one minute	_____	10	
f. Pulled needle out in same path as inserted	_____	5	

PROCEDURE STEPS	STEP PERFORMED	POINTS POSSIBLE	COMMENTS
g. Placed cottonball/gauze square over site	_____	5	
13. Instructed patient to apply gentle pressure to site and elevate arm slightly.	_____	5	
14. Filled specimen tube(s) quickly.	_____	10	
a. Angled flow of blood to run down side of tube	_____	10	
b. Filled tubes in correct order of draw	_____	15	
c. Made blood smears as needed	_____	5	
15. Stood red-stoppered tubes vertically.	_____	5	
a. Did not shake tubes/mixed additives carefully	_____	5	
16. Deposited needle/syringe in sharps container.	_____	5	
17. Assembled specimen tubes/lab form together in biobag.	_____	5	
18. Attended to patient's needs.	_____	5	
a. Applied bandage	_____	5	
19. Discarded disposables in proper containers.	_____	5	
20. Removed gloves/placed in biobag.	_____	5	
a. Washed hands	_____	5	
21. Returned items to proper storage.	_____	5	
22. Recorded procedure in patient's chart.	_____	10	
a. Initialed	_____	5	

EVALUATOR: NOTE TIME COMPLETED _____

ADD POINTS OF STEPS CHECKED   _____ EARNED
TOTAL POINTS POSSIBLE   320 POSSIBLE

Points assigned reflect importance of step to meeting objective: Important = (5)   Essential = (10)   Critical = (15)
Automatic failure results if any of the critical steps are omitted or performed incorrectly.

DETERMINE SCORE (divide points earned by total points possible, multiply results by 100)   _____ SCORE*

Evaluator's Name (print) _____ Signature _____

Comments _____

DOCUMENTATION

Chart the procedure in the patient's medical record.

Date: _____

Charting: _____

_____

_____

_____

Student's Initials: _____

Name _____

Date _____ Score* _____

PROCEDURE 15–12   Obtain Venous Blood with Vacuum Tube

TERMINAL PERFORMANCE OBJECTIVE - Demonstrate the steps necessary for obtaining venous blood using the vacuum tube method.

PROCEDURE STEPS	STEP PERFORMED	POINTS POSSIBLE	COMMENTS
EVALUATOR: Place check mark in space following each step performed satisfactorily			
NOTE TIME BEGAN _____			
1. Identified patient.	_____	10	
2. Washed hands.	_____	5	
3. Assembled necessary items near patient.	_____	5	
4. Completed lab request form.	_____	5	
a. Labeled specimen tube(s)	_____	5	
5. Explained procedure to patient.	_____	5	
a. Asked patient for preferred venipuncture site	_____	5	
6. Positioned patient appropriately.	_____	5	
7. Put on gloves.	_____	5	
8. Secured needle into adapter.	_____	10	
9. Applied tourniquet to patient's upper arm.	_____	5	
a. Placed 3″ above elbow	_____	10	
10. Cleansed site lightly with alcohol/cottonball.	_____	5	
a. Allowed alcohol to air dry/dried with cottonball	_____	5	
11. Asked patient to clench fist to make vein stand up.	_____	5	
12. Took needle guard off.	_____	5	
a. Pointed bevel of needle up	_____	10	
b. Inserted needle tip into vein with quick and steady motion	_____	10	
c. Inserted needle into vein at 15° angle	_____	10	
d. Held skin taut for easier insertion	_____	5	
e. Inserted needle between ¼″ and ½″	_____	15	
13. Held adapter with one hand.	_____	5	
a. Placed index and great fingers of other hand on either side of protruding edges of adapter	_____	5	
b. Pushed vacuum tube completely into adapter with thumb	_____	10	
c. Allowed needle to puncture rubber stopper	_____	15	
d. Asked patient to release clenched fist slowly	_____	5	
e. Released tourniquet within one minute	_____	10	
f. Pulled filled tube out by holding it between			

PROCEDURE STEPS	STEP PERFORMED	POINTS POSSIBLE	COMMENTS
thumb and great finger and pushed against adapter with index finger	_____	5	
g. Filled required number of tubes in correct order	_____	10	
h. Pulled needle out in same path as inserted	_____	5	
i. Placed cottonball/gauze square over site	_____	5	
14. Instructed patient to apply gentle pressure to site and elevate arm slightly.	_____	5	
15. Stood red-stoppered tubes vertically.	_____	5	
a. Did not shake tubes/mixed additives carefully	_____	5	
b. Made blood smear if ordered	_____	5	
16. Deposited needle/syringe in sharps container.	_____	5	
17. Assembled specimen tubes/lab form together in biobag.	_____	5	
18. Attended to patient's needs.	_____	5	
a. Applied bandage	_____	5	
19. Discarded disposables in proper containers.	_____	5	
20. Removed gloves/placed in biobag.	_____	5	
a. Washed hands	_____	5	
21. Returned items to proper storage.	_____	5	
22. Recorded procedure in patient's chart.	_____	5	
a. Initialed	_____	5	

EVALUATOR: NOTE TIME COMPLETED _____

ADD POINTS OF STEPS CHECKED   _____ EARNED
TOTAL POINTS POSSIBLE   290 POSSIBLE

Points assigned reflect importance of step to meeting objective: Important = (5)   Essential = (10)   Critical = (15)
Automatic failure results if any of the critical steps are omitted or performed incorrectly.

DETERMINE SCORE (divide points earned by total points possible, multiply results by 100)   _____ SCORE*

Evaluator's Name (print) _____ Signature _____

Comments _____

DOCUMENTATION

Chart the procedure in the patient's medical record.

Date: _____

Charting: _____

_____

_____

_____

Student's Initials: _____

Name _____

Date _____ Score* _____

PROCEDURE 15–13   Complete an ESR Using the Wintrobe Method

TERMINAL PERFORMANCE OBJECTIVE - Demonstrate all required steps to complete the procedure for an ESR using the Wintrobe method.

PROCEDURE STEPS	STEP PERFORMED	POINTS POSSIBLE	COMMENTS
EVALUATOR: Place check mark in space following each step performed satisfactorily			
NOTE TIME BEGAN _____			
1. Assembled all needed items.	_____	10	
2. Washed hands.	_____	5	
a. Put on gloves	_____	5	
3. Fitted rubber bulb onto large end of glass pipette.	_____	5	
4. Depressed bulb and placed tip of pipette into bottom of specimen tube.	_____	10	
5. Filled pipette with blood by letting up slowly on depressed bulb.	_____	10	
6. Placed tip of filled pipette into Wintrobe tube without touching sides of tube.	_____	10	
7. Pressed bulb and filled Wintrobe tube.	_____	10	
a. Kept tip below meniscus while filling tube to precisely the zero line on tube	_____	15	
8. Set tube into leveled stand.	_____	5	
9. Wrote down slot number.	_____	5	
10. Set timer immediately for one hour.	_____	10	
a. Wrote down exact time	_____	10	
11. Discard disposables.	_____	5	
12. Removed gloves.	_____	5	
a. Washed hands			
13. Returned items to proper storage.	_____	5	
14. Read Wintrobe tube after exactly one hour.	_____	15	
a. Read at meniscus	_____	15	
15. Recorded reading on patient's chart.	_____	5	
a. Initialed	_____	5	

EVALUATOR: NOTE TIME COMPLETED _____

ADD POINTS OF STEPS CHECKED   _____ EARNED

TOTAL POINTS POSSIBLE   170 POSSIBLE

Points assigned reflect importance of step to meeting objective: Important = (5)   Essential = (10)   Critical = (15)

Automatic failure results if any of the critical steps are omitted or performed incorrectly.

DETERMINE SCORE (divide points earned by total points possible, multiply results by 100)   _____ SCORE*

Evaluator's Name (print) _____ Signature _____

Comments _____

DOCUMENTATION

Chart the procedure in the patient's medical record.

Date: _____

Charting: _____

_____

_____

_____

Student's Initials: _____

Name _____

Date _____ Score* _____

PROCEDURE 15–14   Catheterize Urinary Bladder

TERMINAL PERFORMANCE OBJECTIVE - Demonstrate all required steps to perform a urinary bladder catheterization.

PROCEDURE STEPS	STEP PERFORMED	POINTS POSSIBLE	COMMENTS
EVALUATOR: Place check mark in space following each step performed satisfactorily			
NOTE TIME BEGAN _____			
1. Identify patient.	_____	5	
2. Placed catheter kit on Mayo table next to patient.	_____	5	
3. Explained procedure to patient.	_____	5	
4. a. Adjusted lamp	_____	5	
b. Turned lamp on	_____	5	
5. Asked patient to lie back on table.	_____	5	
a. Assisted patient into dorsal recumbent position	_____	10	
b. Assisted patient in positioning her feet in stirrups	_____	10	
6. Draped patient with sheet.	_____	5	
a. Exposed only external genitalia	_____	5	
7. Pulled out foot rest.	_____	5	
8. Opened outer wrapping of sterile kit.	_____	5	
9. Placed sterile towel between patient's knees.	_____	5	
10. Placed sterile plastic sheet under patient's buttocks.	_____	5	
11. Placed catheter kit on foot rest.	_____	5	
12. Asked patient to keep knees apart.	_____	5	
13. Washed and dried hands.	_____	5	
14. Put on sterile latex gloves.	_____	5	
15. Poured antiseptic solution over cotton balls in medicine cups.	_____	10	
16. Opened urine specimen container.	_____	5	
17. Applied sterile lubricant to one of the gauze squares.	_____	5	
18. Spread labia and wiped genitalia with each of the three antiseptic soaked cotton balls.	_____	10	
a. Used front to back motion	_____	10	
b. Discarded onto Mayo table	_____	5	
19. Placed tip of catheter in lubricant and other end of catheter into basin.	_____	5	
20. Held catheter about four inches from lubricated end.	_____	5	
21. Inserted lubricated tip of catheter into urinary meatus gently.	_____	15	
22. Instructed patient to breathe slowly and deeply.	_____	5	
23. Stopped urine flow by closing metal clamps attached to tubing.	_____	10	
24. Positioned end of tube into urine specimen container.	_____	10	

PROCEDURE 15–14 Catheterize Urinary Bladder—continued

PROCEDURE STEPS	STEP PERFORMED	POINTS POSSIBLE	COMMENTS
25. Released clamp to collect specimen.	_____	10	
26. Allowed remainder of urine flow to collect in basin.	_____	5	
a. Measured amount of urine—both specimen and basin	_____	15	
27. Withdrew catheter tube gently.	_____	5	
28. Dried area with sterile gauze squares or cotton balls.	_____	5	
29. Secured lid onto urine specimen container.	_____	5	
30. Placed reusable items in cold water to soak.	_____	5	
31. Removed items from foot rest.	_____	5	
32. Cleaned exam table.	_____	5	
33. Discarded gloves and other disposables.	_____	5	
34. Washed hands.	_____	5	
35. Turned lamp off and returned to usual position.	_____	5	
36. Assisted patient in sitting up or relaxing in a horizontal recumbent position.	_____	5	
37. Labeled specimen (completed request form and attached).	_____	5	
38. Assisted patient from exam table.	_____	5	
39. Recorded procedure and measured amount of urine.	_____	5	
a. Observations and comments	_____	5	
b. Initialed	_____	5	

EVALUATOR: NOTE TIME COMPLETED _____

ADD POINTS OF STEPS CHECKED   _____ EARNED

TOTAL POINTS POSSIBLE   300 POSSIBLE

Points assigned reflect importance of step to meeting objective: Important = (5)   Essential = (10)   Critical = (15)
Automatic failure results if any of the critical steps are omitted or performed incorrectly.

DETERMINE SCORE (divide points earned by total points possible, multiply results by 100)   _____ SCORE*

Evaluator's Name (print) _____ Signature _____

Comments _____

DOCUMENTATION

Chart the procedure in the patient's medical record.

Date: _____

Charting: _____

_____

_____

_____

Student's Initials: _____

Name _____

Date _____ Score* _____

PROCEDURE 15–15   Test Urine with Multistix® 10 SG.

TERMINAL PERFORMANCE OBJECTIVE - Demonstrate the steps required to perform the procedure for using Multistix® 10 SG.

PROCEDURE STEPS	STEP PERFORMED	POINTS POSSIBLE	COMMENTS
EVALUATOR: Place check mark in space following each step performed satisfactorily			
NOTE TIME BEGAN _____			
1. Washed hands.	_____	5	
a. Put on gloves	_____	5	
2. Assembled all needed items.	_____	5	
3. Stirred urine with tongue depressor.	_____	10	
4. Removed cap from bottle.	_____	5	
5. Took reagent strip out without touching test paper end.	_____	5	
6. Placed cap back on bottle securely.	_____	5	
7. Reviewed times given for reading each test on bottle.	_____	5	
8. Dipped test paper end of reagent strip into urine specimen.	_____	5	
9. Removed strip by touching its edge against inside of container to remove excess urine.	_____	5	
10. Began timing test immediately.	_____	15	
11. Placed reagent strip next to color chart.	_____	10	
12. Read each test section at proper time.	_____	15	
13. Discarded disposables in proper receptacle.	_____	5	
14. Returned items to proper storage.	_____	5	
15. Removed gloves.	_____	5	
a. Washed hands	_____	5	
16. Recorded results of each test section on patient's chart.	_____	15	

EVALUATOR: NOTE TIME COMPLETED _____

ADD POINTS OF STEPS CHECKED   _____ EARNED
TOTAL POINTS POSSIBLE   130 POSSIBLE

Points assigned reflect importance of step to meeting objective: Important = (5)   Essential = (10)   Critical = (15)
Automatic failure results if any of the critical steps are omitted or performed incorrectly.

DETERMINE SCORE (divide points earned by total points possible, multiply results by 100)   _____ SCORE*

Evaluator's Name (print) _____   Signature _____

Comments _____

DOCUMENTATION

Chart the procedure in the patient's medical record.

Date: _____

Charting: _____

_____

_____

_____

Student's Initials: _____

Name _____

Date _____ Score* _____

PROCEDURE 15–16 Determine Glucose Content of Urine with Clinitest Tablet

TERMINAL PERFORMANCE OBJECTIVE - Demonstrate the steps in the procedure for using Clinitest tablets to determine the glucose content of urine.

PROCEDURE STEPS	STEP PERFORMED	POINTS POSSIBLE	COMMENTS
EVALUATOR: Place check mark in space following each step performed satisfactorily			
NOTE TIME BEGAN _____			
1. Washed hands.	_____	5	
a. Put on gloves	_____	5	
2. Assembled needed items.	_____	5	
3. Stirred urine with tongue depressor.	_____	5	
4. Filled dropper halfway with urine.	_____	5	
5. Held test tube near top between thumb and index finger.	_____	5	
6. Released five drops of urine into test tube.	_____	10	
7. Rinsed dropper.	_____	5	
8. Half filled dropper with water.	_____	10	
9. Released ten drops water into test tube.	_____	10	
10. Mixed gently.	_____	5	
11. Set test tube in rack.	_____	5	
12. Opened bottle.	_____	5	
13. Shook out one Clinitest tablet into bottle cap.	_____	10	
14. Dropped one tablet into test tube from cap.	_____	10	
15. Recapped bottle.	_____	5	
16. Watched reaction of tablet and urine-water mixture.	_____	15	
17. Began 15 second timing immediately when boiling stopped.	_____	15	
18. Held test tube at top.	_____	10	
19. Tilted test tube back and forth to mix contents.	_____	10	
20. Compared color of contents to color chart to read results.	_____	15	
21. Recorded results as % of milligrams/deciliter on patient's chart.	_____	15	
a. Initialed	_____	5	
22. Rinsed test tube with cold water.	_____	5	
23. Washed and dried test tube and dropper.	_____	5	

PROCEDURE 15–16   Determine Glucose Content of Urine with Clinitest Tablet—continued

PROCEDURE STEPS	STEP PERFORMED	POINTS POSSIBLE	COMMENTS
24. Discarded disposables in proper receptacle.	_____	5	
25. Removed gloves.	_____	5	
a. Washed hands	_____	5	
26. Returned items to proper storage.	_____	5	

EVALUATOR: NOTE TIME COMPLETED _____

ADD POINTS OF STEPS CHECKED

TOTAL POINTS POSSIBLE

_____ EARNED

220 POSSIBLE

Points assigned reflect importance of step to meeting objective: Important = (5)   Essential = (10)   Critical = (15)
Automatic failure results if any of the critical steps are omitted or performed incorrectly.

DETERMINE SCORE (divide points earned by total points possible, multiply results by 100)   _____ SCORE*

Evaluator's Name (print) _____ Signature _____

Comments _____

DOCUMENTATION

Chart the procedure in the patient's medical record.

Date: _____

Charting: _____

_____

_____

_____

Student's Initials: _____

Name _____

Date _____ Score* _____

PROCEDURE 15–17   Obtain Urine Sediment for Microscopic Examination

TERMINAL PERFORMANCE OBJECTIVE - Demonstrate all steps required in the procedure for obtaining urine sediment for microscopic examination.

PROCEDURE STEPS	STEP PERFORMED	POINTS POSSIBLE	COMMENTS
EVALUATOR: Place check mark in space following each step performed satisfactorily			
NOTE TIME BEGAN _____			
1. Washed hands.	_____	5	
a. Put on gloves	_____	5	
2. Assembled needed items.	_____	5	
3. Stirred urine with tongue depressor.	_____	10	
4. Poured equal amounts (100c) of urine into two tubes.	_____	5	
5. Placed test tubes on opposite sides of centrifuge.	_____	5	
6. Turned timer past time desired and then back to set time (3 minutes).	_____	5	
7. Removed test tube after centrifuge had come to a complete stop.	_____	5	
8. Poured off supernatant.	_____	10	
9. Tapped bottom of test tube gently against counter or palm of hand to mix sediment.	_____	10	
10. Obtained sediment with pipette from test tube.	_____	15	
11. Placed sediment in center of slide with frosted end.	_____	15	
12. Placed cover glass over sediment on slide.	_____	5	
13. Allowed sediment to settle.	_____	5	
14. Placed slide on stage of microscope.	_____	5	
15. Viewed slide under low power objective to scan.	_____	5	
a. Used dim light	_____	5	
16. Changed objective to high power.	_____	15	
17. Viewed at least ten fields.	_____	10	
18. Turned light off.	_____	5	
19. Recorded microscopic observations.	_____	15	
a. Initialed	_____	5	
20. Rinsed, washed and dried glass items.	_____	5	
21. Discarded disposables in proper receptacle.	_____	5	

PROCEDURE STEPS	STEP PERFORMED	POINTS POSSIBLE	COMMENTS
22. Removed gloves.	_____	5	
a. Washed hands	_____	5	
23. Returned items to proper storage.	_____	5	
EVALUATOR: NOTE TIME COMPLETED _____			

ADD POINTS OF STEPS CHECKED   _____ EARNED

TOTAL POINTS POSSIBLE   195 POSSIBLE

Points assigned reflect importance of step to meeting objective: Important = (5)   Essential = (10)   Critical = (15)
Automatic failure results if any of the critical steps are omitted or performed incorrectly.

DETERMINE SCORE (divide points earned by total points possible, multiply results by 100)   _____ SCORE*

Evaluator's Name (print) _____ Signature _____

Comments _____

DOCUMENTATION

Chart the procedure in the patient's medical record.

Date: _____

Charting: _____

_____

_____

_____

Student's Initials: _____

Name _____

Date _____ Score* _____

PROCEDURE 15–18   Instruct Patient to Collect Sputum Specimen

---

TERMINAL PERFORMANCE OBJECTIVE - Demonstrate all steps required in the procedure for instructing a patient in the collection of a sputum specimen for analysis.

PROCEDURE STEPS	STEP PERFORMED	POINTS POSSIBLE	COMMENTS
EVALUATOR: Place check mark in space following each step performed satisfactorily			
NOTE TIME BEGAN _____			
1. Assembled items next to patient.	_____	10	
2. Wrote patient's name on specimen cup label.	_____	10	
3. Completed lab request form.	_____	5	
4. Explained physician's orders to patient.	_____	10	
a. Wrote instructions out/gave printed instructions to patient	_____	15	
5. Instructed patient to:			
a. Expel only those secretions of first AM coughing episode into center of cup	_____	15	
b. Fill cup one-half full	_____	10	
c. Seal with cover	_____	5	
d. Write time and date on label and request form	_____	10	
e. Take to lab/medical office as soon as possible	_____	10	
f. Secure lab request form to specimen container with tape or rubber band	_____	5	
g. Refrigerate if she/he cannot take within two hours	_____	10	
6. Record what instructions were given to patient.	_____	5	
a. Initialed	_____	5	
EVALUATOR: NOTE TIME COMPLETED _____			

ADD POINTS OF STEPS CHECKED   _____ EARNED

TOTAL POINTS POSSIBLE   125 POSSIBLE

Points assigned reflect importance of step to meeting objective: Important = (5) Essential = (10) Critical = (15)
Automatic failure results if any of the critical steps are omitted or performed incorrectly.

DETERMINE SCORE (divide points earned by total points possible, multiply results by 100)   _____ SCORE*

Evaluator's Name (print) _____ Signature _____

Comments _____

DOCUMENTATION

Chart the procedure in the patient's medical record.

Date: _____

Charting: _____ __

_____

_____

_____

Student's Initials: _____

Name _____

Date _____ Score* _____

PROCEDURE 15–19   Instruct Patient to Collect a Stool Specimen

TERMINAL PERFORMANCE OBJECTIVE - Demonstrate the steps required in the procedure for instructing a patient in the collection of an adequate stool specimen for laboratory analysis.

PROCEDURE STEPS	STEP PERFORMED	POINTS POSSIBLE	COMMENTS
EVALUATOR: Place check mark in space following each step performed satisfactorily			
NOTE TIME BEGAN _____			
1. Assembled items next to patient.	_____	10	
2. Identified patient.	_____	10	
3. Explained physician's orders.	_____	10	
4. Gave printed instructions or wrote out.	_____	10	
5. Wrote information on label of specimen cups and lab request form.	_____	5	
6. Instructed patient to:			
a. Obtain small amount of stool from next bowel movement with tongue depressor	_____	15	
b. Place specimen in container	_____	10	
c. Secure cup with cover	_____	5	
d. Write date and time of specimen on label	_____	5	
e. Write time and date on request form and attach request form to specimen container	_____	5	
f. Take to lab/medical office as soon as possible	_____	10	
g. Refrigerate specimen if she/he cannot take within two hours	_____	10	
7. Explained when report would be available.	_____	5	
8. Recorded that instructions were given on patient's chart.	_____	15	
a. Initialed	_____	5	

EVALUATOR: NOTE TIME COMPLETED _____

ADD POINTS OF STEPS CHECKED   _____ EARNED

TOTAL POINTS POSSIBLE   130 POSSIBLE

Points assigned reflect importance of step to meeting objective: Important = (5)   Essential = (10)   Critical = (15)

Automatic failure results if any of the critical steps are omitted or performed incorrectly.

DETERMINE SCORE (divide points earned by total points possible, multiply results by 100)   _____ SCORE*

Evaluator's Name (print) _____ Signature _____

Comments _____

DOCUMENTATION

Chart the procedure in the patient's medical record.

Date: _____

Charting: _____

_____

_____

_____

Student's Initials: _____

Name _____

Date _____ Score* _____

PROCEDURE 15–20   Perform a Hemoccult® Sensa® Test

TERMINAL PERFORMANCE OBJECTIVE - Demonstrate each step required in the Hemoccult® Sensa® testing procedure.

PROCEDURE STEPS	STEP PERFORMED	POINTS POSSIBLE	COMMENTS
EVALUATOR: Place check mark in space following each step performed satisfactorily			
NOTE TIME BEGAN _____			
1. Washed hands.	_____	5	
2. Put on gloves.	_____	5	
3. Assembled items needed for testing on counter.	_____	10	
4. Opened test slide of Hemoccult paper slide.	_____	10	
5. Removed cap from bottle of developer.	_____	5	
6. Placed 2 drops of developer on each of three sections:			
a. A	_____	15	
b. B	_____	15	
c. Control	_____	15	
7. Began timing immediately for 60 seconds.	_____	15	
8. Watched closely for any change of color at 30 seconds.	_____	5	
9. Compared test with control and read results after 60-second time period.	_____	15	
10. Recorded results on patient's chart.	_____	15	
a. Initialed	_____	5	
11. Discarded disposables.	_____	5	
12. Returned items to proper storage.	_____	5	
13. Removed gloves.	_____	5	
a. Washed hands	_____	5	
EVALUATOR: NOTE TIME COMPLETED _____			

ADD POINTS OF STEPS CHECKED   _____ EARNED

TOTAL POINTS POSSIBLE   155 POSSIBLE

Points assigned reflect importance of step to meeting objective: Important = (5)   Essential = (10)   Critical = (15)
Automatic failure results if any of the critical steps are omitted or performed incorrectly.

DETERMINE SCORE (divide points earned by total points possible, multiply results by 100)   _____ SCORE*

Evaluator's Name (print) _____ Signature _____

Comments _____

DOCUMENTATION

Chart the procedure in the patient's medical record.

Date: _____

Charting: _____

_____

_____

_____ _____

Student's Initials: _____ _____

Name _____

Date _____ Score* _____

PROCEDURE 15–21   Prepare Bacteriological Smear

TERMINAL PERFORMANCE OBJECTIVE - Demonstrate the steps of the procedure for preparing a bacteriological smear for microscopic analysis.

PROCEDURE STEPS	STEP PERFORMED	POINTS POSSIBLE	COMMENTS
EVALUATOR: Place check mark in space following each step performed satisfactorily			
NOTE TIME BEGAN _____			
1. Assembled all needed items.	_____	10	
2. Penciled patient's name on frosted end of glass slide.	_____	10	
3. Completed lab request form.	_____	5	
4. Washed hands.	_____	5	
a. Put on gloves	_____	5	
5. Prepared smear(s):	_____	5	
a. Held slide with thumb and great finger	_____	5	
b. Rolled swab containing specimen evenly over two-thirds of slide	_____	15	
6. Lit bunsen burner.	_____	5	
a. Adjusted flame	_____	5	
7. Held frosted part of slide with forceps or thumb and index finger.	_____	5	
8. Passed smear (side up) of slide through blue flame two or three times.	_____	15	
9. Turned burner off.	_____	5	
10. Placed heat-fixed smear on staining rack or Placed on stage of microscope for observation.	_____	10	
11. Discarded used disposables in proper receptacle.	_____	5	
12. Returned items to proper storage.	_____	5	
13. Removed gloves.	_____	5	
a. Washed hands	_____	5	
14. Recorded procedure on patient's chart	_____	5	
a. Initialed	_____	5	
EVALUATOR: NOTE TIME COMPLETED _____			

ADD POINTS OF STEPS CHECKED

TOTAL POINTS POSSIBLE

_____ EARNED

135 POSSIBLE

Points assigned reflect importance of step to meeting objective: Important = (5)   Essential = (10)   Critical = (15)
Automatic failure results if any of the critical steps are omitted or performed incorrectly.

DETERMINE SCORE (divide points earned by total points possible, multiply results by 100)   _____ SCORE*

Evaluator's Name (print) _____ Signature _____

Comments _____

DOCUMENTATION

Chart the procedure in the patient's medical record.

Date: _____

Charting: _____

_____

_____

_____

Student's Initials: _____

Name _____

Date _____ Score* _____

PROCEDURE 15–22   Obtain a Throat Culture

TERMINAL PERFORMANCE OBJECTIVE - Demonstrate the steps required to perform the procedure for obtaining a throat culture.

PROCEDURE STEPS	STEP PERFORMED	POINTS POSSIBLE	COMMENTS
EVALUATOR: Place check mark in space following each step performed satisfactorily			
NOTE TIME BEGAN _____			
1. Identified patient.	_____	5	
2. Washed hands.	_____	10	
a. Put on gloves	_____	5	
b. Assembled needed items near patient	_____	5	
3. Labeled culture plate.	_____	5	
a. Completed lab request form if required	_____	10	
4. Explained procedure to patient.	_____	5	
5. Assisted patient into comfortable position.	_____	5	
a. Asked for assistance if child.	_____	5	
6. Opened sterile swab.	_____	5	
7. Asked patient to open mouth wide.	_____	5	
8. Examined patient's throat visually with light.	_____	10	
9. Depressed tongue with sterile tongue depressor.	_____	15	
10. Asked patient to say "ahh."	_____	15	
11. Inserted sterile swab to back of throat.	_____	5	
12. Rolled swab over area to obtain specimen.	_____	15	
13. Removed swab and depressor from patient's mouth.	_____	10	
14. Attended to patient; offered tissue.	_____	10	
15. Applied specimen to agar of petri dish in pattern.	_____	15	
16. Placed lid on dish.	_____	5	
a. Secured with tape	_____	5	
17. Discarded disposables in proper receptacle.	_____	5	
18. Placed culture dish in incubator bottom up or Attached request form and sent to lab.	_____	5	
19. Removed gloves.	_____	5	
a. Washed hands	_____	5	

PROCEDURE STEPS	STEP PERFORMED	POINTS POSSIBLE	COMMENTS
20. Recorded procedure in patient's chart.	_____	5	
a. Initialed	_____	5	

EVALUATOR: NOTE TIME COMPLETED _____

ADD POINTS OF STEPS CHECKED   _____ EARNED
TOTAL POINTS POSSIBLE   200 POSSIBLE

Points assigned reflect importance of step to meeting objective: Important = (5)   Essential = (10)   Critical = (15)
Automatic failure results if any of the critical steps are omitted or performed incorrectly.

DETERMINE SCORE (divide points earned by total points possible, multiply results by 100)   _____ SCORE*

Evaluator's Name (print) _____ Signature _____

Comments _____

DOCUMENTATION

Chart the procedure in the patient's medical record.

Date: _____

Charting: _____

_____

_____

_____

Student's Initials: _____

PROCEDURE 15–23   Prepare Gram Stain

TERMINAL PERFORMANCE OBJECTIVE - Demonstrate the steps of the procedure for preparing a Gram stain.

PROCEDURE STEPS	STEP PERFORMED	POINTS POSSIBLE	COMMENTS
EVALUATOR: Place check mark in space following each step performed satisfactorily			
NOTE TIME BEGAN _____			
1. Assembled all needed items on counter.	_____	10	
2. Washed hands.	_____	5	
a. Put apron/gloves on	_____	5	
3. Placed heat-fixed slide on staining rack.	_____	5	
4. Opened crystal violet dye.	_____	5	
5. Filled dropper.	_____	5	
6. Applied over entire specimen area of slide.	_____	10	
7. Timed for sixty seconds.	_____	10	
8. Held frosted end with forceps.	_____	5	
9. Tipped slide to allow stain to run off into tray.	_____	5	
10. Washed slide with water from top to bottom.	_____	10	
11. Placed slide flat on rack.	_____	5	
12. Filled dropper with Gram's iodine.	_____	10	
13. Applied over entire specimen area.	_____	10	
14. Tipped slide to allow stain to run off.	_____	5	
15. Refilled dropper with Gram's iodine.	_____	10	
16. Applied to entire specimen area.	_____	10	
a. Timed for sixty seconds	_____	5	
17. Tipped slide to allow stain to run off.	_____	5	
18. Washed slide with water.	_____	10	
19. Applied alcohol/acetone with dropper until purple color in excess runoff was gone.	_____	15	
20. Washed with water immediately.	_____	10	
21. Applied Safranin solution with dropper.	_____	10	
22. Immediately washed with water.	_____	10	
23. Held slide by frosted end.	_____	5	
24. Wiped excess solution from underneath.	_____	5	

PROCEDURE STEPS	STEP PERFORMED	POINTS POSSIBLE	COMMENTS
25. Held slide on its side and tapped onto paper towel to remove excess.	_____	5	
26. Allowed slide to air dry or Blotted slide carefully between two paper towels.	_____	5	
27. Applied small drop of immersion oil to specimen.	_____	5	
a. Placed cover glass on slide	_____	5	
28. Placed slide on stage of microscope to view.	_____	5	
a. Turned light source on to view	_____	5	
29. Discarded disposables in proper receptacle.	_____	5	
30. Washed used items.	_____	5	
31. Returned items to proper storage.	_____	5	
a. Replaced caps on bottles immediately after use	_____	5	
32. Removed gloves.	_____	5	
a. Washed hands	_____	5	
33. Recorded procedure and results on patient's chart.	_____	5	
a. Initialed	_____	15	

EVALUATOR: NOTE TIME COMPLETED _____

ADD POINTS OF STEPS CHECKED   _____ EARNED

TOTAL POINTS POSSIBLE   280 POSSIBLE

Points assigned reflect importance of step to meeting objective: Important = (5)   Essential = (10)   Critical = (15)
Automatic failure results if any of the critical steps are omitted or performed incorrectly.

DETERMINE SCORE (divide points earned by total points possible, multiply results by 100)   _____ SCORE*

Evaluator's Name (print) _____ Signature _____

Comments _____

DOCUMENTATION

Chart the procedure in the patient's medical record.

Date: _____

Charting: _____

_____

_____

_____

Student's Initials: _____

Name _____

Date _____ Score* _____

PROCEDURE 16–1   Perform a Scratch Test

TERMINAL PERFORMANCE OBJECTIVE - Demonstrate each of the steps required in the scratch test procedure.

PROCEDURE STEPS	STEP PERFORMED	POINTS POSSIBLE	COMMENTS
EVALUATOR: Place check mark in space following each step performed satisfactorily			
NOTE TIME BEGAN _____			
1. Identified patient.	_____	10	
2. Assembled all needed items next to patient.	_____	10	
3. Washed hands.	_____	5	
4. Put on gloves.	_____	5	
5. Explained procedure to patient.	_____	5	
6. Assisted patient into comfortable position.	_____	5	
7. Prepared test site with alcohol pad.	_____	5	
a. Allowed to air dry	_____	5	
8. Marked site(s) with initials or number of extract in pen.	_____	10	
a. Spaced adequately (about 1½″ to 2″ between each)	_____	10	
9. Applied small drop of extract onto site.	_____	10	
a. Repeated for each extract ordered	_____	10	
10. Removed sterile needle or lancet without contaminating it.	_____	15	
a. Made one-eighth inch scratch in surface of skin at site.	_____	15	
11. Began timing for 20 minutes.	_____	15	
12. Checked each site as soon as 20-minute period was up.	_____	15	
a. Cleaned each site with alcohol pad	_____	10	
b. Did not wash off extract identification	_____	15	
13. Washed hands.	_____	5	
14. Compared reaction sites with package insert drawing or measured reaction sites in centimeters.	_____	15	
15. Recorded test results on patient's chart.	_____	15	
a. Initialed	_____	5	
b. Attended to patient	_____	5	
16. Discarded disposables in proper receptacle.	_____	5	

PROCEDURE STEPS	STEP PERFORMED	POINTS POSSIBLE	COMMENTS
17. Returned items to proper storage area.	_____	5	
18. Removed gloves.	_____	5	
a. Washed hands	_____	5	

EVALUATOR: NOTE TIME COMPLETED _____

ADD POINTS OF STEPS CHECKED   _____ EARNED

TOTAL POINTS POSSIBLE   240 POSSIBLE

Points assigned reflect importance of step to meeting objective: Important = (5)   Essential = (10)   Critical = (15)
Automatic failure results if any of the critical steps are omitted or performed incorrectly.

DETERMINE SCORE (divide points earned by total points possible, multiply results by 100)   _____ SCORE*

Evaluator's Name (print) _____ Signature _____

Comments _____ _____

DOCUMENTATION

Chart the procedure in the patient's medical record.

Date: _____

Charting: _____

_____

_____

_____

Student's Initials: _____

PROCEDURE 16–2   Apply a Patch Test

TERMINAL PERFORMANCE OBJECTIVE - Demonstrate each of the steps required in carrying out the skin patch test, including the forty-eight hour recheck.

PROCEDURE STEPS	STEP PERFORMED	POINTS POSSIBLE	COMMENTS
EVALUATOR: Place check mark in space following each step performed satisfactorily			
NOTE TIME BEGAN _____			
1. Identified patient.	_____	10	
2. Assembled items next to patient.	_____	10	
3. Washed hands.	_____	5	
4. Put on gloves.	_____	5	
5. Explained procedure to patient.	_____	5	
6. Assisted patient into comfortable sitting position.	_____	5	
7. Cleaned test site with alcohol pad.	_____	5	
a. Allowed to air dry	_____	5	
8. Applied substance to test site.	_____	10	
9. Secured substance to test site with non-allergic tape.	_____	15	
10. Recorded date, time, substance, and area tested on patient's chart.	_____	15	
a. Initialed	_____	5	
11. Scheduled patient to return in 48 hours for check.	_____	5	
12. Instructed patient to keep test area clean and dry.	_____	10	
13. Removed gloves.	_____	5	
a. Washed hands	_____	5	
When patient returned after 48 hours:			
14. Washed hands.	_____	5	
a. Put on gloves	_____	5	
15. Removed patch.	_____	5	
16. Read results of test.	_____	15	
17. Removed gloves.	_____	5	
a. Washed hands	_____	5	

PROCEDURE STEPS	STEP PERFORMED	POINTS POSSIBLE	COMMENTS
Recorded results on patient's chart.	_____	5	
a. Initialed	_____	5	
EVALUATOR: NOTE TIME COMPLETED _____			

ADD POINTS OF STEPS CHECKED   _____ EARNED

TOTAL POINTS POSSIBLE   170 POSSIBLE

Points assigned reflect importance of step to meeting objective: Important = (5)   Essential = (10)   Critical = (15)
Automatic failure results if any of the critical steps are omitted or performed incorrectly.

DETERMINE SCORE (divide points earned by total points possible, multiply results by 100)   _____ SCORE*

Evaluator's Name (print) _____ Signature _____

Comments _____

DOCUMENTATION

Chart the procedure in the patient's medical record.

Date: _____

Charting: _____

_____

_____

_____

Student's Initials: _____

Name _____

Date _____ Score* _____

PROCEDURE 16–3   Obtain a Standard 12-Lead Electrocardiogram

TERMINAL PERFORMANCE OBJECTIVE - Demonstrate each of the steps required in obtaining a standard 12-lead ECG reading.

PROCEDURE STEPS	STEP PERFORMED	POINTS POSSIBLE	COMMENTS
EVALUATOR: Place check mark in space following each step performed satisfactorily			
NOTE TIME BEGAN _____			
1. Identified patient.	_____	5	
2. Plugged in ECG machine to electrical outlet, away from known electrical interference.	_____	5	
3. Assembled electrodes.	_____	5	
a. Attached to straps	_____	5	
b. Applied electrolyte pads	_____	5	
4. Turned machine on.	_____	5	
5. Washed hands.	_____	5	
6. Asked patient to disrobe from waist up and remove clothing from lower legs.	_____	5	
7. Explained procedure to patient.	_____	5	
8. Assisted patient to table.	_____	5	
a. Asked patient to lie down.	_____	5	
b. Covered patient with drape sheet.	_____	5	
c. Pulled out foot rest.	_____	5	
d. Adjusted pillow under patient's head.	_____	5	
Note: For computerized electrocardiographs:			
a. Applied limb and chest lead wires by clipping to disposable electrodes.	_____	15	
b. Pressed "auto" to run complete 12-lead recording.	_____	10	
c. Removed patient cable and proceeded with step 28.	_____	5	
9. Placed chest strap with hard plastic end under left side of patient's back.	_____	5	
a. Weighed end at patient's right side.	_____	5	
10. Placed upper limb electrodes on outer fleshy area of upper arms.	_____	10	
a. Pointed connectors of electrodes toward shoulders.	_____	5	
b. Moved straps one space tighter than relaxed.	_____	5	
11. Placed lower limb electrodes on inner fleshy area of lower legs.	_____	5	
a. Pointed connectors toward upper part of body	_____	5	

PROCEDURE STEPS	STEP PERFORMED	POINTS POSSIBLE	COMMENTS
12. Connected lead wire tips to electrodes, all pointing downward.	_____	5	
13. Placed power cord directed away from patient.	_____	5	
14. Placed chest electrode under chest strap.	_____	5	
a. Placed electrolyte side up	_____	5	
15. Turned lead selector switch to STD.	_____	5	
a. Adjusted stylus to center of graph paper.	_____	5	
16. Moved record switch to 25 mm/second position.	_____	10	
a. Ran for a few seconds to adjust centering	_____	5	
b. Made standardization mark correctly	_____	5	
c. Turned off	_____	5	
17. Turned lead selector switch to Lead I.	_____	15	
a. Ran 8″–12″ of tracing.	_____	15	
b. Proceeded to run 8″–12″ of Leads II and III.	_____	15	
18. Ran 4″–6″ of leads aVR, aVL and aVF.	_____	15	
19. Paused between leads to allow machine to adjust automatically.	_____	5	
20. Made standardization mark at the beginning of each lead.	_____	5	
21. Marked each lead appropriately with correct code marking.	_____	15	
22. Placed chest electrode in proper positions, V1–V6.	_____	15	
a. Standardized each lead	_____	5	
b. Ran 4″–6″ of each	_____	5	
c. Marked each lead correctly	_____	15	
d. Turned switch to AMP off when changing electrode position	_____	5	
e. Paused a few seconds between leads to allow stylus to adjust	_____	5	
23. Turned lead selector switch back to STD slowly.	_____	5	
a. Ran tracing out until only baseline appears	_____	5	
24. Turned machine off.	_____	5	
25. Tore tracing from machine.	_____	5	
a. Marked immediately with patient's name, age, date	_____	10	
b. Initialed	_____	5	
26. Rolled or loosely overlapped tracing and secured with paper clip.	_____	5	
27. Removed tips of lead wires from limb electrodes.	_____	5	
a. Removed chest electrode and strap	_____	5	
b. Removed limb straps from patient	_____	5	

PROCEDURE 16–3   Obtain a Standard 12-Lead Electrocardiogram—continued

PROCEDURE STEPS	STEP PERFORMED	POINTS POSSIBLE	COMMENTS
c. Instructed patient to wash areas well	_____	5	
28. Removed electrolyte from areas with warmed towel; dried area.	_____	5	
a. Discarded in proper receptacle	_____	5	
29. Assisted patient to sitting position.	_____	5	
a. Assisted patient down from table	_____	5	
b. Assisted to dress prn	_____	5	
30. Changed table paper and pillow cover.	_____	5	
a. Discarded disposables	_____	5	
31. Washed hands.	_____	5	
32. Placed tracing in patient's chart.	_____	5	
a. Initialed ECG order in chart	_____	5	
b. Placed tracing in appropriate area for physician to read or Mounted tracing/placed in patient's chart for physician to read.	_____	5	
33. Recorded any unusual findings or observations on patient's chart.	_____	10	

EVALUATOR: NOTE TIME COMPLETED _____

ADD POINTS OF STEPS CHECKED   _____ EARNED
TOTAL POINTS POSSIBLE   455 POSSIBLE Steps 1–33
                                             140 *Steps 1–8; 28–33

Points assigned reflect importance of step to meeting objective: Important = (5)   Essential = (10)   Critical = (15)
Automatic failure results if any of the critical steps are omitted or performed incorrectly.
DETERMINE SCORE (divide points earned by total points possible, multiply results by 100)   _____ SCORE*

Evaluator's Name (print) _____ Signature _____

Comments _____

DOCUMENTATION
Chart the procedure in the patient's medical record.

Date: _____

Charting: _____
_____
_____
_____

Student's Initials: _____

Name _____

Date _____ Score* _____

PROCEDURE 16–4   Holter Monitoring

TERMINAL PERFORMANCE OBJECTIVE - Demonstrate the steps of the procedure for hooking up a patient for the Holter monitor.

PROCEDURE STEPS	STEP PERFORMED	POINTS POSSIBLE	COMMENTS
EVALUATOR: Place check mark in space following each step performed satisfactorily			
NOTE TIME BEGAN _____			
1. Identified patient.	_____	5	
2. Explained procedure to patient.	_____	5	
3. Asked patient to remove clothing from the waist up.	_____	5	
4. Provided drape sheet.	_____	5	
5. Assisted patient to end of exam table.	_____	5	
6. Washed hands.	_____	5	
7. Assembled equipment and supplies near patient.	_____	5	
8. Tested Holter monitor for proper function.	_____	15	
9. Used shaving cream and razor to remove excess hair from patient's chest.	_____	10	
10. Rinsed, dried, and used alcohol on electrode sites.	_____	5	
11. Rubbed each site vigorously with gauze squares.	_____	10	
12. Applied electrodes/lead wires.	_____	15	
a. Made good contact	_____	15	
b. Secured electrodes with tape	_____	10	
13. Placed belt with recorder around patient's waist.	_____	10	
a. Advised patient in care of recorder	_____	10	
14. Assisted patient in dressing.	_____	5	
15. Instructed patient to perform routine activities.	_____	5	
a. Advised not to bathe in tub or shower	_____	10	
16. Recorded date and time monitor began on patient's chart.	_____	15	
a. Recorded in patient's diary	_____	10	
17. Instructed patient to record symptoms in diary.	_____	10	
18. Gave patient return appointment time in 24 hours.	_____	10	
19. When patient returned:			
a. Assisted patient in disrobing	_____	5	
b. Removed electrodes and wires	_____	5	

PROCEDURE STEPS	STEP PERFORMED	POINTS POSSIBLE	COMMENTS
c. Placed cassette in computerized ECG for printout of tracing	_____	15	
d. Placed diary and recording of ECG in patient's chart	_____	10	
e. Initialed	_____	5	

EVALUATOR: NOTE TIME COMPLETED _____

ADD POINTS OF STEPS CHECKED   _____ EARNED
TOTAL POINTS POSSIBLE   240 POSSIBLE

Points assigned reflect importance of step to meeting objective: Important = (5)   Essential = (10)   Critical = (15)
Automatic failure results if any of the critical steps are omitted or performed incorrectly.

DETERMINE SCORE (divide points earned by total points possible, multiply results by 100)   _____ SCORE*

Evaluator's Name (print) _____ Signature _____

Comments _____

DOCUMENTATION

Chart the procedure in the patient's medical record.

Date: _____

Charting: _____

_____

_____

_____

Student's Initials: _____

Name _____

Date _____ Score* _____

PROCEDURE 17–1   Prepare Skin for Minor Surgery

TERMINAL PERFORMANCE OBJECTIVE - Demonstrate each of the steps required in the skin prep procedure for minor surgery.

PROCEDURE STEPS	STEP PERFORMED	POINTS POSSIBLE	COMMENTS
EVALUATOR: Place check mark in space following each step performed satisfactorily			
NOTE TIME BEGAN _____			
1. Washed hands.	_____	5	
2. Assembled all necessary items.	_____	10	
3. Identified patient.	_____	5	
a. Explained procedure to patient	_____	5	
4. Asked patient to remove necessary clothing.	_____	5	
a. Instructed patient where to put clothing	_____	5	
b. Assisted patient as necessary	_____	5	
5. Positioned patient appropriately.	_____	5	
a. Draped patient appropriately	_____	5	
6. Positioned Mayo table over patient near surgical site.	_____	5	
7. Positioned gooseneck lamp over site.	_____	5	
8. Placed gauze squares in soapy solution.	_____	10	
a. Used one at a time to soap area to be shaved.	_____	10	
b. Discarded each in basin after use	_____	10	
9. Used scissors to clip hair as necessary.	_____	10	
10. Shaved hair placing razor at 30° angle.	_____	10	
a. Held skin taut while shaving	_____	10	
b. Shaved in direction hair grows	_____	15	
c. Wiped hair and soap from razor with tissues	_____	10	
d. Swished razor through soapy water	_____	5	
e. Shook excess water from razor	_____	5	
f. Repeated steps 10 a through e as necessary	_____	15	
11. Removed all soap and hair from site with sterile gauze and water.	_____	10	
a. Dried area with sterile gauze squares	_____	5	
12. Applied antiseptic solution to site with sterile gauze.	_____	15	
a. Applied in a circular motion from center outward	_____	10	

PROCEDURE STEPS	STEP PERFORMED	POINTS POSSIBLE	COMMENTS
13. Covered skin prep area with sterile drape sheet.	_____	10	
a. Instructed patient not to touch site/tray	_____	5	
14. Discarded disposable items in proper container.	_____	5	
15. Returned reusable items to proper storage.	_____	5	
16. Removed gloves and discarded properly.	_____	5	
17. Washed hands.	_____	5	
18. Initialed procedure completed.	_____	5	
19. Attended to patient comfort.	_____	5	

EVALUATOR: NOTE TIME COMPLETED _____

ADD POINTS OF STEPS CHECKED   _____ EARNED

TOTAL POINTS POSSIBLE   255 POSSIBLE

Points assigned reflect importance of step to meeting objective: Important = (5)   Essential = (10)   Critical = (15)
Automatic failure results if any of the critical steps are omitted or performed incorrectly.

DETERMINE SCORE (divide points earned by total points possible, multiply results by 100)   _____ SCORE*

Evaluator's Name (print) _____ Signature _____

Comments _____

DOCUMENTATION

Chart the procedure in the patient's medical record.

Date: _____

Charting: _____

_____

_____

_____

Student's Initials: _____

Name _____

Date _____ Score* _____

PROCEDURE 17–2   Put on Sterile Gloves

TERMINAL PERFORMANCE OBJECTIVE - Demonstrate the correct method of putting on sterile gloves.

PROCEDURE STEPS	STEP PERFORMED	POINTS POSSIBLE	COMMENTS
EVALUATOR: Place check mark in space following each step performed satisfactorily			
NOTE TIME BEGAN _____			
1. Selected appropriate size gloves.	_____	10	
2. Removed jewelry.	_____	5	
3. Performed surgical scrub.	_____	10	
a. Used nail brush	_____	5	
b. Thoroughly dried hands	_____	5	
4. Opened sterile gloves without contaminating them.	_____	15	
a. Placed package on counter with cuffs of gloves toward body	_____	10	
5. Grasped cuff with finger and thumb of non-dominant hand.	_____	10	
a. Inserted dominant hand in glove	_____	10	
b. Pulled glove onto dominant hand by pulling cuff with non-dominant hand	_____	10	
6. Placed gloved fingers under cuff of other glove.	_____	15	
a. Inserted hand into glove	_____	10	
b. Pushed up on folded cuff	_____	10	
7. Placed gloved fingers under each cuff to smooth gloves over wrists	_____	15	
a. Checked gloves for tears and holes.	_____	10	
8. Kept hands above waist level.	_____	10	
a. Did not touch anything other than sterile items.	_____	10	
9. Removed gloves by pulling outside cuff with thumb and fingers.	_____	10	
a. Pulled gloves off inside out	_____	5	
b. Did not touch contaminated side	_____	5	

PROCEDURE STEPS	STEP PERFORMED	POINTS POSSIBLE	COMMENTS
10. Placed gloves in biohazard bag.	_____	5	
EVALUATOR: NOTE TIME COMPLETED _____			

ADD POINTS OF STEPS CHECKED   _____ EARNED
TOTAL POINTS POSSIBLE   195 POSSIBLE

Points assigned reflect importance of step to meeting objective: Important = (5)   Essential = (10)   Critical = (15)
Automatic failure results if any of the critical steps are omitted or performed incorrectly.

DETERMINE SCORE (divide points earned by total points possible, multiply results by 100)   _____ SCORE*

Evaluator's Name (print) _____ Signature _____

Comments _____

Name _____

Date _____ Score* _____

PROCEDURE 17–3   Assist with Minor Surgery

TERMINAL PERFORMANCE OBJECTIVE - Demonstrate each of the steps required in assisting with minor surgery.

PROCEDURE STEPS	STEP PERFORMED	POINTS POSSIBLE	COMMENTS
EVALUATOR: Place check mark in space following each step performed satisfactorily			
NOTE TIME BEGAN _____			
1. Identified patient.	_____	10	
2. Washed hands.	_____	5	
3. Assembled appropriate items on Mayo tray (sterile packs).	_____	15	
a. Positioned next to treatment table	_____	10	
b. Checked expiration dates of items	_____	10	
4. Explained procedure to patient.	_____	5	
a. Obtained signature on consent form	_____	5	
b. Advised patient to empty bladder	_____	5	
c. Took vital signs and recorded	_____	5	
d. Instructed patient to disrobe as indicated for procedure	_____	10	
e. Advised where to put belongings	_____	5	
5. Assisted patient to treatment table.	_____	5	
a. Positioned patient	_____	10	
6. Performed skin prep procedure.	_____	10	
7. Draped patient appropriately.	_____	5	
8. Placed sterile towel on Mayo tray.	_____	5	
a. Put sterile gloves on	_____	10	
b. Opened sterile items at tabs	_____	10	
c. Placed items in order of use	_____	10	
d. Covered with sterile towel	_____	10	
e. Removed gloves	_____	5	
f. Washed hands	_____	5	
9. When physician was ready to begin:			
a. Removed cover		5	
b. Handed physician sterile gloves	_____	5	
c. Wiped top of vial with alcohol	_____	5	
d. Held anesthetic vial for doctor	_____	5	
10. Washed hands and regloved to assist.	_____	10	
a. Mopped with sterile gauze	_____	15	
b. Handed sterile items to physician PRN	_____	15	

PROCEDURE STEPS	STEP PERFORMED	POINTS POSSIBLE	COMMENTS
c. Opened specimen container for biopsy	_____	15	
d. Clipped suture PRN	_____	10	
11. Cleaned and bandaged surgery site.	_____	5	
a. Asked patient if allergic to adhesive	_____	5	
12. Removed gloves.	_____	5	
a. Washed hands	_____	5	
13. Assisted patient to sitting position.	_____	5	
a. And then from table	_____	5	
14. Provided patient education.	_____	5	
a. Care of site	_____	5	
b. Return visit appointment given	_____	5	
15. Regloved to clean up room.	_____	5	
a. Discarded disposables in biohazardous waste container	_____	5	
b. Rinsed instruments in cool water and placed in detergent solution to soak	_____	5	
16. Removed gloves.	_____	5	
a. Washed hands	_____	5	
17. Restocked room	_____	5	

EVALUATOR: NOTE TIME COMPLETED _____

ADD POINTS OF STEPS CHECKED   _____ EARNED
TOTAL POINTS POSSIBLE   330 POSSIBLE

Points assigned reflect importance of step to meeting objective: Important = (5)   Essential = (10)   Critical = (15)
Automatic failure results if any of the critical steps are omitted or performed incorrectly.

DETERMINE SCORE (divide points earned by total points possible, multiply results by 100)   _____ SCORE*

Evaluator's Name (print) _____ Signature _____

Comments _____

DOCUMENTATION

Chart the procedure in the patient's medical record.

Date: _____

Charting: _____

_____

_____

_____

Student's Initials: _____

Name _____

Date _____ Score* _____

PROCEDURE 17–4 Assisting with Suturing a Laceration

TERMINAL PERFORMANCE OBJECTIVE - Demonstrate each of the steps required in the procedure to assist with suturing a laceration.

PROCEDURE STEPS	STEP PERFORMED	POINTS POSSIBLE	COMMENTS
EVALUATOR: Place check mark in space following each step performed satisfactorily			
NOTE TIME BEGAN _____			
1. Washed hands.	_____	5	
2. Assembled all necessary items.	_____	10	
3. Identified patient.	_____	5	
a. Explained procedure to patient	_____	5	
b. Advised patient to empty bladder	_____	5	
4. Took and recorded patient's vital signs.	_____	5	
5. Asked/assisted patient in removing clothing.	_____	5	
a. Explained where to store clothing	_____	5	
6. Positioned patient appropriately.	_____	10	
7. Performed skin prep of site.	_____	15	
8. Draped patient appropriately.	_____	10	
9. Assembled unsterile items on Mayo tray.	_____	10	
10. Answered patient's questions.	_____	5	
11. Opened sterile pack on Mayo tray.	_____	5	
a. Handled sterile towel from underneath	_____	10	
b. Dropped sterile items on sterile field as appropriate	_____	15	
12. Put PPE and sterile gloves on.	_____	15	
13. Arranged sterile items in order of use.	_____	15	
a. Covered sterile field with sterile towel	_____	5	
14. Removed gloves.	_____	5	
a. Washed hands	_____	5	
In Assisting physician with actual procedure:			
15. Removed cover from set-up.	_____	5	
16. Handed sterile gloves to physician.	_____	10	
17. Held vial of anesthetic for physician.	_____	5	
a. Wiped top of vial with alcohol pad	_____	5	
18. Washed hands.	_____	5	
a. Put on sterile gloves	_____	15	
19. Handed sterile items to physician as needed.	_____	15	
20. Mopped excess blood from site/sterile gauze.	_____	15	
21. Clipped sutures as directed by physician.	_____	15	

PROCEDURE 17–4   Assisting with Suturing a Laceration—continued

PROCEDURE STEPS	STEP PERFORMED	POINTS POSSIBLE	COMMENTS
22. Assisted with cleaning site.	_____	15	
a. Bandaged site appropriately	_____	10	
b. Asked if patient has adhesive allergy	_____	10	
c. Regloved as necessary	_____	5	
d. Disposed of soiled items in biohazardous bag	_____	5	
e. Washed hands	_____	5	
23. Administered tetanus toxoid as directed by physician.	_____	5	
24. Assisted patient in sitting.	_____	5	
a. Assisted patient in dressing	_____	5	
b. Assisted patient from exam table	_____	5	
25. Instructed patient in caring for suture site.	_____	5	
26. Provided return appointment.	_____	10	
27. Put on gloves to clean up room.	_____	5	
a. Placed disposables in biobag/sharps	_____	10	
b. Rinsed instruments in cool water	_____	5	
c. Placed instruments in detergent solution	_____	5	
28. Removed gloves/PPE.	_____	5	
a. Placed soiled disposables in biobag	_____	5	
b. Washed hands	_____	5	
29. Restocked treatment room.	_____	5	
30. Recorded procedure in patient's chart.	_____	5	
a. Initialed	_____	5	

EVALUATOR: NOTE TIME COMPLETED _____

ADD POINTS OF STEPS CHECKED   _____ EARNED
TOTAL POINTS POSSIBLE   400 POSSIBLE

Points assigned reflect importance of step to meeting objective: Important = (5)   Essential = (10)   Critical = (15)
Automatic failure results if any of the critical steps are omitted or performed incorrectly.

DETERMINE SCORE (divide points earned by total points possible, multiply results by 100)   _____ SCORE*

Evaluator's Name (print) _____ Signature _____

Comments _____

DOCUMENTATION

Chart the procedure in the patient's medical record.

Date: _____

Charting: _____

_____

_____

_____

Student's Initials: _____

Name _____

Date _____ Score* _____

PROCEDURE 17–5   Remove Sutures

TERMINAL PERFORMANCE OBJECTIVE - Demonstrate the steps required in removing sutures.

PROCEDURE STEPS	STEP PERFORMED	POINTS POSSIBLE	COMMENTS
EVALUATOR: Place check mark in space following each step performed satisfactorily			
NOTE TIME BEGAN _____			
1. Identified patient.	_____	5	
2. Washed hands.	_____	5	
3. Placed Mayo tray next to treatment table.	_____	5	
a. Assembled items on tray	_____	5	
4. Asked about condition of suture site.	_____	5	
a. If laceration/ask about booster	_____	5	
b. Took vital signs and recorded	_____	5	
c. Recorded other information	_____	5	
5. Asked patient to remove appropriate clothing if necessary.	_____	10	
6. Assisted patient to treatment table.	_____	5	
a. Into position and draped as necessary	_____	10	
b. Explained procedure	_____	5	
7. Washed hands.	_____	5	
a. Put gloves on	_____	5	
8. Removed bandage/inspected site.	_____	10	
9. Soaked to remove bandage if stuck.	_____	10	
10. Advised physician to check the site.	_____	10	
11. Followed doctor's orders to remove sutures.	_____	15	
a. Opened sterile pack of instruments	_____	15	
b. Used thumb forceps to grasp knot of suture and pull up	_____	15	
c. Placed tip of suture removal scissors next to skin to clip suture	_____	15	
d. Pulled suture toward the incision	_____	15	
e. Continued until all sutures were removed.	_____	15	
12. Applied antiseptic solution to site.	_____	10	
a. Allowed to air dry	_____	5	
b. Applied steri-strips or butterfly closures PRN.	_____	15	

PROCEDURE STEPS	STEP PERFORMED	POINTS POSSIBLE	COMMENTS
c. Bandaged as necessary.	_____	10	
d. Asked patient if allergic to adhesive	_____	10	
13. Removed gloves.	_____	5	
a. Washed hands	_____	5	
14. Provided patient education.	_____	5	
15. Cleaned room.	_____	5	
a. Cared for instruments (Glove PRN)	_____	5	
16. Recorded information on patient's chart.	_____	5	
a. Initialed	_____	5	

EVALUATOR: NOTE TIME COMPLETED _____

ADD POINTS OF STEPS CHECKED   _____ EARNED
TOTAL POINTS POSSIBLE   285 POSSIBLE

Points assigned reflect importance of step to meeting objective: Important = (5)   Essential = (10)   Critical = (15)
Automatic failure results if any of the critical steps are omitted or performed incorrectly.

DETERMINE SCORE (divide points earned by total points possible, multiply results by 100)   _____ SCORE*

Evaluator's Name (print) _____ Signature _____

Comments _____

DOCUMENTATION

Chart the procedure in the patient's medical record.

Date: _____

Charting: _____

_____

_____

_____

Student's Initials: _____

Name _____

Date _____ Score* _____

PROCEDURE 18–1   Obtain and Administer Oral Medication

TERMINAL PERFORMANCE OBJECTIVE - Demonstrate the steps required to obtain the ordered oral medication and administer it to the patient.

PROCEDURE STEPS	STEP PERFORMED	POINTS POSSIBLE	COMMENTS
EVALUATOR: Place check mark in space following each step performed satisfactorily			
NOTE TIME BEGAN _____			
1. Read order of medication and compared it with medication in storage area.	_____	10	
a. Obtained ordered medication	_____	15	
2. Calculated dosage if necessary.	_____	15	
3. Washed hands.	_____	5	
4. Removed bottle cap.	_____	5	
a. Placed cap inside-up on counter	_____	5	
b. Poured desired amount into cap and then into medicine cup	_____	15	
or			
If liquid; poured desired amount directly into medicine cup at eye level.	_____	15	
5. Placed medicine on tray.	_____	5	
a. Placed cup of water on tray (if medicine is in pill or capsule form)	_____	5	
6. Read label of medicine container again.	_____	10	
a. Took medicine to patient	_____	10	
7. Identified patient.	_____	5	
8. Explained procedure to patient.	_____	15	
9. Observed patient taking medication.	_____	15	
a. Reported any reaction or problem to the physician	_____	10	
10. Read label of medication container again.	_____	10	
11. Discarded disposables.	_____	5	
12. Returned items to proper storage.	_____	5	
13. Recorded medication information on patient's chart.	_____	15	
a. Initialed	_____	5	
EVALUATOR: NOTE TIME COMPLETED _____			

ADD POINTS OF STEPS CHECKED   _____ EARNED
TOTAL POINTS POSSIBLE   185 POSSIBLE

Points assigned reflect importance of step to meeting objective: Important = (5)   Essential = (10)   Critical = (15)
Automatic failure results if any of the critical steps are omitted or performed incorrectly.

DETERMINE SCORE (divide points earned by total points possible, multiply results by 100)   _____ SCORE*

Evaluator's Name (print) _____ Signature _____

Comments _____

DOCUMENTATION

Chart the procedure in the patient's medical record.

Date: _____

Charting: _____

_____

_____

_____

Student's Initials: _____

Name _____

Date _____ Score* _____

PROCEDURE 18–2   Withdraw Medication from an Ampule

TERMINAL PERFORMANCE OBJECTIVE - Demonstrate each of the steps required to withdraw medication from an ampule.

PROCEDURE STEPS	STEP PERFORMED	POINTS POSSIBLE	COMMENTS
EVALUATOR: Place check mark in space following each step performed satisfactorily			
NOTE TIME BEGAN _____			
1. Washed hands.	_____	5	
2. Placed sterile gauze square over middle of ampule.	_____	5	
3. Held ampule between thumb and index finger of one hand.	_____	10	
4. Flicked pointed end of ampule with index finger to release medicine into bottom of ampule.	_____	15	
5. Grasped tip of ampule and snapped off.	_____	15	
a. Discarded tip of ampule	_____	10	
6. Secured needle and syringe by turning barrel to right while holding guard.	_____	10	
7. Expelled air from syringe.	_____	10	
8. Inserted tip of needle below line of liquid in ampule without touching sides.	_____	15	
9. Drew ordered amount of medicine into barrel of syringe.	_____	15	
a. Avoided air from entering by keeping tip of needle below line of liquid	_____	15	
10. Removed needle without touching sides of ampule.	_____	15	
11. Replaced needle guard without contaminating needle (scoop method).	_____	5	
12. Placed filled syringe on medicine tray.	_____	5	
13. Discarded disposables in proper receptacle.	_____	5	
EVALUATOR: NOTE TIME COMPLETED _____			

ADD POINTS OF STEPS CHECKED   _____ EARNED

TOTAL POINTS POSSIBLE   155 POSSIBLE

Points assigned reflect importance of step to meeting objective: Important = (5)   Essential = (10)   Critical = (15)

Automatic failure results if any of the critical steps are omitted or performed incorrectly.

DETERMINE SCORE (divide points earned by total points possible, multiply results by 100)   _____ SCORE*

Evaluator's Name (print) _____ Signature _____

Comments _____

Name _____

Date _____ Score* _____

PROCEDURE 18–3   Withdraw Medication from a Vial

TERMINAL PERFORMANCE OBJECTIVE - Demonstrate each of the steps required to withdraw medication from a vial.

PROCEDURE STEPS	STEP PERFORMED	POINTS POSSIBLE	COMMENTS
EVALUATOR: Place check mark in space following each step performed satisfactorily			
NOTE TIME BEGAN _____			
1. Washed hands.	_____	5	
2. Calculated dosage.	_____	15	
3. Cleaned rubber-topped vial with alcohol pad.	_____	10	
4. Secured needle onto syringe by holding needle guard and turning barrel of syringe to the right.	_____	10	
5. Removed needle guard without contaminating the needle.	_____	10	
6. Pulled back on plunger to fill syringe with same amount of air as medication ordered.	_____	10	
7. Held syringe at barrel.	_____	10	
8. Held vial upside down.	_____	10	
9. Inserted needle into rubber top and pushed plunger in, expelling air into vial.	_____	15	
10. Pulled back plunger to allow desired amount of medication to enter syringe.	_____	15	
a. Kept needle below level of medication in vial to avoid air bubbles	_____	15	
b. Flicked barrel of syringe to release air bubbles into hub of syringe and pushed plunger to release	_____	15	
11. Pulled needle out of vial without contaminating it.	_____	10	
12. Replaced needle guard.	_____	5	
13. Placed filled syringe on medicine tray.	_____	5	
a. Placed alcohol on tray	_____	5	
EVALUATOR: NOTE TIME COMPLETED _____			

ADD POINTS OF STEPS CHECKED   _____ EARNED

TOTAL POINTS POSSIBLE   165 POSSIBLE

Points assigned reflect importance of step to meeting objective: Important = (5)   Essential = (10)   Critical = (15)
Automatic failure results if any of the critical steps are omitted or performed incorrectly.

DETERMINE SCORE (divide points earned by total points possible, multiply results by 100)   _____ SCORE*

Evaluator's Name (print) _____ Signature _____

Comments _____

Name _____

Date _____ Score* _____

PROCEDURE 18–4   Administer Intradermal Injection

TERMINAL PERFORMANCE OBJECTIVE - Demonstrate each of the steps required in administering an intradermal injection.

PROCEDURE STEPS	STEP PERFORMED	POINTS POSSIBLE	COMMENTS
EVALUATOR: Place check mark in space following each step performed satisfactorily			
NOTE TIME BEGAN _____			
1. Washed hands.	_____	5	
2. Read order.	_____	5	
3. Prepared syringe with ordered amount of medicine.	_____	15	
4. Replaced needle guard.	_____	10	
5. Placed medicine on tray.	_____	5	
6. Compared medicine order with patient's chart.	_____	15	
7. Identified patient.	_____	5	
8. Explained procedure to patient.	_____	5	
9. Placed medicine tray near patient.	_____	5	
10. Used alcohol pad to clean injection site.	_____	10	
a. Allowed alcohol to air dry	_____	5	
11. Removed needle guard without contaminating it.	_____	15	
12. Held patient's skin taut between thumb and index finger to steady area to be injected.	_____	5	
13. Inserted needle at 10°–15° angle.	_____	10	
a. Held bevel of needle up	_____	15	
14. Expelled medicine from syringe.	_____	15	
a. Caused wheal to develop	_____	15	
15. Removed needle quickly.	_____	10	
a. At same angle as insertion	_____	10	
b. Wiped site with gauze pad	_____	5	
c. Did not massage site	_____	10	
16. Observed patient.	_____	10	
a. Timed reaction	_____	15	
17. Gave patient instructions/answered questions.	_____	5	
18. Applied bandage.	_____	5	
19. Discarded disposables in sharps container including intact syringe and needle.	_____	5	

PROCEDURE STEPS	STEP PERFORMED	POINTS POSSIBLE	COMMENTS
20. Returned items to proper storage.	_____	5	
21. Recorded information on patient's chart.	_____	15	
a. Initialed	_____	5	

EVALUATOR: NOTE TIME COMPLETED _____

ADD POINTS OF STEPS CHECKED   _____ EARNED
TOTAL POINTS POSSIBLE   260 POSSIBLE

Points assigned reflect importance of step to meeting objective: Important = (5)   Essential = (10)   Critical = (15)
Automatic failure results if any of the critical steps are omitted or performed incorrectly.

DETERMINE SCORE (divide points earned by total points possible, multiply results by 100)   _____ SCORE*

Evaluator's Name (print) _____ Signature _____

Comments _____

DOCUMENTATION

Chart the procedure in the patient's medical record.

Date: _____

Charting: _____

_____

_____

_____

Student's Initials: _____

PROCEDURE 18–5 Administer Subcutaneous Injection

TERMINAL PERFORMANCE OBJECTIVE - Demonstrate each of the steps required in administering a subcutaneous injection.

PROCEDURE STEPS	STEP PERFORMED	POINTS POSSIBLE	COMMENTS
EVALUATOR: Place check mark in space following each step performed satisfactorily			
NOTE TIME BEGAN _____			
1. Compared orders with medication.	_____	10	
2. Washed hands.	_____	5	
3. Prepared syringe.	_____	10	
a. Replaced needle guard	_____	5	
4. Placed filled syringe on medicine tray.	_____	10	
5. Compared medication order with patient's chart.	_____	15	
6. Identified patient.	_____	5	
7. Explained procedure to patient.	_____	5	
8. Asked patient to remove necessary clothing.	_____	10	
9. Used alcohol pad to clean injection site.	_____	10	
10. Removed needle guard without contaminating it.	_____	15	
11. Held skin at injection site taut.	_____	5	
12. Held syringe securely with bevel of needle down.	_____	10	
13. Inserted needle at 45° angle.	_____	15	
14. Held barrel of syringe with one hand.	_____	10	
a. Aspirated with other hand	_____	15	
b. Determined if in a blood vessel	_____	15	
15. Pushed plunger of syringe to release medication.	_____	15	
16. Pulled needle out at same angle as insertion.	_____	10	
17. Wiped site with alcohol pad.	_____	5	
18. Placed dry cotton ball on site.	_____	5	
a. Massaged area gently	_____	5	
19. Observed patient for possible reaction.	_____	5	
20. Reported any reaction to physician.	_____	10	
21. Advised patient to remain for 20 minutes.	_____	10	
22. Answered questions from patient.	_____	5	
23. Applied bandage.	_____	5	
24. Discarded disposables including intact syringe and needle in sharps container.	_____	5	

PROCEDURE 18–5   Administer Subcutaneous Injection—continued

PROCEDURE STEPS	STEP PERFORMED	POINTS POSSIBLE	COMMENTS
25. Returned items to proper storage.	_____	5	
26. Recorded information on patient's chart.	_____	5	
a. Initialed	_____	5	
EVALUATOR: NOTE TIME COMPLETED _____			

ADD POINTS OF STEPS CHECKED   _____ EARNED

TOTAL POINTS POSSIBLE   265 POSSIBLE

Points assigned reflect importance of step to meeting objective: Important = (5)   Essential = (10)   Critical = (15)
Automatic failure results if any of the critical steps are omitted or performed incorrectly.

DETERMINE SCORE (divide points earned by total points possible, multiply results by 100)   _____ SCORE*

Evaluator's Name (print) _____ Signature _____

Comments _____

DOCUMENTATION

Chart the procedure in the patient's medical record.

Date: _____

Charting: _____

_____

_____

_____

Student's Initials: _____

Name _____

Date _____ Score* _____

PROCEDURE 18–6   Administer Intramuscular Injection

TERMINAL PERFORMANCE OBJECTIVE - Demonstrate each of the steps required in administering an intramuscular injection.

PROCEDURE STEPS	STEP PERFORMED	POINTS POSSIBLE	COMMENTS
EVALUATOR: Place check mark in space following each step performed satisfactorily			
NOTE TIME BEGAN _____			
1. Washed hands.	_____	5	
2. Read label of medication.	_____	5	
3. Compared with order.	_____	10	
4. Prepared syringe with ordered amount of medication.	_____	15	
5. Replaced needle guard.	_____	5	
6. Placed filled syringe on medicine tray.	_____	10	
7. Compared medication order with patient's chart.	_____	15	
8. Identified patient.	_____	5	
9. Explained procedure to patient.	_____	5	
10. Asked patient to remove necessary clothing.	_____	5	
11. Cleaned injection site with alcohol pad.	_____	10	
a. Allowed to air dry	_____	5	
12. Removed needle guard.	_____	10	
13. Secured injection site between thumb and index finger.	_____	10	
14. Grasped syringe as a dart.	_____	10	
15. Inserted needle at 90° angle.	_____	15	
16. Aspirated syringe.	_____	15	
a. Determined if in a blood vessel	_____	15	
17. Pushed plunger of syringe to release medication.	_____	15	
18. Pulled needle out at angel of insertion.	_____	10	
19. Wiped injection site with alcohol pads.	_____	5	
20. Gently massaged area with dry cotton ball.	_____	5	
21. Observed patient for reaction.	_____	10	
22. Reported any reaction to physician.	_____	10	
23. Applied bandage.	_____	5	
24. Discarded disposables including intact syringe and needle in sharps container.	_____	5	

PROCEDURE 18–6   Administer Intramuscular Injection—continued

PROCEDURE STEPS	STEP PERFORMED	POINTS POSSIBLE	COMMENTS
25. Washed and sterilized reusable items.	_____	5	
26. Returned items to proper storage.	_____	5	
27. Recorded information on patient's chart.	_____	5	
a. Initialed	_____	5	

EVALUATOR: NOTE TIME COMPLETED _____

ADD POINTS OF STEPS CHECKED   _____ EARNED
TOTAL POINTS POSSIBLE   255 POSSIBLE

Points assigned reflect importance of step to meeting objective: Important = (5)   Essential = (10)   Critical = (15)
Automatic failure results if any of the critical steps are omitted or performed incorrectly.

DETERMINE SCORE (divide points earned by total points possible, multiply results by 100)   _____ SCORE*

Evaluator's Name (print) _____ Signature _____

Comments _____

DOCUMENTATION

Chart the procedure in the patient's medical record.

Date: _____

Charting: _____

_____

_____

_____

Student's Initials: _____

Name _____

Date _____ Score* _____

PROCEDURE 18–7   Administer Intramuscular Injection by Z-Tract Method

TERMINAL PERFORMANCE OBJECTIVE - Demonstrate each of the steps required in administering an intramuscular injection by Z-tract method.

PROCEDURE STEPS	STEP PERFORMED	POINTS POSSIBLE	COMMENTS
EVALUATOR: Place check mark in space following each step performed satisfactorily			
NOTE TIME BEGAN _____			
1. Washed hands.	_____	5	
2. Read label of medication.	_____	10	
3. Compared with order.	_____	15	
4. Prepared syringe with ordered amount of medication.	_____	15	
5. Replaced needle guard.	_____	5	
6. Placed filled syringe on medicine tray.	_____	5	
7. Compared medication order with patient's chart.	_____	15	
8. Identified patient.	_____	5	
9. Explained procedure to patient.	_____	5	
10. Asked patient to remove necessary clothing.	_____	10	
11. Cleaned injection site with alcohol pad.	_____	10	
a. Allowed to air dry	_____	5	
12. Removed needle guard.	_____	5	
13. Read package insert instructions of medication.	_____	10	
14. Used sterile gauze square to displace skin/tissues throughout injection.	_____	10	
15. Inserted needle at 90° angle.	_____	15	
16. Used fingers to pull back on plunger to aspirate while holding barrel of syringe with thumb and ring finger.	_____	15	
17. Pushed plunger of syringe to slowly expel medication.	_____	15	
18. Waited a few seconds before withdrawing needle.	_____	15	
19. Removed needle quickly in same path as entered.	_____	10	
20. Let go of displaced skin/tissue immediately after needle is withdrawn to cover needle path.	_____	15	
21. Covered injection site with alcohol pad.	_____	5	
a. Held in place a few seconds	_____	5	
b. Did not massage injection site	_____	10	
22. Observed patient for reaction.	_____	10	

PROCEDURE STEPS	STEP PERFORMED	POINTS POSSIBLE	COMMENTS
23. Reported any reaction to physician.	_____	5	
24. Applied bandage.	_____	5	
25. Discarded disposables including intact syringe and needle in sharps container.	_____	5	
26. Washed and sterilized reusable items.	_____	5	
27. Returned items to proper storage.	_____	5	
28. Recorded information on patient's chart.	_____	5	
a. Initialed	_____	5	

EVALUATOR: NOTE TIME COMPLETED _____

ADD POINTS OF STEPS CHECKED   _____ EARNED
TOTAL POINTS POSSIBLE   280 POSSIBLE

Points assigned reflect importance of step to meeting objective: Important = (5)   Essential = (10)   Critical = (15)
Automatic failure results if any of the critical steps are omitted or performed incorrectly.

DETERMINE SCORE (divide points earned by total points possible, multiply results by 100)   _____ SCORE*

Evaluator's Name (print) _____ Signature _____

Comments _____

DOCUMENTATION

Chart the procedure in the patient's medical record.

Date: _____

Charting: _____

_____

_____

_____

Student's Initials: _____

Name _____

Date _____ Score* _____

PROCEDURE 19–1   Give Mouth-to-Mouth Resuscitation

TERMINAL PERFORMANCE OBJECTIVE - In a course taught by a certified instructor, using a training mannequin, demonstrate mouth-to-mouth resuscitation. Perform the steps as instructed following recommended standard precautions.

PROCEDURE STEPS	STEP PERFORMED	POINTS POSSIBLE	COMMENTS
EVALUATOR: Place check mark in space following each step performed satisfactorily			
NOTE TIME BEGAN _____			
1. Determined whether unresponsive victim is breathing.	_____	15	
2. Positioned victim on back on firm surface.	_____	5	
3. Rescuer was positioned at victim's side near head and shoulders.	_____	5	
4. Opened airway, if not effective, continued with procedure.	_____	15	
5. Checked for mouth obstruction.	_____	10	
6. Demonstrated procedure to remove obstruction.	_____	15	
7. Used head tilt-chin lift maneuver thereby moving tongue from back of throat. If not effective, continued with procedure.	_____	15	
8. Pinched victim's nostrils together with fingers of one hand while placing heel of hand on forehead to keep the head tilted.	_____	10	
9. Took a deep breath and then sealed mouth over victim's and breathed two slow breaths into the victim's mouth. Took a breath after each ventilation.	_____	15	
10. Turned head to one side, felt and listened for return of air. Watched chest for movement. If not effective, lifted chin, tilted head, tried again.	_____	15	
11. If inflation had not occurred, gave cycles of 12 breaths per minute. Watched for return of breathing.	_____	15	
12. Continued cycles till breathing restored, assistance arrived, or exhausted.	_____	10	
13. Recorded and initialed procedure on patient's chart.	_____		
EVALUATOR: NOTE TIME COMPLETED _____			

ADD POINTS OF STEPS CHECKED   _____ EARNED
TOTAL POINTS POSSIBLE   155 POSSIBLE

Points assigned reflect importance of step to meeting objective: Important = (5)   Essential = (10)   Critical = (15)
Automatic failure results if any of the critical steps are omitted or performed incorrectly.

DETERMINE SCORE (divide points earned by total points possible, multiply results by 100)   _____ SCORE*

Evaluator's Name (print) _____ Signature _____

Comments _____

DOCUMENTATION

Chart the procedure in the patient's medical record.

Date: _____

Charting: _____

_____

_____

_____

Student's Initials: _____

Name _____

Date _____ Score* _____

PROCEDURE 19–2   Give Cardiopulmonary Resuscitation (CPR) to Adults

TERMINAL PERFORMANCE OBJECTIVE - In a course taught by a certified instructor, and using a training mannequin, demonstrate the procedure performing each step, following recommended precautions.

PROCEDURE STEPS	STEP PERFORMED	POINTS POSSIBLE	COMMENTS
EVALUATOR: Place check mark in space following each step performed satisfactorily			
NOTE TIME BEGAN _____			
1. Gently shook victim and asked "Are you OK?"	_____	10	
2. If no response, called or sent someone for help.	_____	15	
3. Positioned mannequin on floor.	_____	5	
4. Rescuer was positioned at victim's side near head.	_____	5	
5. Opened airway, if not effective, continued with procedure.	_____	15	
6. Checked for mouth obstruction.	_____	5	
7. Positioned victim to open airway; pinched nostrils together with fingers while placing heel of hand on forehead to maintain head tilt.	_____	10	
8. Took a deep breath, sealed mouth over victim's and breathed two slow breaths into victim's mouth. Took a breath after each ventilation.	_____	15	
9. Turned head to one side, listened, and felt for return of air. Watched chest for movement.	_____	5	
10. Checked for carotid pulse, allowed up to 10 seconds.	_____	15	
11. If victim had a pulse, continued mouth-to-mouth respiration at rate of one breath every five seconds, if no pulse, began chest compressions.	_____	—	
12. Identified location for chest compressions and positioned hands.			
a. Located lower rib cage	_____	5	
b. Followed up to sternum	_____	5	
c. Placed two index fingers at lower end of sternum	_____	5	
d. Placed heel of hand nearest head next to fingers	_____	5	
e. Positioned other hand over hand on sternum, locked fingers	_____	10	
f. Held fingers away from body	_____	10	
13. Rose on knees, shoulder width apart.	_____	5	
a. Directly over sternum	_____	5	
b. Locked elbows	_____	5	

PROCEDURE 19–2   Give Cardiopulmonary Resuscitation (CPR) to Adults—continued

PROCEDURE STEPS	STEP PERFORMED	POINTS POSSIBLE	COMMENTS
14. Used a smooth, even motion to push straight down on chest and compressed about 1″ to 2″ for a count of fifteen compressions.	_____	15	
15. Gave two ventilations.	_____	15	
16. Repeated four cycles: Pause, checked for breathing and carotid pulse.	_____	15	
17. If no pulse, resumed compressions and ventilations.	_____	—	
18. Paused every few minutes to check for pulse and respirations.	_____	—	
19. Continued CPR until victim recovered, help arrived, victim was pronounced dead, or you became exhausted.	_____	—	
20. Cleaned mannequin as instructed.	_____	10	
21. Recorded and initialed procedure on patient's chart.	_____	10	

EVALUATOR: NOTE TIME COMPLETED _____

ADD POINTS OF STEPS CHECKED   _____ EARNED

TOTAL POINTS POSSIBLE   220 POSSIBLE

Points assigned reflect importance of step to meeting objective: Important = (5)   Essential = (10)   Critical = (15)
Automatic failure results if any of the critical steps are omitted or performed incorrectly.

DETERMINE SCORE (divide points earned by total points possible, multiply results by 100)   _____ SCORE*

Evaluator's Name (print) _____ Signature _____

Comments _____

DOCUMENTATION

Chart the procedure in the patient's medical record.

Date: _____

Charting: _____

_____

_____

_____

Student's Initials: _____

Name _____

Date _____ Score* _____

PROCEDURE 19–3   Give Cardiopulmonary Resuscitation (CPR) to Infants and Children

TERMINAL PERFORMANCE OBJECTIVE - In a course taught by a certified instructor, using a training mannequin, demonstrate the procedure as instructed, performing each step, and following standard precautions.

PROCEDURE STEPS	STEP PERFORMED	POINTS POSSIBLE	COMMENTS
EVALUATOR: Place check mark in space following each step performed satisfactorily			
NOTE TIME BEGAN _____			
1. Gently shook and called to a child or flicked bottom of foot of an infant to check for consciousness.	_____	5	
2. Called to another person to phone 911 or local emergency service and began resuscitation.	_____	15	
3. Placed infant or child on back on firm surface.	_____	5	
4. Tipped victim's head back and lifted chin to open airway.	_____	15	
5. Listened and watched and felt for breathing.	_____	10	
6. If no breathing was observed, gave two slow breaths, one to two seconds each.	_____	15	
7. Checked carotid pulse for up to 10 seconds.	_____	15	
a. Child at carotid location	_____	10	
b. Infants at mid upper arm over brachial	_____	10	
8. If pulse, continue one ventilation.	_____	10	
a. Every 3 seconds for infant			
b. Every 4 seconds for child			
9. If no pulse was present, started cardiac compression.			
a. Infant—Two fingers, mid-sternum, depress 1 inch; 100 times per minute.	_____	15	
b. Child—Adult position, one hand, depressed 1 inch to 1½ inches, 80–100 times per minute.	_____	15	
10. Did ten cycles of compressions and breaths.	_____	15	
11. Checked for pulse and breathing for up to 5 seconds.	_____	5	
12. If alone, summoned help.	_____	15	

PROCEDURE STEPS	STEP PERFORMED	POINTS POSSIBLE	COMMENTS
13. If there was no pulse, gave one breath and continued cycle until help arrived.	_____	10	
14. Sanitized the mannequin.	_____	5	
15. Recorded and initialed procedure on patient's chart.	_____	10	

EVALUATOR: NOTE TIME COMPLETED _____

ADD POINTS OF STEPS CHECKED   _____ EARNED
TOTAL POINTS POSSIBLE   200 POSSIBLE

Points assigned reflect importance of step to meeting objective: Important = (5)   Essential = (10)   Critical = (15)
Automatic failure results if any of the critical steps are omitted or performed incorrectly.

DETERMINE SCORE (divide points earned by total points possible, multiply results by 100)   _____ SCORE*

Evaluator's Name (print) _____ Signature _____

Comments _____

DOCUMENTATION

Chart the procedure in the patient's medical record.

Date: _____

Charting: _____

_____

_____

_____

Student's Initials: _____

Name _____

Date _____ Score* _____

PROCEDURE 19–4   Clean Wound Areas

TERMINAL PERFORMANCE OBJECTIVE - Provided with all necessary equipment and supplies, demonstrate cleaning wounds, following procedure steps and standard precautions.

PROCEDURE STEPS	STEP PERFORMED	POINTS POSSIBLE	COMMENTS
EVALUATOR: Place check mark in space following each step performed satisfactorily			
NOTE TIME BEGAN _____			
1. Assembled equipment and materials.	_____	5	
2. Washed hands and put on gloves.	_____	10	
3. Grasped gauze sponges with sponge forceps.	_____	5	
4. Dipped into warm detergent water.	_____	5	
5. Washed wound and wound area to remove microorganisms and any foreign matter.			
a. Avoided further injury from instrument	_____	10	
b. Worked from inner to outer area, 2″ to 3″ beyond wound	_____	15	
6. Irrigated wound thoroughly with sterile water.	_____	15	
7. Blotted wound dry with sterile gauze.	_____	10	
8. Covered with dry sterile dressing and bandaged in place.	_____	15	
9. Instructed patient to call physician immediately if evidence of infection developed.	_____	15	
10. Cleaned up work area. Placed all used materials and gloves in the biohazardous waste bag and into proper receptacle for safe disposal.	_____	5	
11. Washed hands.	_____	5	
12. Recorded and initialed procedure on patient's chart.	_____	10	
EVALUATOR: NOTE TIME COMPLETED _____			

ADD POINTS OF STEPS CHECKED   _____ EARNED
TOTAL POINTS POSSIBLE   125 POSSIBLE

Points assigned reflect importance of step to meeting objective: Important = (5)   Essential = (10)   Critical = (15)
Automatic failure results if any of the critical steps are omitted or performed incorrectly.

DETERMINE SCORE (divide points earned by total points possible, multiply results by 100)   _____ SCORE*

Evaluator's Name (print) _____ Signature _____

Comments _____

DOCUMENTATION

Chart the procedure in the patient's medical record.

Date: _____

Charting: _____

_____

_____

_____

Student's Initials: _____

Name _____

Date _____ Score* _____

PROCEDURE 19–5   Apply Bandage in Recurrent Turn to Finger

TERMINAL PERFORMANCE OBJECTIVE - Provided with all necessary equipment and supplies, apply recurrent turn bandage following procedure steps and standard precautions.

PROCEDURE STEPS	STEP PERFORMED	POINTS POSSIBLE	COMMENTS
EVALUATOR: Place check mark in space following each step performed satisfactorily			
NOTE TIME BEGAN _____			
1. Washed hands. Put on gloves if appropriate.	_____	5	
2. Assembled supplies.	_____	5	
3. Covered injury with dressing.	_____	10	
4. Secured dressing with bandage of gauze.			
a. Start at proximal end, palm side	_____	5	
b. Go to proximal end, back of hand	_____	5	
c. Repeat desired times	_____	5	
5. Held recurrent turns in place with spiral turns.	_____	10	
6. Secured by tying off gauze at proximal end of finger.	_____	10	
7. Discarded contaminated materials and gloves if used in biohazardous waste bag.	_____	15	
8. Washed hands.	_____	5	
9. Recorded and initialed procedure in patient's chart.	_____	10	

EVALUATOR: NOTE TIME COMPLETED _____

ADD POINTS OF STEPS CHECKED

TOTAL POINTS POSSIBLE

_____ EARNED

85 POSSIBLE

Points assigned reflect importance of step to meeting objective: Important = (5)   Essential = (10)   Critical = (15)
Automatic failure results if any of the critical steps are omitted or performed incorrectly.

DETERMINE SCORE (divide points earned by total points possible, multiply results by 100)   _____ SCORE*

Evaluator's Name (print) _____ Signature _____

Comments _____

DOCUMENTATION

Chart the procedure in the patient's medical record.

Date: _____

Charting: _____

_____

_____

_____

Student's Initials: _____

Name _____

Date _____ Score* _____

PROCEDURE 19–6   Apply Bandage in Open or Closed Spiral

TERMINAL PERFORMANCE OBJECTIVE - Provided with all necessary equipment and supplies, apply open and closed spiral bandage so dressing is secure, following procedural steps and standard precautions.

PROCEDURE STEPS	STEP PERFORMED	POINTS POSSIBLE	COMMENTS
EVALUATOR: Place check mark in space following each step performed satisfactorily			
NOTE TIME BEGAN _____			
1. Washed hands. Put on gloves if appropriate.	_____	5	
2. Assembled needed supplies.	_____	5	
3. Carefully opened dressing, without contaminating, and placed over wound area.	_____	10	
4. Anchored bandage by placing end of bandage on bias at starting point.	_____	5	
5. Encircled part, allowing corner of bandage end to protrude.	_____	5	
6. Turned down protruding tip of bandage.	_____	5	
7. Encircled part again.	_____	5	
8. Continued to encircle area to be covered with spiral turns spaced so that they do not overlap. *OR* Formed closed spiral by continuing to encircle with overlapping spiral turns until all open spaces were covered.	_____	5	
9. Completed bandage by tying off or taping in place.	_____	5	
a. Tape if used, must be in opposite direction to body movement. Subtract 10 pts if applied incorrectly	_____		
10. Discarded contaminated materials and gloves if used in biohazardous waste bag.	_____	15	
11. Washed hands.	_____	5	
12. Recorded and initialed procedure on patient's chart.	_____	10	
EVALUATOR: NOTE TIME COMPLETED _____			

ADD POINTS OF STEPS CHECKED   _____ EARNED
TOTAL POINTS POSSIBLE   80 POSSIBLE

Points assigned reflect importance of step to meeting objective: Important = (5)   Essential = (10)   Critical = (15)
Automatic failure results if any of the critical steps are omitted or performed incorrectly.

DETERMINE SCORE (divide points earned by total points possible, multiply results by 100)   _____ SCORE*

Evaluator's Name (print) _____ Signature _____

Comments _____

DOCUMENTATION

Chart the procedure in the patient's medical record.

Date: _____

Charting: _____

_____

_____

_____

Student's Initials: _____

Name _____

Date _____ Score* _____

PROCEDURE 19–7 Apply Figure-Eight Bandage to Hand and Wrist

TERMINAL PERFORMANCE OBJECTIVE - Provided with all necessary equipment and materials, apply a figure-eight bandage to the hand and wrist neatly to secure dressing following procedure steps and standard precautions.

PROCEDURE STEPS	STEP PERFORMED	POINTS POSSIBLE	COMMENTS
EVALUATOR: Place check mark in space following each step performed satisfactorily			
NOTE TIME BEGAN _____			
1. Washed hands. Put on gloves if appropriate.	_____	5	
2. Assembled needed supplies.	_____	5	
3. Applied dressing. Did not contaminate any part that would touch wound area.	_____	10	
4. Anchored bandage with one or two turns around palm of hand.	_____	5	
5. Rolled gauze diagonally across front of wrist and in figure-eight pattern around the hand.	_____	10	
6. Tied off at the wrist. Avoided constricting circulation.	_____	15	
7. Discarded contaminated materials and gloves if used in biohazardous waste bag.	_____	15	
8. Washed hands.	_____	5	
9. Recorded and initialed procedure on patient's chart.	_____	10	
EVALUATOR: NOTE TIME COMPLETED _____			

ADD POINTS OF STEPS CHECKED   _____ EARNED
TOTAL POINTS POSSIBLE   80 POSSIBLE

Points assigned reflect importance of step to meeting objective: Important = (5)   Essential = (10)   Critical = (15)
Automatic failure results if any of the critical steps are omitted or performed incorrectly.

DETERMINE SCORE (divide points earned by total points possible, multiply results by 100)   _____ SCORE*

Evaluator's Name (print) _____ Signature _____

Comments _____

DOCUMENTATION

Chart the procedure in the patient's medical record.

Date: _____

Charting: _____

_____

_____

_____

Student's Initials: _____

Name _____

Date _____ Score* _____

PROCEDURE 19–8   Apply Cravat Bandage to Forehead, Ear, or Eyes

TERMINAL PERFORMANCE OBJECTIVE - Provided with all necessary equipment and supplies, apply a cravat bandage to the head following procedure steps and standard precautions.

PROCEDURE STEPS	STEP PERFORMED	POINTS POSSIBLE	COMMENTS
EVALUATOR: Place check mark in space following each step performed satisfactorily			
NOTE TIME BEGAN _____			
1. Washed hands. Put on gloves if appropriate.	_____	5	
2. Assembled needed supplies.	_____	5	
3. Carefully placed dressing over wound taking care not to contaminate area which would be over wound.	_____	15	
4. Placed center of cravat over dressing.	_____	5	
5. Took ends around to opposite side of head and crossed them. Did not tie.	_____	5	
6. Brought ends back to starting point and tied.	_____	10	
7. Discarded contaminated materials and gloves, if used, in biohazardous waste bag.	_____	15	
8. Washed hands.	_____	5	
9. Recorded and initialed procedure on patient's chart.	_____	10	

EVALUATOR: NOTE TIME COMPLETED _____

ADD POINTS OF STEPS CHECKED   _____ EARNED
TOTAL POINTS POSSIBLE   75 POSSIBLE

Points assigned reflect importance of step to meeting objective: Important = (5)   Essential = (10)   Critical = (15)
Automatic failure results if any of the critical steps are omitted or performed incorrectly.

DETERMINE SCORE (divide points earned by total points possible, multiply results by 100)   _____ SCORE*

Evaluator's Name (print) _____ Signature _____

Comments _____

DOCUMENTATION

Chart the procedure in the patient's medical record.

Date: _____

Charting: _____

_____

_____

_____

Student's Initials: _____

PROCEDURE 19–9   Apply Triangular Bandage to Head

TERMINAL PERFORMANCE OBJECTIVE - Provided with all necessary equipment and supplies, apply a triangular bandage to the head following procedure steps and standard precautions so the dressing is neat and secure.

PROCEDURE STEPS	STEP PERFORMED	POINTS POSSIBLE	COMMENTS
EVALUATOR: Place check mark in space following each step performed satisfactorily			
NOTE TIME BEGAN _____			
1. Washed hands. Put on gloves if appropriate.	_____	5	
2. Assembled needed supplies.	_____	5	
3. Carefully placed dressing over wound area without contaminating.	_____	15	
4. Folded a hem about two inches wide along base of bandage.	_____	10	
5. With hem on outside, placed bandage on head so that middle of base was on forehead close to eyebrows and point hangs down back.	_____	10	
6. Brought two ends around head above ears and crossed them just below occipital prominence at back of head.	_____	10	
7. Drew ends snugly around head and tied them in center of forehead.	_____	5	
8. Steadied head with one hand and with other hand drew point down firmly behind to hold dressing securely against head.	_____	10	
9. Grasped point and tucked it into area where bandage ends crossed.	_____	5	
10. Discarded contaminated materials and gloves if used in biohazardous waste bag.	_____	15	
11. Washed hands.	_____	5	
12. Recorded and initialed procedure on patient's chart.	_____	10	
EVALUATOR: NOTE TIME COMPLETED _____			

ADD POINTS OF STEPS CHECKED   _____ EARNED
TOTAL POINTS POSSIBLE   105 POSSIBLE

Points assigned reflect importance of step to meeting objective: Important = (5)   Essential = (10)   Critical = (15)
Automatic failure results if any of the critical steps are omitted or performed incorrectly.

DETERMINE SCORE (divide points earned by total points possible, multiply results by 100)   _____ SCORE*

Evaluator's Name (print) _____ Signature _____

Comments _____

DOCUMENTATION

Chart the procedure in the patient's medical record.

Date: _____

Charting: _____

_____

_____

_____

Student's Initials: _____

Name _____

Date _____ Score* _____

PROCEDURE 20–1 Apply Arm Sling

TERMINAL PERFORMANCE OBJECTIVE - Provided with the necessary equipment, demonstrate the steps in the procedure for applying an arm sling so that the arm is supported properly and the sling is correctly tied.

PROCEDURE STEPS	STEP PERFORMED	POINTS POSSIBLE	COMMENTS
EVALUATOR: Place check mark in space following each step performed satisfactorily			
NOTE TIME BEGAN _____			
1. Washed hands.	_____	5	
2. Placed one end of triangle bandage over shoulder on uninjured side and let other end hang down over chest.	_____	15	
3. Pulled point behind elbow of injured arm.	_____	5	
4. Pulled end of bandage which was hanging down up around injured arm and over shoulder.	_____	5	
5. Raised end until hand rested 4″ to 5″ above elbow.	_____	15	
6. Tied ends at side of neck; checked hand.	_____	15	
7. Closed point end at elbow.	_____	15	
a. Folded neatly and pin or			
b. Tied knot in cloth to make sling snug at elbow			
8. Extended fingers slightly beyond edge of sling.	_____	15	
9. Recorded and initialed procedure on patient's chart.	_____	10	
EVALUATOR: NOTE TIME COMPLETED _____			

ADD POINTS OF STEPS CHECKED   _____ EARNED
TOTAL POINTS POSSIBLE   100 POSSIBLE

Points assigned reflect importance of step to meeting objective: Important = (5)   Essential = (10)   Critical = (15)
Automatic failure results if any of the critical steps are omitted or performed incorrectly.

DETERMINE SCORE (divide points earned by total points possible, multiply results by 100)   _____ SCORE*

Evaluator's Name (print) _____ Signature _____

Comments _____

DOCUMENTATION

Chart the procedure in the patient's medical record.

Date: _____

Charting: _____

_____

_____

_____

Student's Initials: _____

Name _____

Date _____ Score* _____

PROCEDURE 20–2   Use a Cane

TERMINAL PERFORMANCE OBJECTIVE - Provided with a cane, demonstrate adjusting the length of a cane and provide patient with instruction to properly and safely use a cane. The cane will be the appropriate length and the patient will demonstrate correct usage.

PROCEDURE STEPS	STEP PERFORMED	POINTS POSSIBLE	COMMENTS
EVALUATOR: Place check mark in space following each step performed satisfactorily			
NOTE TIME BEGAN _____			
1. Identified patient and confirmed physician's orders.	_____	5	
2. Assembled equipment. Checked cane for intact rubber tip.	_____	10	
3. Adjusted height of cane.			
a. Elbow flexed at 25° to 30° angle	_____	15	
b. Handle just below hip on strong side	_____	15	
4. Demonstrated use of cane—moving cane forward with injured extremity.	_____	15	
5. Allowed patient to practice the procedure.	_____	5	
6. Demonstrated going up stairs and had patient practice (Uninjured extremity up first).	_____	15	
7. Demonstrate going down stairs and had patient practice (Uninjured extremity down first).	_____	15	
8. Rechecked cane height.	_____	5	
9. Ensured correct usage.	_____	15	
10. Recorded and initialed procedure on patient's chart.	_____	10	

EVALUATOR: NOTE TIME COMPLETED _____

ADD POINTS OF STEPS CHECKED   _____ EARNED

TOTAL POINTS POSSIBLE   125 POSSIBLE

Points assigned reflect importance of step to meeting objective: Important = (5)   Essential = (10)   Critical = (15)
Automatic failure results if any of the critical steps are omitted or performed incorrectly.

DETERMINE SCORE (divide points earned by total points possible, multiply results by 100)   _____ SCORE*

Evaluator's Name (print) _____ Signature _____

Comments _____

DOCUMENTATION

Chart the procedure in the patient's medical record.

Date: _____

Charting: _____

_____

_____

_____

Student's Initials: _____

PROCEDURE 20–3   Use Crutches

TERMINAL PERFORMANCE OBJECTIVE - Provided with all necessary equipment and supplies, adjust the length of the crutches and demonstrate the steps of this procedure to instruct a patient in the correct use of crutches. The crutches will be the correct length and the patient will be able to demonstrate the proper and safe use of crutches.

PROCEDURE STEPS	STEP PERFORMED	POINTS POSSIBLE	COMMENTS
EVALUATOR: Place check mark in space following each step performed satisfactorily			
NOTE TIME BEGAN _____			
1. Identified patient and confirmed physician's orders.	_____	5	
2. Assembled equipment. Made sure crutches were intact (hand pads and rubber tips) and stable.	_____	5	
3. Stabilized patient upright near wall or chair for support.	_____	10	
4. Adjusted length of crutches.			
a. Elbows with 30° bend	_____	15	
b. Pads 2″ below axilla	_____	15	
5. Explained proper usage to patient.			
a. Supported weight on hands	_____	15	
b. Took small steps	_____	10	
c. Stood on uninjured extremity, swung injured extremity with crutches	_____	15	
6. Demonstrated proper use of crutches for gait ordered.	_____	15	
7. Allowed patient to practice the procedure to ensure correct use.	_____	10	
8. Recorded and initialed procedure on patient's chart.	_____	10	
EVALUATOR: NOTE TIME COMPLETED _____			

ADD POINTS OF STEPS CHECKED   _____ EARNED
TOTAL POINTS POSSIBLE   125 POSSIBLE

Points assigned reflect importance of step to meeting objective: Important = (5)   Essential = (10)   Critical = (15)
Automatic failure results if any of the critical steps are omitted or performed incorrectly.

DETERMINE SCORE (divide points earned by total points possible, multiply results by 100)   _____ SCORE*

Evaluator's Name (print) _____ Signature _____

Comments _____

DOCUMENTATION

Chart the procedure in the patient's medical record.

Date: _____

Charting: _____

_____

_____

_____

Student's Initials: _____

Name _____

Date _____ Score* _____

PROCEDURE 20–4   Use a Walker

TERMINAL PERFORMANCE OBJECTIVE - Provided with a walker, adjust it to the appropriate height and demonstrate the steps in the procedure to instruct a patient in the proper use of a walker. The patient will be able to demonstrate the safe and correct use of a walker.

PROCEDURE STEPS	STEP PERFORMED	POINTS POSSIBLE	COMMENTS
EVALUATOR: Place check mark in space following each step performed satisfactorily			
NOTE TIME BEGAN _____			
1. Identified patient and confirmed physician's orders.	_____	5	
2. Assembled equipment. Checked walker for rubber tips, pads at handles, and stability.	_____	10	
3. Stabilized patient upright near wall or chair for support.	_____	10	
4. Adjusted walker to fit patient			
a. Handles hip level	_____	15	
b. Elbows bent 25–30°	_____	15	
5. Positioned the walker around the patient.	_____	5	
6. Instructed patient to pick up the walker and move it slightly forward and walk into it.	_____	10	
7. Demonstrated the correct use of a walker.	_____	15	
8. Had patient practice the procedure.	_____	5	
9. Observed patient and was ready to assist in case of possible fall until able to use safely and correctly.	_____	10	
10. Recorded and initialed procedure on patient's chart.	_____	10	
EVALUATOR: NOTE TIME COMPLETED _____			

ADD POINTS OF STEPS CHECKED   _____ EARNED

TOTAL POINTS POSSIBLE   110 POSSIBLE

Points assigned reflect importance of step to meeting objective: Important = (5)   Essential = (10)   Critical = (15)
Automatic failure results if any of the critical steps are omitted or performed incorrectly.

DETERMINE SCORE (divide points earned by total points possible, multiply results by 100)   _____ SCORE*

Evaluator's Name (print) _____ Signature _____

Comments _____

DOCUMENTATION

Chart the procedure in the patient's medical record.

Date: _____

Charting: _____

_____

_____

_____

Student's Initials: _____

Name _____

Date _____ Score* _____

PROCEDURE 20–5 Assist Patient from Wheelchair to Examination Table

TERMINAL PERFORMANCE OBJECTIVE - Provided with necessary equipment, demonstrate the steps in the procedure for assisting a patient from wheelchair to examination table in a safe manner.

PROCEDURE STEPS	STEP PERFORMED	POINTS POSSIBLE	COMMENTS
EVALUATOR: Place check mark in space following each step performed satisfactorily			
NOTE TIME BEGAN _____			
1. Unlocked wheels of chair and wheeled patient to examination room.	_____	5	
2. Positioned chair as near as possible to place where patient should sit on table.	_____	5	
3. Lowered table to chair level or provided stool.	_____	5	
4. Locked wheels on chair.	_____	15	
5. Folded footrests back.	_____	10	
6. Assumed stable position in front of patient.	_____	10	
7. Assisted patient to stand; side step or pivot to front of table.	_____	15	
8. Assisted patient to sitting position on table.	_____	10	
9. Helped adjust position and recline for examination.	_____	5	
10. Placed pillow under head.	_____	5	
11. Draped as appropriate.	_____	5	
12. Unlocked chair wheels and moved chair out of way.	_____	5	
EVALUATOR: NOTE TIME COMPLETED _____			

ADD POINTS OF STEPS CHECKED _____ EARNED

TOTAL POINTS POSSIBLE 95 POSSIBLE

Points assigned reflect importance of step to meeting objective: Important = (5) Essential = (10) Critical = (15)
Automatic failure results if any of the critical steps are omitted or performed incorrectly.

DETERMINE SCORE (divide points earned by total points possible, multiply results by 100) _____ SCORE*

Evaluator's Name (print) _____ Signature _____

Comments _____

Name _____

Date _____ Score* _____

PROCEDURE 20–6   Assist Patient from Examination Table to Wheelchair

TERMINAL PERFORMANCE OBJECTIVE - Provided with a wheelchair and an examination table, demonstrate the steps in the procedure, in order, to assist the patient from examination table to wheelchair in a safe manner.

PROCEDURE STEPS	STEP PERFORMED	POINTS POSSIBLE	COMMENTS
EVALUATOR: Place check mark in space following each step performed satisfactorily			
NOTE TIME BEGAN _____			
1. Repositioned chair and locked wheels.	_____	15	
2. Assisted patient to sitting position on table.	_____	10	
3. Assisted to redress as needed.	_____	5	
4. Supported patient while assisting to step onto floor or stepstool (if stool—assisted to step onto floor).	_____	15	
5. Side-stepped or pivoted patient to position in front of chair.	_____	15	
6. Instructed patient to reach back to chair arms while helping lower patient into chair.	_____	15	
7. Adjusted footrests.	_____	10	
8. Unlocked wheels and returned patient to consultation or reception room.	_____	5	
EVALUATOR: NOTE TIME COMPLETED _____			

ADD POINTS OF STEPS CHECKED   _____ EARNED
TOTAL POINTS POSSIBLE   90 POSSIBLE

Points assigned reflect importance of step to meeting objective: Important = (5)   Essential = (10)   Critical = (15)
Automatic failure results if any of the critical steps are omitted or performed incorrectly.

DETERMINE SCORE (divide points earned by total points possible, multiply results by 100)   _____ SCORE*

Evaluator's Name (print) _____   Signature _____

Comments _____

CERTIFICATE OF COMPLETION

CERTIFIES THAT

_____

NAME

Has successfully completed the study of

MEDICAL ASSISTING

ADMINISTRATIVE AND CLINICAL COMPETENCIES

_____

DATE

_____

INSTRUCTOR

_____

SCHOOL

_____

DIRECTOR